Neurology of the Newborn Infant

Guest Editor

ADRÉ J. DU PLESSIS, MBChB, MPH

CLINICS IN PERINATOLOGY

www.perinatology.theclinics.com

December 2009 • Volume 36 • Number 4

SAUNDERS an imprint of ELSEVIER, Inc.

W.B. SAUNDERS COMPANY
A Division of Elsevier Inc.

Elsevier, Inc. ● 1600 John F. Kennedy Blvd. ● Suite 1800 ● Philadelphia, PA 19103-2899

http://www.theclinics.com

CLINICS IN PERINATOLOGY Volume 36, Number 4
December 2009 ISSN 0095-5108, ISBN-10: 1-4377-1401-3, ISBN-13: 978-1-4377-1401-2

Editor: Carla Holloway
Developmental Editor: Donald Mumford

Clinics in Perinatology (ISSN 0095-5108) is published quarterly by Elsevier Inc., 360 Park Avenue South, New York, NY 10010-1710. Months of issue are March, June, September, and December. Business and Editorial Offices: 1600 John F. Kennedy Blvd., Ste. 1800, Philadelphia, PA 19103-2899. Customer Service Office: 3251 Riverport Lane, Maryland Heights, MO 63043. Periodicals postage paid at New York, NY and additional mailing offices. Subscription prices are $239.00 per year (US individuals), $347.00 per year (US institutions), $281.00 per year (Canadian individuals), $441.00 per year (Canadian institutions), $345.00 per year (foreign individuals), $441.00 per year (foreign institutions) $116.00 per year (US students), and $168.00 per year (Canadian and foreign students). Foreign air speed delivery is included in all Clinics subscription prices. All prices are subject to change without notice. **POSTMASTER:** Send address changes to *Clinics in Perinatology*, Elsevier Health Sciences Division, Subscription Customer Service, 3251 Riverport Lane, Maryland Heights, MO 63043. **Customer Service: Telephone: 1-800-654-2452** (U.S. and Canada); **1-314-447-8871** (outside U.S. and Canada). **Fax: 1-314-447-8029. E-mail: journalscustomerservice-usa@elsevier.com** (for print support); **journalsonlinesupport-usa@elsevier.com** (for online support).

Reprints. For copies of 100 or more, of articles in this publication, please contact the Commercial Reprints Department, Elsevier Inc., 360 Park Avenue South, New York, NY 10010-1710. Tel. (212) 633-3812; Fax: (212) 482-1935; email: reprints@elsevier.com.

Clinics in Perinatology is also publilshed in Spanish by McGraw-Hill Interamericana Editores S.A., P.O. Box 5-237, 06500 Mexico D.F., Mexico.

Clinics in Perinatology is covered in *MEDLINE/PubMed (Index Medicus) Current Contents, Excepta Medica, BIOSIS and ISI/BIOMED.*

Printed and bound in the United Kingdom
Transferred to Digital Print 2011

Contributors

GUEST EDITOR

ADRÉ J. DU PLESSIS, MBChB, MPH
Associate Professor of Neurology, Harvard Medical School; Associate in Neurology and Director of Fetal-Neonatal Neurology, Children's Hospital Boston, Boston, Massachusetts

AUTHORS

HAIM BASSAN, MD
Pediatric Neurology Unit, Neonatal Neurology Service, Dana Children's Hospital, Tel Aviv Sourasky Medical Center, Sackler Faculty of Medicine, Tel Aviv University, Tel Aviv, Israel

ALI FATEMI, MD
Assistant Professor of Neurology and Pediatrics, Kennedy Krieger Institute, Johns Hopkins Medical Institutions, Baltimore, Maryland

DONNA M. FERRIERO, MD
Department of Pediatrics; Department of Neurology; Neonatal Brain Disorders Laboratory, University of California, San Francisco, California

FERNANDO F. GONZALEZ, MD
Department of Pediatrics; Neonatal Brain Disorders Laboratory, University of California, San Francisco, California

GORM GREISEN, MD, DMSc
Professor and Head of the Department of Neonatology, Department of Neonatology, Rigshospitalet, Copenhagen, Denmark

HENRIK HAGBERG, MD, PhD
Department of Obstetrics and Gynecology, Perinatal Center, Sahlgrenska Academy at University of Gothenburg, Gothenburg, Sweden; Department of Obstetrics, Institute of Reproductive and Developmental Biology, Imperial College London, London, United Kingdom

GREGORY L. HOLMES, MD
Professor of Medicine and Pediatrics, Department of Neurology, Center for Neuroscience at Dartmouth, Dartmouth-Hitchcock Medical Center, Dartmouth Medical School, Lebanon, New Hampshire

FRANCES E. JENSEN, MD
Professor of Neurology, Director of Epilepsy Research, Children's Hospital Boston, Boston, Massachusetts

MICHAEL V. JOHNSTON, MD
Blum-Moser Chair for Pediatric Neurology, Kennedy Krieger Institute; Professor
of Neurology, Pediatrics, and Physical Medicine and Rehabilitation, Johns Hopkins
Medical Institutions, Baltimore, Maryland

CATHERINE LIMPEROPOULOS, PhD
Assistant Professor, Department of Neurology and Neurosurgery; Department
of Pediatrics, School of Physical and Occupational Therapy, McGill University; Pediatric
Neurology, Montreal Children's Hospital, Montreal, Quebec, Canada; Fetal-Neonatal
Neurology Research Group, Department of Neurology, Children's Hospital Boston,
Harvard Medical School, Boston, Massachusetts

CARINA MALLARD, PhD
Department of Neuroscience and Physiology, Perinatal Center, Sahlgrenska
Academy at University of Gothenburg, Gothenburg, Sweden

LAURA R. MENT, MD
Professor of Pediatrics and Neurology, Department of Pediatrics, Yale University
School of Medicine, New Haven, Connecticut

ELIZA MYERS, MD
Clinical Fellow, Department of Pediatrics, Yale University School of Medicine,
New Haven, Connecticut

SHAHAB NOORI, MD
Department of Pediatrics, Section of Neonatal-Perinatal Medicine, The Children's
Hospital, College of Medicine, The University of Oklahoma Health Sciences Center,
Oklahoma City, Oklahoma

ISTVAN SERI, MD, PhD
Division of Neonatal Medicine, Department of Pediatrics, Center for Fetal and Neonatal
Medicine, Keck School of Medicine, University of Southern California; Department of
Pediatrics, The Los Angeles County + University of Southern California Medical Center,
Los Angeles, California

THEODORA A. STAVROUDIS, MD
Division of Neonatal Medicine, Department of Pediatrics, Center for Fetal and
Neonatal Medicine, Keck School of Medicine; Department of Pediatrics, The Los Angeles
County + University of Southern California Medical Center, Los Angeles, California

XIAOYANG WANG, MD, PhD
Department of Neuroscience and Physiology, Perinatal Center, Sahlgrenska
Academy at University of Gothenburg, Gothenburg, Sweden; Department of Pediatrics,
the Third Affiliated Hospital of Zhengzhou University, Zhengzhou, China

MARY ANN WILSON, PhD
Associate Professor of Neurology and Neuroscience, Kennedy Krieger Institute,
Johns Hopkins Medical Institutions, Baltimore, Maryland

MARTIN WOLF, PhD
Privatdozent and Head of Biomedical Optics Research Laboratory, Clinic of Neonatology,
University Hospital Zurich, Zurich, Switzerland

Contents

Little is known about the effect on clinically relevant outcomes of the complex hemodynamic changes occurring during adaptation to extrauterine life in preterm neonates, particularly in very low birth weight neonates. As cardiovascular adaptation in this extremely vulnerable patient population is complicated by immaturity of all organ systems, especially that of the cardiorespiratory, central nervous, and endocrine systems, maladaptation has been suspected, but not necessarily proven, to contribute to mortality and long-term morbidities. This article describes recent advances in the understanding of hemodynamic changes in very low birth weight neonates during postnatal transition, and reviews the complex and developmentally regulated interaction between systemic and cerebral hemodynamics and the effect of this interaction on clinically relevant outcomes.

New discoveries in neonatal imaging, cerebral monitoring, and hemodynamics, and greater understanding of inflammatory and genetic mechanisms involved in intracranial hemorrhage (ICH) in the preterm infant are creating opportunities for innovative early detection and prevention approaches. This article covers the spectrum of ICH in the preterm infant, including germinal matrix intraventricular hemorrhage, its complications, and associated phenomena, such as the emerging role of cerebellar hemorrhage. The overall aim of this article is to review the current knowledge of the mechanisms, diagnosis, outcome, and management of preterm ICH; to revisit the origins from which they develop; and to discuss future expectations.

The toll-like receptors (TLRs) are a family of microbe-sensing receptors on peripheral immune cells. TLRs have also been discovered to be present in the brain, particularly in circumventricular organs, microglia, and astrocytes. Some TLRs are strongly expressed in the embryonic brain and TLR3 and TLR8 have been implicated in neurogenesis and neurite outgrowth in the developing brain, whereas TLR2 and TLR4 have been shown to regulate adult neurogenesis. TLR2 and TLR4 also play a role in acute ischemic brain injury in the adult, although no neuroprotection was observed following perinatal hypoxic-ischemic injury. These findings suggest that different TLRs have specific roles in the immature and adult brain following brain damage.

Preterm birth has been defined as one of the major public health problems of this decade, preterm neonates being at high risk for neurodevelopmental disabilities. As preterm survival rates increase, the next great imperative for perinatal medicine is to understand and prevent the serious adverse neurodevelopmental outcomes of preterm birth. The challenge for neonatologists and neurologists alike is identifying early markers of outcome in the prematurely born. This article reviews current trends in prevalence, mortality, and morbidity, and the present status of outcome data for cognitive and neurosensory neurodevelopmental dysfunctions in preterm infants. New neuroimaging modalities and analysis tools are contributing to the understanding of neurologic sequelae of preterm birth by providing microstructural evidence of injury sustained by the preterm brain.

Recent studies in survivors of extreme prematurity point to an increased prevalence of a previously underrecognized atypical social-behavioral profile strongly suggestive of an autism spectrum disorder. Prospective studies that incorporate early autism screening and autism diagnostic testing are needed to better delineate the sensitivity and specificity of early signs of autism in ex-premature children. Advances in neonatal MRI techniques capable of quantitative structural and functional measurements will also provide important insights into the effects of prematurity itself, and prematurity-related brain injury on the genesis of autism spectrum disorders in this population. Available evidence linking prematurity and autism spectrum disorders is reviewed in this article.

This article reviews tissue oximetry and imaging to study the preterm and newborn infant brain by near-infrared spectroscopy. These two technologies are now advanced; nearly 100 reports on their use in newborn infants have been published, and commercial instruments are available. The precision of oximetry, however, is a limitation for its clinical use of assessing cerebral oxygenation. Imaging of brain function needs very well defined protocols for sensory stimulation as well as signal analysis to provide meaningful results.

that the sequelae of seizures are strongly age dependent; seizures will affect the developing and plastic neuronal circuitry much differently than the fixed circuitry of the mature brain. Seizures at an early developmental stage can dramatically affect the construction of networks, resulting in severe and permanent handicaps in some patients. In the young brain, the long-lasting detrimental consequences of seizures are caused by an alteration of developmental programs rather than by neuronal cell loss, as occurs in adults. In animal models, neonatal seizures result in decreases in neurogenesis, sprouting of mossy fibers, and long-standing changes in signaling properties. Seizures in rat pups are also associated with abnormalities in firing patterns of single cells in the hippocampus. Furthermore, these anatomic and physiologic changes correlate well with behavioral dysfunction.

GOAL STATEMENT

The goal of *Clinics in Perinatology* is to keep practicing neonatologists and maternal-fetal medicine specialists up to date with current clinical practice in perinatology by providing timely articles reviewing the state of the art in patient care.

ACCREDITATION

The *Clinics in Perinatology* is planned and implemented in accordance with the Essential Areas and Policies of the Accreditation Council for Continuing Medical Education (ACCME) through the joint sponsorship of the University of Virginia School of Medicine and Elsevier. The University of Virginia School of Medicine is accredited by the ACCME to provide continuing medical education for physicians.

The University of Virginia School of Medicine designates this educational activity for a maximum of 15 *AMA PRA Category 1 Credits*™ for each issue, 60 credits per year. Physicians should only claim credit commensurate with the extent of their participation in the activity.

The American Medical Association has determined that physicians not licensed in the US who participate in this CME activity are eligible for a maximum of 15 *AMA PRA Category 1 Credits*™ for each issue, 60 credits per year.

Credit can be earned by reading the text material, taking the CME examination online at http://www.theclinics.com/home/cme, and completing the evaluation. After taking the test, you will be required to review any and all incorrect answers. Following completion of the test and evaluation, your credit will be awarded and you may print your certificate.

FACULTY DISCLOSURE/CONFLICT OF INTEREST

The University of Virginia School of Medicine, as an ACCME accredited provider, endorses and strives to comply with the Accreditation Council for Continuing Medical Education (ACCME) Standards of Commercial Support, Commonwealth of Virginia statutes, University of Virginia policies and procedures, and associated federal and private regulations and guidelines on the need for disclosure and monitoring of proprietary and financial interests that may affect the scientific integrity and balance of content delivered in continuing medical education activities under our auspices.

The University of Virginia School of Medicine requires that all CME activities accredited through this institution be developed independently and be scientifically rigorous, balanced and objective in the presentation/discussion of its content, theories and practices.

All authors/editors participating in an accredited CME activity are expected to disclose to the readers relevant financial relationships with commercial entities occurring within the past 12 months (such as grants or research support, employee, consultant, stock holder, member of speakers bureau, etc.). The University of Virginia School of Medicine will employ appropriate mechanisms to resolve potential conflicts of interest to maintain the standards of fair and balanced education to the reader. Questions about specific strategies can be directed to the Office of Continuing Medical Education, University of Virginia School of Medicine, Charlottesville, Virginia.

The faculty and staff of the University of Virginia Office of Continuing Medical Education have no financial affiliations to disclose.

The authors/editors listed below have identified no professional or financial affiliations for themselves or their spouse/partner:
Haim Bassan, MD; Robert Boyle, MD (Test Author); Adré J. du Plessis, MBChB, MPH (Guest Editor); Ali Fatemi, MD; Donna M. Ferriero, MD; Fernando F. Gonzalez, MD; Gorm Greisen, MD, DMSc; Henrik Hagberg, MD, PhD; Carla Holloway (Acquisitions Editor); Frances E. Jensen, MD; Michael V. Johnston, MD; Catherine Limperopoulos, PhD; Carina Mallard, PhD; Laura R. Ment, MD; Eliza Myers, MD; Shahab Noori, MD; Theodora A. Stavroudis, MD; Xiaoyang Wang, MD, PhD; Mary Ann Wilson, PhD; and, Martin Wolf, PhD.

The authors/editors listed below identified the following professional or financial affiliations for themselves or their spouse/partner:
Gregory L. Holmes, MD is an industry funded research/investigator and serves on the Advisory Committee for Johnson & Johnson and Ersai.
Istvan Seri, MD, PhD is a consultant and serves on the Advisory Board for Dey LP, and is an industry funded research/investigator for Somanetics Inc.

Disclosure of Discussion of Non-FDA Approved Uses for Pharmaceutical Products and/or Medical Devices.
The University of Virginia School of Medicine, as an ACCME provider, requires that all faculty presenters identify and disclose any off-label uses for pharmaceutical and medical device products. The University of Virginia School of Medicine recommends that each physician fully review all the available data on new products or procedures prior to clinical use.

TO ENROLL

To enroll in the Clinics in Perinatology Continuing Medical Education program, call customer service at 1-800-654-2452 or visit us online at www.theclinics.com/home/cme. The CME program is available to subscribers for an additional fee of $195.00

FORTHCOMING ISSUES

RECENT ISSUES

THE CLINICS ARE NOW AVAILABLE ONLINE!

Access your subscription at:
www.theclinics.com

Preface

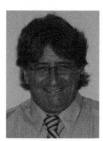

Adré J. du Plessis, MBChB, MPH
Guest Editor

Neonatal neurology began to emerge as a clinical discipline in the 1970s, pioneered by a small cadre of neurologists and neonatologists from around the world. Foremost among these was Joseph Volpe, whose seminal work, "Neurology of the Newborn" galvanized the field. During those early years, the number of presentations on the newborn brain at national academic meetings could be counted on one hand. Over the subsequent 3 decades, however, neonatal neurology has grown into one of the most vibrant subspecialties in newborn medicine, with major meetings now dedicating entire sessions and special interest groups to the newborn brain.

There are several reasons for the remarkable growth in neonatal neurology. First, advances in neonatal critical care have resulted in dramatic decreases in mortality, shifting the focus from survival to the quality of survival of these at-risk infants, which is in turn inextricably linked to their neurologic integrity. Advances in basic neuroscience are opening a host of exciting new pathways for understanding the immature brain and are holding out the promise of emerging neuroprotective modalities. Furthermore, innovative neurodiagnostic techniques, particularly in neuroimaging, now interrogate the structure and function of the neonatal nervous system at the time of acute injury, when the expressiveness of that system is limited. These advances have created a platform from which neuroscience discoveries may translate to clinical benefit. Not surprisingly, these exciting developments have attracted many bright researchers and clinicians to the field and have amplified debates around emerging issues.

The goal of this edition of *Clinics in Perinatology* is to provide clinicians with an updated foundation in areas that continue to challenge the field of neonatal neurology and an orientation to its recently emerging issues.

Drs. Noori, Stavroudis, and Seri tackle the reinvigorated debate on the role of hemodynamic factors in prematurity-related brain injury. Despite the widely held notion that blood pressure disturbances are an important cause of brain injury in this population, human data to support this relationship are surprisingly sparse. Blood pressure, however, is only part of a complex hemodynamic interplay that determines tissue blood flow. Current inability to measure cerebral and systemic blood flow (cardiac output) continuously at the bedside remains the major impediment to developing

doi:10.1016/j.clp.2009.09.001
perinatology.theclinics.com

rational hemodynamic management strategies, particularly in sick premature infants (see Wolf and Greisen elsewhere in this issue).

In recent years, the clinical and research focus in prematurity-related brain injury has been largely on parenchymal, mainly white matter, injury. Intracranial hemorrhage and its complications remain an important cause of brain injury, however, particularly in premature infants. Dr. Bassan provides a detailed review of the pathogenetic mechanisms, diagnostic challenges, and long-term outcomes of the various hemorrhagic lesions, including cerebellar hemorrhage, and their complications. In addition, he discusses the frustrating lack of strategies for the prevention of intracranial hemorrhage and associated secondary mechanisms of brain injury.

The relationship between inflammation and hypoxia-ischemia/reperfusion injury is complex and dynamic, perhaps nowhere more so than in the brain. A large body of experimental and epidemiologic data has implicated infection-inflammation in neonatal brain injury, whereas inflammation is now known to mediate brain injury after a variety of insults, including hypoxia-ischemia/reperfusion. Toll-like receptors are critical pattern-recognition components of the innate immune system and have now been identified on certain brain cells, including microglia and astrocytes. Further complicating understanding of their role in injury (and counteracting their injurious action) is recent evidence that toll-like receptors are involved in normal brain development. Drs. Mallard, Wang, and Hagberg review recent insights into this potentially important pathway of brain injury.

Drs. Myers and Ment review the changing trends in survival and outcome of premature infants, with special focus on the postsurfactant/antenatal era since 1995. Issues reviewed include the slow increase in the incidence of premature birth, the suggestion that the survival rates might be approaching a plateau, and the interesting role of gender on outcome. The unreliable prognostic value of functional outcome testing in the early, preschool years is discussed and contrasted with stability of prognostic factors in school-age and adolescent years. The unreliability of early functional testing for prediction of long-term outcome highlights the need for reliable early measures of brain structure by advanced MRI that reliably predict long-term functional outcome.

Aberrant responses to insults during critical phases of brain development are thought to underlie the disturbed social-behavioral phenotypes seen in survivors of extreme prematurity. Several studies have described these aberrant behavioral patterns, which seem to fit the rubric of autistic spectrum behaviors. Dr. Limperopoulos reviews the emerging evidence supporting a connection between prematurity and autistic spectrum disorders. In addition, she reviews data that link this apparent prematurity-related autistic syndrome to disturbances in cerebellar injury and subsequent growth.

Near-infrared spectroscopy, a bedside technique for measuring tissue oxygenation, arrived on the scene 30 years ago and seemed to fill the enormous gap in the ability to detect developing cerebral hypoxemia. There have been many difficulties with the technique, however, and fundamental assumptions regarding its use have not been resolved. The potential benefits and limitations of the technique are discussed critically by Drs. Wolf and Greisen.

Understanding of the mechanisms underlying hypoxic-ischemic/reperfusion injury in the immature brain has advanced significantly in recent years and is reviewed by Drs. Fatemi, Wilson, and Johnston. Dr. Johnston has been at the forefront of this field since the early descriptions of excitotoxicity as mediator of brain injury and thus as a target for intervention. Dr. Johnston and colleagues provide a broad and detailed review of the understanding of the fundamental mechanisms of hypoxic-ischemic brain injury over the years.

After appearing so tantalizingly within reach 20 years ago with the initial unfolding of the excitoxicity hypothesis, safe and effective neuroprotection has been difficult to translate from the laboratory to infants. Only induced hypothermia seems to have survived the journey from bench to bedside. Drs. Gonzalez and Ferriero discuss these challenges and the current status of neuroprotection strategies for the immature brain. In addition to discussing agents against neuronal hypoxic-ischemic/reperfusion injury, these authors address potential interventions for protection of other, non-neuronal cells against a broader spectrum of insults. They also discuss exciting new developments in the protective effects of growth factors (including erythropoietin), stem cell therapies, antioxidants, antiexcitotoxicity, and anti-inflammatory approaches while emphasizing the importance of combination protocols.

Neonatal seizures remain the most common and obvious clinical manifestation of central nervous system injury in term and preterm infants. What is clear about neonatal seizures is that they have significantly different etiologic profiles from those in adults and also fail to respond to the anticonvulsant medications used in adults. As she reviews the unique etiologic and diagnostic challenges in this area, Dr. Jensen directly addresses the fact that treatment for neonatal seizures has not changed in several decades. Her presentation of the latest basic science findings regarding age-specific seizure mechanisms and of the new therapeutic options being driven by these discoveries offers an early view that possibilities for significant change now exist in this critical arena.

Supplementing the update on neonatal seizures by Dr. Jensen is a review of the longstanding debate regarding the ability of neonatal seizures to cause or extend brain injury independent of their triggering etiology. Dr. Holmes discusses intriguing recent discoveries showing that during critical periods of brain development, seizures may have distributed sublethal effects on neuronal populations and neural systems, resulting in longstanding aberrant connectivity and synaptogenesis, thereby disrupting normal developmental programs. These data further highlight the urgent need for reliable antiseizure agents in this immature population.

The previous edition of *Clinics in Perinatology* focused on fetal neurology as an emerging clinical field. Naturally, the development of the nervous system from fetal to preterm or term infancy forms a continuum. The bridge between these two life phases remains one of the least understood periods in the human lifespan. The need to know as much as possible about fetal and neonatal neurology, in particular about the transitional period that connects the two, warrants further development of the special areas of expertise that this and the previous edition of *Clinics in Perinatology* have showcased.

I am once again extremely grateful to Elsevier for the invitation to serve as guest editor for a subject that has been a career-long passion. I am also deeply grateful to the collaborating authors for the uniformly superb reviews that they put together despite their overextended work lives. Finally, I again owe an enormous debt of gratitude to Shaye Moore and Carla Holloway for their dedicated supervision of all aspects of this project.

Adré J. du Plessis, MBChB, MPH
Department of Neurology, Fegan 11
Children's Hospital Boston
300 Longwood Avenue
Boston, MA 02115, USA

E-mail address:
adre.duplessis@childrens.harvard.edu

Systemic and Cerebral Hemodynamics During the Transitional Period After Premature Birth

Shahab Noori, MD[a], Theodora A. Stavroudis, MD[b,c],
Istvan Seri, MD, PhD[b,c],*

KEYWORDS

- Prematurity • Cerebral blood flows • Systemic blood flow
- CNS injury • Autoregulation • Vital organs • Outcomes

During the complex process of cardiovascular adaptation, the parallel circuit of the fetal circulation changes to the postnatal circulation in which the systemic and pulmonary circuits function in series. As the lungs become the organ of gas exchange at delivery, the systemic and pulmonary circulations separate and, in the healthy term neonate, fetal channels functionally close within a few hours or up to 48 hours after birth.[1] However, in the preterm neonate, especially in the very low birth weight (VLBW) neonate (gestational age <30 wk and a birth weight <1500 g), this process is complicated by immaturity in general and by the immaturity of the cardiorespiratory, central nervous, and endocrine systems in particular.[1–4] This article discusses the hemodynamic changes in the VLBW neonate during postnatal transition and reviews the interaction between systemic and cerebral hemodynamics, and the effect of this interaction on clinically relevant outcomes in this extremely vulnerable patient population.

DEFINITION OF NEONATAL SHOCK IN THE TRANSITIONAL PERIOD

When cardiovascular impairment does occur in the transitional period, the newborn may present with only the early compensated phase of shock, or its condition may

[a] Section of Neonatal-Perinatal Medicine, Department of Pediatrics, The Children's Hospital, College of Medicine, The University of Oklahoma Health Sciences Center, 1200 Everett Drive, 7th Floor North Pavilion, Oklahoma City, OK 73104-5047, USA
[b] USC Division of Neonatal Medicine, Department of Pediatrics, Center for Fetal and Neonatal Medicine, Children's Hospital, Los Angeles, Keck School of Medicine, University of Southern California, 4650 Sunset Boulevard, Mailstop #31, Los Angeles, CA 90027, USA
[c] Department of Pediatrics, The LAC+USC Medical Center, Keck School of Medicine, University of Southern California, 2051 Marengo Street, Los Angeles, CA 90033, USA
* Corresponding author. USC Division of Neonatal Medicine, Center for Fetal and Neonatal Medicine, Children's Hospital, Los Angeles, Keck School of Medicine, University of Southern California, 4650 Sunset Boulevard, Mailstop #31, Los Angeles, CA 90027.
E-mail address: iseri@chla.usc.edu (I. Seri).

Clin Perinatol 36 (2009) 723–736
doi:10.1016/j.clp.2009.07.015   perinatology.theclinics.com
0095-5108/09/$ – see front matter © 2009 Elsevier Inc. All rights reserved.

further deteriorate and develop into the uncompensated phase of shock (see later discussion). Shock is defined as "a state of cellular energy failure resulting from an inability of tissue oxygen delivery to satisfy tissue oxygen demand."[5,6] From a pathophysiologic standpoint, 3 phases of shock have been identified.[7–9]

In the compensated phase, complex neuroendocrine compensatory mechanisms maintain perfusion and oxygen delivery to the vital organs (brain, heart, and adrenal glands) in the normal range at the expense of decreased perfusion to the rest of the organs (nonvital organs). This state is achieved by vasodilation in the vessels of the vital organs and vasoconstriction in the vascular beds of the nonvital organs in response to a decrease in perfusion pressure or oxygen delivery.[10,11] Blood pressure (BP) is maintained within the normal range and heart rate increases, whereas systemic perfusion in general may be somewhat decreased during this phase. As perfusion of nonvital organs is decreased as a result of compensatory vasoconstriction in their vascular beds, there are clinical signs of compromised nonvital organ function, such as decreased urine output. In addition, evidence of poor peripheral perfusion may also be detected, such as cold extremities and prolonged capillary refill time.

In the uncompensated phase, the infant develops hypotension because of failure of the neuroendocrine mechanisms to compensate for the worsening low cardiac output state, and thus perfusion of all organs, including the vital organs, becomes compromised, and lactic acidosis develops.

If treatment is ineffective, failure of organ function develops and shock enters its irreversible phase, in which permanent damage to organs occurs and interventions will be ineffective to reverse the patient's condition.

Thus, timely recognition and prompt treatment of circulatory compromise are important. However, at present there is no evidence that treatment of neonatal hypotension improves outcome.[12] In addition, the gestational and postnatal age-dependent normal blood pressure (BP) range is not known in the preterm neonate during transition,[13] hindering prompt recognition of the different phases of shock. Hence, it is crucial to decipher the hemodynamic changes during the transitional period with a special focus on the interaction between systemic and cerebral hemodynamics, so that survival and long-term neurodevelopmental outcome can be improved. Recent advances in our ability to monitor systemic and cerebral, renal, intestinal, and muscle blood flow, and tissue oxygenation and brain function at the bedside hold the promise of achieving a better understanding of the complex hemodynamic changes during transition.[14] These advances will then hopefully lead to the development of targeted interventions and, thus, better outcomes.

CARDIOVASCULAR ADAPTATION TO EXTRAUTERINE LIFE IN THE VLBW NEONATE

The fetus develops under relatively hypoxemic conditions compared with the level of oxygenation after delivery.[15] In utero, the placenta is the organ of gas exchange, the site of transport processes between the mother and the fetus, and the source of several hormones vital for normal intrauterine development and peri- and postnatal adaptation during labor and after delivery. As a result of the low vascular resistance of the placenta, the high vascular resistance of the fluid-filled fetal lungs, and the presence of the fetal channels, the fetal circulation functions as a parallel circuit, with right-to-left shunting of relatively oxygenated blood through the foramen ovale (FO) and less well saturate blood across the ductus arteriosus. The right ventricle plays a dominant role in maintaining the combined cardiac output of the parallel circulation.[16] The unique features of the fetal circulation ensure that the brain and myocardium receive the most highly oxygenated blood in the fetus.[15]

When the low-resistance placenta is separated from the fetal circulation at birth, a sudden increase in systemic vascular resistance (SVR) occurs, to which the left ventricle of the heart must immediately adapt. The stress on the myocardium is usually not a problem in late preterm and term neonates, as they have achieved appropriate levels of myocardial structural and functional maturity, and autonomic nervous system and endocrine function. Therefore, these neonates are able to sustain appropriate systemic perfusion to meet the increased oxygen demand during and after transition from fetal to extrauterine life. However, the absolute brain blood flow, assessed by ultrasound as the sum of blood flow through the 4 arteries supplying the brain,[17] increases more during the first 2 days after delivery than during the ensuing 12 days, even in preterm infants with gestational ages between 32 and 35 weeks. This finding indicates that the more pronounced increase in cerebral blood flow (CBF) from the first to the second postnatal day is part of the normal hemodynamic transition to extrauterine life.[17] The slope of the increase in CBF during the first 2 days is steeper in preterm neonates with a gestational age of 28 to 32 weeks.[17] It is not known whether the trend of a larger increase in CBF immediately after delivery would hold for patients less than 28 weeks old.

The myocardium of the very preterm neonate has limited capacity, and, according to one of the leading hypotheses explaining the pathophysiology of transitional circulatory compromise in the very preterm neonate, the sudden increase in SVR following cord clamping may result in transient myocardial dysfunction and thus decreased systemic perfusion.[18] Because compensatory mechanisms are immature, the decrease in systemic perfusion may result in decreases in CBF, and thus oxygen delivery, to the brain early in the process. Decreased oxygen delivery to the brain may then result in injury in the central nervous system (CNS) in general, and in the white matter (WM) in particular, because blood flow to the WM in the human neonate is extremely low even under normal conditions.[19] Moreover, available findings indicate that, even without appreciable injury to the CNS during the period of relative systemic hypoperfusion during postnatal transition, the initial decrease in systemic perfusion is followed by an improvement in the cardiovascular status and reperfusion of the organs. This hypoperfusion-reperfusion cycle may result in injury to the brain in the form of peri-/intraventricular hemorrhage (PIVH).[20,21] Thus, it seems that the initial ischemia and the ensuing reperfusion have the potential to cause injury to the immature brain. In addition to these direct hemodynamic changes, oxidative injury and the decreased capacity of the VLBW neonate to control nonspecific inflammatory processes are believed also to play an important role in the pathophysiology of brain injury in the VLBW neonate during the period of transition to extrauterine life.[22]

Evidence for the Role of Myocardial Immaturity and the Sudden Increase in SVR in the Development of the Ischemia-reperfusion Cycle

The major challenge in obtaining accurate information on systemic perfusion and its effect on CBF and cerebral oxygen delivery lies in the fact that the fetal channels remain open in most preterm neonates during the transitional period.[1,2] As mentioned earlier, the parallel circuit of the fetal circulation must change into the mature circulation after delivery, so that the systemic and pulmonary circuits are completely separated and the cardiovascular system functions as a circulation in series.[9,23,24] However, when this process is compromised by ongoing ductal patency, as occurs in 50% to 70% of VLBW neonates,[1,2] the increase in SVR and BP, combined with the gradual decrease in the pulmonary vascular resistance (PVR), results in an increasing pattern of left-to-right shunting across the ductus arteriosus (DA).[1,4] In most VLBW neonates, PVR initially decreases rapidly, for physiologic and nonphysiologic reasons.[1] Physiologic mechanisms playing the most prominent role in the postnatal drop in PVR include the mechanical effects of initiation of air breathing on PVR and the increased postnatal oxygenation-associated direct, paracrine, and endocrine vasodilation.[25] Nonphysiologic reasons include surfactant administration or the inappropriate targeting of higher arterial oxygen saturations.[1,26] With the left-to-right ductal shunting, pulmonary overcirculation develops and left ventricular output (LVO), the gold standard of bedside assessment of systemic perfusion, cannot be used as a measure of systemic perfusion in these VLBW neonates (**Fig. 1**).[27] Indeed under these circumstances, the LVO measures systemic perfusion and ductal blood flow. Unfortunately, in several studies investigating the post-transitional changes in systemic perfusion or the effects of vasopressors, inotropes, and lusitropes on cardiovascular function, this fact has not been consistently acknowledged.[28,29] Therefore, the conclusions drawn in many of these studies[27] need to be carefully reevaluated. However, more recent studies have acknowledged this problem and used right ventricular output (RVO) to assess systemic perfusion in the VLBW neonate during the transitional period.[30–33] However, as left-to-right shunting across a nonconstricting patent ductus arteriosus (PDA) increases over the course of the first 12 to 36 hours, left atrial volume and pressure continue to increase, and, in many cases, this situation leads to the development of a significant left-to-right shunt across the FO.[27] The left-to-right shunt through the patent foramen ovale (PFO) will then render the use of RVO as a measure of systemic blood flow inaccurate, as RVO now represents systemic inflow and PFO flow.[27] Unfortunately, because neither PDA nor PFO flow can be accurately estimated with functional echocardiography, there is no acceptable conventional measure to assess systemic blood flow in these patients. To circumvent this problem, Evans and Kluckow[34] suggested the use of superior vena cava (SVC) flow as a measure of upper body blood flow in preterm neonates with the fetal channels open. These investigators and their colleagues showed that low SVC flow is

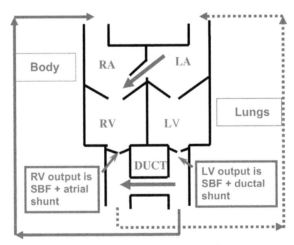

Fig. 1. The effect of left-to-right shunting across the PDA and PFO on LVO and RVO measurements. LVO consists of total pulmonary venous return and ductal blood flow, whereas RVO represents systemic venous return and left-to-right shunting through the PFO. SBF indicates systemic blood flow. (*From* Kluckow M and Seri I. Clinical presentations of neonatal shock: the VLBW infant during the first postnatal day. In: Hemodynamics and cardiology. Neonatal questions and controversies. Kleinman CS, Seri I, editors. Philadelphia: Saunders Elsevier; 2008. p. 147–77; with permission.)

associated with poor short- and long-term outcomes.[35] In addition, the findings obtained by the use of SVC flow have provided novel insights into the mechanisms of transitional hemodynamics, including the observation that PIVH occurs in many patients as systemic blood flow improves and reperfusion of the brain takes place.[20,36] This finding supports the role of the ischemia-reperfusion cycle in the pathophysiology of PIVH (see later discussion).[27,36] Other investigators using near infrared spectroscopy (NIRS) to assess changes in oxygen delivery and consumption in the brain in VLBW neonates during the first 3 to 4 postnatal days have come to similar conclusions.[37,38] The use of SVC flow measurements has remained more a research than a clinical tool[39] because of its vulnerability to error and the technical difficulties associated with its use as a surrogate measure of systemic blood flow.

The original findings using SVC flow as a surrogate measure of systemic blood flow during the transitional period with the fetal channels open revealed that 50% to 70% of very immature infants (gestational age of <27 weeks) may have significant decreases in SVC flow during the first 3 to 36 postnatal hours.[20,34] A more recent study from the same group found a lower incidence (approximately 20%) of low SVC flow, and the investigators speculated that improvements in the peri- and postnatal management of these infants may have contributed to the decrease in the incidence of catastrophically low SVC flows.[33]

Evidence for Additional Factors Playing a Role in the Ischemia-reperfusion Cycle During Transition

Based on these findings, it was proposed that systemic and thus cerebral hypoperfusion is primarily due to the inability of the immature myocardium to cope with the sudden increase in the SVR.[18,20,27,36] The hypoperfusion is then followed by myocardial adaptation and improvement in systemic blood flow, with the associated reperfusion playing a role in the development of PIVH in the very preterm neonate. Thus, it seemed plausible that by minimizing or preventing the occurrence of the initial hypoperfusion, reperfusion will not take place, and CNS outcomes will improve. Therefore, a randomized placebo-controlled blinded clinical trial was undertaken to investigate whether the use of milrinone to minimize or prevent the increase in SVR immediately after delivery would be associated with a decrease in the incidence of systemic hypoperfusion and perhaps PIVH.[33] However, after obtaining information on the pharmacokinetics, and thus the appropriate dosing of milrinone in the preterm neonate,[40] this interventional trial showed no improvement in the incidence of SVC flow used as a surrogate of systemic blood flow. Although these findings are disappointing, they underscore the complexity of the pathophysiology of cardiovascular compromise in the very preterm neonate, and suggest that the theory that systemic and cerebral hypoperfusion and reperfusion occur solely because of myocardial immaturity in the face of the sudden postnatal increase in SVR may be overly simplistic. In addition, there is a debate about the occurrence or severity of the proposed initial vasoconstriction as evidence also suggests that, at least in preterm neonates with chorioamnionitis, vasodilation and hyperdynamic myocardial function are the predominant characteristic features of the transitional circulation early after delivery.[41,42] Studies on microvascular perfusion also support the presence of vasodilation, although the timing of the event needs to be further characterized using laser-Doppler or side-stream dark field imaging technology.[43]

Assignment of vital organ blood flow regulation
Several indirect lines of evidence obtained in human neonates suggest that the assignment of the circulation of the forebrain to a high-priority vascular bed may not be

complete in the extremely preterm neonate at birth.[38,44,45] This hypothesis is supported by findings of CBF regulation in developing animals, in which the ability of the vascular bed of the forebrain to vasodilate in response to hypoxia/hypoperfusion lags far behind that of the hindbrain.[44,45] In fact, studies on dog pups indicate that the forebrain vessels vasoconstrict as the vessels of nonvital organs, while the vessels of the hindbrain vasodilate in response to exposure to hypoxia (**Fig. 2**).[45] The teleologic explanation for these observations may be that the forebrain does not contribute to survival of the fetus during early gestation. The finding that CBF autoregulation also develops in the brainstem first and in the forebrain only later in gestation[44] supports the notion that the developmentally regulated difference in the importance for fetal existence and wellbeing between the hind- and forebrain affects the timing of the development of the blood flow autoregulatory functions and vital organ assignment characteristics in these parts of the brain.

The identification of vital organs with high-priority vascular beds can be traced back to studies of diving physiology, in which an organism has to adapt to the gradual development of oxygen-limiting conditions when submerged under water for prolonged periods of time. In these circumstances, blood flow becomes centralized through vasoconstriction in nonvital organs, and is directed through vasodilation toward the brain, heart, and adrenal glands (vital organs). Thus, as described earlier, in an attempt to sustain vital organ function, the vessels of the vital organs respond to decreased perfusion pressure or oxygen delivery with vasodilation (high-priority

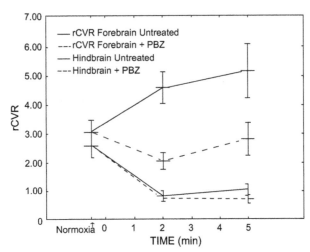

Fig. 2. Changes in regional cerebral vascular resistance (rCVR) during asphyxia in newborn dogs. rCVR in the forebrain (cortical regions) and hindbrain (pons, medulla and spinal cord) of untreated and phenoxybenzamine (PBZ)-treated newborn dogs. During normoxia, hindbrain and forebrain rCVR are not different. After 2 to 5 minutes of asphyxia in untreated dogs, rCVR in the hindbrain decreases, whereas in the forebrain it increases ($P<.05$). In the forebrain, PBZ (a non-selective α-receptor antagonist) restores the vasodilatory response to hypoxia expected to occur in a mature vital organ, whereas it does not further alter rCVR in the hindbrain, suggesting that maximum vasodilation in response to hypoxia is achieved in this region of the brain. See text for details. (*From* Hernandez MJ, Hawkins RA, Brennan RW. Sympathetic control of regional cerebral blood flow in the asphyxiated newborn dog. In: Cerebral blood flow, effects of nerves and neurotransmitters. Heistad DD, Marcus ML editors. New York: Elsevier; 1982. p. 359–66; with permission.)

vascular beds), whereas the vessels of the nonvital organs with low-priority vascular beds vasoconstrict. Indeed, the diving reflex has been demonstrated in the late-gestation fetus when a hypoxic insult activates a chain of events leading to redistribution of blood flow to the brain, adrenal glands, and heart, and away from the lungs, gastrointestinal tract, kidney, and skin (nonvital organs).[8,15] As mentioned earlier, because the various stages of organ development likely have an influence on what is vital for the organism at a given gestational age, it is conceivable that the forebrain does not attain vital organ assignment from a blood flow regulatory standpoint until later in gestation.[38,44,45] The cellular mechanisms of the assignment of vital and nonvital organ status from a blood flow regulatory standpoint are poorly understood.

In summary, one can speculate that the proposed diminished capacity or failure of the forebrain vessels to vasodilate when the very preterm neonate faces the complex process of cardiovascular transition may contribute to hypoperfusion of the forebrain when the patient is in the compensated phase of shock. As this phase is difficult to recognize immediately after delivery, forebrain hypoperfusion and, on adaptation of the newborn to the extrauterine environment, the ensuing reperfusion can occur completely unnoticed. In addition, there is little one can do about this process at present other than attempt to prevent the occurrence of additional stressful events for the very preterm neonate during the initial period of postnatal transition.

AUTOREGULATION OF CBF AND THE EFFECT OF CHANGES IN $PaCO_2$

Autoregulation is the result of a myogenic reflex whereby the arteries constrict when transmural pressure increases, and dilate when there is a decrease in pressure. The reflex thus results in almost unchanged blood flow within a range of arterial BPs.[46,47]

Available findings suggest that autoregulation of CBF is present in the normotensive very preterm neonate.[46,48] However, the autoregulatory BP range is believed to be narrow in neonates, especially in preterm infants. Findings in the instrumented fetal lamb model indicate that the lower limit and the range of the CBF autoregulatory BP increase as gestational age advances.[49,50] However, the more immature the animal, the closer the mean BP runs to the lower elbow of the BP autoregulatory curve, suggesting that even small decreases in BP may render the cerebral perfusion pressure passive.[49]

Several studies, using mostly ultrasound or NIRS, have examined the relationship between the state of CBF autoregulation and the development of CNS pathology in preterm neonates.[46] The findings of these studies suggest an association but do not prove causation between CBF variability, with its limited or compromised autoregulation, and clinically relevant neurodevelopmental outcomes (see later discussion).

Autoregulation is significantly affected by factors other than BP, such as by changes in $PaCO_2$.[46,47,50] Indeed, the CO_2-CBF reactivity is more robust than pressure-flow reactivity, so a 1-mm Hg change in $PaCO_2$ results in a 4% change in CBF, whereas a 1-mm Hg change in BP is estimated to be associated with a 1% change in CBF only.[47,50] As hypo- and hypercapnia-induced arterial vasoconstriction and dilation respectively are mediated through changes induced by CO_2 in the perivascular pH,[47,50] and because the tight junctions of the blood-brain barrier restrict the diffusion of bicarbonate to buffer the changes in H^+ concentration,[47,50] CBF is affected more and for a longer time by changes in $PaCO_2$ than is blood flow in other organs. The reason for the prolonged effects of changes in $PaCO_2$ is that it takes several hours for bicarbonate concentration to equilibrate.[47,50] Perivascular pH exerts its effect on smooth muscle function via its direct effect on potassium conductance, and thus on the membrane potential of arterial smooth muscle cells.[47] Changes in membrane potential in turn affect the function of voltage-gated calcium channels and thus calcium availability within the smooth muscle cell, leading to vasoconstriction or vaso-dilation with increased or decreased availability of intracellular calcium, respectively.[51,52] BP also alters smooth muscle cell membrane conductance, but, as discussed above, its effect is limited compared with that of CO_2.

Because the very preterm neonate has difficulties maintaining appropriate gas exchange without support, and because CO_2 is such a potent regulator of CBF, changes in $Paco_2$ during resuscitation and mechanical ventilation are associated with CNS pathology. Indeed, a $Paco_2$ less than 30 mm Hg for 30 minutes or more is associated with a significant increase in periventricular leukomalacia (PVL) and cerebral palsy,[53,54] whereas marked hypercapnea or fluctuation in $Paco_2$ are associated with increased incidence of PIVH in very preterm neonates.[55–57]

ASSOCIATION BETWEEN SYSTEMIC HYPOTENSION, HYPOPERFUSION, AND THEIR TREATMENT AND NEURODEVELOPMENTAL IMPAIRMENT IN THE VLBW NEONATE

Due to several factors, it has been difficult to ascertain the effect of hypotension or its treatment on brain injury or neurodevelopmental impairment. First, because of the documented association between hypotension and brain injury, and because improvements in systemic and cerebral hemodynamics (ie, oxygen delivery) are believed to protect against brain injury, common practice has been to treat hypotension.[58–62] As a result, there are no prospective studies evaluating the effect of untreated hypotension on clinically relevant short- and long-term outcomes. Second, hypotension frequently occurs during the transition to postnatal life, especially in less-mature preterm neonates, so developmentally regulated factors such as myocardial dysfunction, vital organ assignment, PDA, and factors associated with the treatment of these neonates, such as high positive airway pressure, likely play a role in the development of brain injury. In addition, sick preterm infants with hypotension are also more likely to present with a dysregulated nonspecific inflammatory process, irrespective of their hemodynamic status. As increased production of inflammatory cytokines and oxygen free radicals are believed to be the common pathway of brain injury caused by ischemia-reperfusion and inflammation,[54] it is difficult, if not impossible, to identify the independent contribution of systemic hypotension versus inflammation to poor neurodevelopmental outcomes. As mentioned earlier, a gestational and postnatal age-dependent definition of hypotension based on physiology, pathophysiology, and clinically relevant outcome measures is lacking.[13] That hypotension, as currently defined, may not be predictive of early brain injury[8,63] is especially important when examining the association between hypotension (and its treatment) and neurodevelopmental impairment.

Indeed, there are limited and mostly retrospective data on the long-term outcome of hypotensive preterm infants, as most studies on the subject have focused on the association between hypotension and PIVH. A retrospective study has documented an association between the duration of hypotension in VLBW infants and adverse neurodevelopmental outcome at 24 months of age.[59] In a more recent large prospective study, in which hypotension was defined as a mean BP less than 30 mm Hg in very preterm neonates, hypotensive infants had a significant increase in adverse neurologic outcome at term.[64] After adjustment for gestational age, PVL, and bronchopulmonary dysplasia, hypotension was still associated with an approximately 2-fold increase in neurologic morbidity.[64] Furthermore, a few retrospective studies have recently raised concerns by finding an association between treated hypotension and poor outcomes.[65–67] In one of these studies, extremely low birth weight (ELBW) infants who were treated for hypotension had an increased rate of delayed motor development and hearing loss compared with their nonhypotensive counterparts.[65] However, it remains unclear whether hypotension, its treatment, or both were responsible for the documented association. The other retrospective study[66] compared hospital outcome in 3 groups of ELBW infants: normotensive neonates, and hypotensive patients with and without poor perfusion. Hypotension was defined as a mean BP less than gestational age. Hypotensive patients with signs of poor perfusion had significantly higher mortality and lower rates of survival without severe brain injury or surgical gastrointestinal problems compared with the other 2 groups. One interpretation of the findings of this retrospective study is that hypotensive preterm infants without evidence of hypoperfusion may not necessarily be at high risk for mortality and selected morbidities. However, as mortality rate was high (approximately 72%) in the hypotensive patients with poor perfusion, another interpretation may be that the delay in treatment of uncompensated shock in this vulnerable patient population is associated with progression of shock to the irreversible phase, and thus with high mortality. When examining the potential benefit or harm of the treatment of hypotension, lumping all hypotensive patients into 1 group regardless of their response to the treatment is a significant and common limitation in these studies. This point is important, as the findings of the only prospective randomized clinical trial available on this subject showed that hypotensive VLBW neonates had a higher rate of severe PIVH than nonhypotensive controls.[67] However, this difference disappeared when only the hypotensive patients who responded to vasopressors/inotropes were compared with the control group. Furthermore, the study found no association between abnormal ultrasound findings and the use of vasopressors/inotropes (dopamine or epinephrine). At 2- to 3-year follow-up, there was no difference in the rate of abnormal neurologic status, developmental delay, or combined adverse outcome between the survivors of the hypotensive and control groups. Although the results of this study provide some reassurance about the safety and potential benefits of the careful use of vasopressors/inotropes for the treatment of hypotension, the small sample size and the lack of an untreated hypotensive group limit the scope for generalization from the findings.

It remains unclear whether the choice of vasopressor/inotropes used for the treatment of hypotension in the VLBW neonate has an effect on clinically relevant CNS outcomes. A recent meta-analysis found no difference between dopamine and dobutamine on neonatal mortality, incidence of PVL, or severe PIVH.[68] Similarly, the available data do not show a difference in death or neurodevelopmental outcome at 3 years of age in preterm infants treated with dopamine or dobutamine for low SVC blood flow.[69] However, the limited available data and the inherent weaknesses associated with the use of meta-analysis preclude us from drawing firm conclusions on this subject.

Because of the routine use of BP and serum lactic acid measurements in clinical practice, most studies have evaluated hypotension or metabolic acidosis as predictors of neurodevelopmental outcome. Because of the limitations in our ability to determine systemic and organ blood flows, especially during the transitional period, few studies have evaluated the role of brain or upper body blood flow on short- or long-term outcomes. As discussed earlier, preterm infants have low CBF in the first day of postnatal life.[19,20,36–38,46,70] However, by the second day after birth, CBF increases. Several investigators, using various methods, have demonstrated that preterm infants who subsequently develop PIVH have a more exaggeratedly low CBF during the first day of life.[17,20,21,27,71,72] However, an association between early hypotension and PVL is less well documented. Other than the possible role in the pathogenesis of PIVH, low

CBF may also adversely affect neurodevelopment independent of the development of PIVH. Indeed, preterm infants with low SVC flow during early postnatal transition have been shown to have a higher rate of mortality and neurodevelopmental impairments at 3 years of age.[35,69] However, these findings need to be confirmed using continuous and direct assessment of brain blood flow or tissue oxygen delivery. Indeed, recent advances in technology, especially in NIRS combined with the use of amplitude-integrated electroencephalography, show promise in improving our ability to assess the interaction between hypotension and brain perfusion and function, and to study the effect of hypotension and its treatment on long-term outcome.

SUMMARY

In the VLBW neonate during the transitional period, complex interactions exist between systemic blood flow, BP, and CBF, and between alterations in CBF and short- and long-term neurodevelopmental sequelae. Developmentally regulated immaturity of cardiovascular adaptive mechanisms, such as the immaturity of myocardial and autonomic nervous system functions, vital organ assignment, and oxygen demand and delivery coupling, represent the most important hemodynamic factors that limit the capacity of the very preterm neonate to adapt to the extrauterine environment without a significant risk of injury to the brain. In addition to these hemodynamic factors, inflammation and other factors play a significant and often synergistic role in the development of CNS injury in this extremely vulnerable patient population.

REFERENCES

1. Noori S, Seri I. The VLBW neonate with a hemodynamically significant patent ductus arteriosus during the first postnatal week. In: Kleinman CS, Seri I, editors. Hemodynamics and cardiology. Neonatal questions and controversies. Philadelphia: Saunders Elsevier; 2008. p. 178–94.
2. Reller MD, Rice MJ, McDonald RW. Review of studies evaluating ductal patency in the premature infant. J Pediatr 1993;122:S59–62.
3. Clyman RI, Waleh N, Black SM, et al. Regulation of ductus arteriosus patency by nitric oxide in fetal lambs: the role of gestation, oxygen tension, and vasa vasorum. Pediatr Res 1998;43:633–44.
4. Evans N, Malcolm G, Osborn D, et al. Diagnosis of patent ductus arteriosus in preterm infants. NeoReviews 2004;5:e86–97.
5. Noori S, Seri I. Etiology, pathophysiology, and phases of neonatal shock. In: Kleinman CS, Seri I, editors. Hemodynamics and cardiology. Neonatal questions and controversies. Philadelphia: Saunders Elsevier; 2008. p. 3–18.
6. Singer M. Cellular dysfunction in sepsis. Clin Chest Med 2008;29:655–60.
7. Zaritsky A, Chernow B. The use of catecholamines in pediatrics. J Pediatr 1984; 105:341–50.
8. McLean CW, Cayabyab R, Noori S, et al. Cerebral circulation and hypotension in the premature infant – diagnosis and treatment. In: Perlman JM, editor. Controversies in neonatal neurology. Philadelphia: Saunders Elsevier; 2008. p. 3–26.
9. Iwamoto HS. Cardiovascular effects of acute hypoxia and asphyxia. In: Hanson MA, Spencer JAD, Rodeck CH, editors. Fetus and neonate. Physiology and clinical application, The circulation, vol. 1. Cambridge (UK): Cambridge University Press; 1993. p. 197–214.
10. Sheldon RE, Peeters LL, Jones MD, et al. Redistribution of cardiac output and oxygen delivery in the hypoxemic fetal lamb. Am J Obstet Gynecol 1979;135:1071–8.

11. Shah P, Riphagen S, Beyene J, et al. Multiorgan dysfunction in infants with post-asphyxial hypoxic-ischaemic encephalopathy. Arch Dis Child Fetal Neonatal Ed 2004;89(2):F152–5.
12. Barrington KJ, Dempsey EM. Cardiovascular support in the preterm: treatments in search of indications. J Pediatr 2006;148:289–91.
13. Engle WD. Definition of normal blood pressure range: the elusive target. In: Kleinman CS, Seri I, editors. Hemodynamics and cardiology. Neonatal questions and controversies. Philadelphia: Saunders Elsevier; 2008. p. 39–65.
14. Cayabyab R, McLean CW, Seri I. Definition of hypotension and assessment of hemodynamics in the preterm neonate. J Perinatol 2009;29(Suppl 2):S58–62.
15. Wilkening RB, Meschia G. Fetal oxygen uptake, oxygenation, and acid-base balance as a function of uterine blood flow. Am J Physiol 1983;244:H749–55.
16. Clyman RI, Heymann MA, editors. Maternal-fetal Medicine. Philadelphia: WB Saunders CO; 1999. p. 249.
17. Kehrer M, Blumenstock G, Ehehalt S, et al. Development of cerebral blood flow volume in preterm neonates during the first two weeks of life. Pediatr Res 2005;58:927–30.
18. Evans N. Assessment and support of the preterm circulation. Early Hum Dev 2006;82:803–10.
19. Greisen G, Børch K. White matter injury in the preterm neonate: the role of perfusion. Dev Neurosci 2001;23:209–12.
20. Kluckow M, Evans N. Low superior vena cava flow and intraventricular hemorrhage in preterm infants. Arch Dis Child Fetal Neonatal Ed 2000;82:F188–94.
21. Osborn DA, Evans N, Kluckow M. Hemodynamic and antecedent risk factors of early and late periventricular/intraventricular hemorrhage in premature infants. Pediatrics 2003;112:33–9.
22. Volpe JJ. Postnatal sepsis, necrotizing entercolitis, and the critical role of systemic inflammation in white matter injury in premature infants. J Pediatr 2008;153:160–3.
23. Davies JM, Tweed WA. The regional distribution and determinants of myocardial blood flow during asphyxia in the fetal lamb. Pediatr Res 1984;18:764–7.
24. Kiserud T, Acharya G. The fetal circulation. Prenat Diagn 2004;24:1049–59.
25. Faro R, Moreno L, Hislop AA, et al. Pulmonary endothelium dependent vasodilation emerges after birth in mice. Eur J Pharmacol 2007;567:240–4.
26. Kluckow M, Evans N. Ductal shunting, high pulmonary blood flow, and pulmonary hemorrhage. J Pediatr 2000;137:68–72.
27. Kluckow M, Seri I. Clinical presentations of neonatal shock: the VLBW infant during the first postnatal day. In: Kleinman CS, Seri I, editors. Hemodynamics and cardiology. Neonatal questions and controversies. Philadelphia: Saunders Elsevier; 2008. p. 147–77.
28. Roze JC, Tohier C, Maingueneau C, et al. Response to dobutamine and dopamine in the hypotensive very preterm infant. Arch Dis Child 1993;69: 59–63.
29. Lundstrøm K, Pryds O, Greisen G. The hemodynamic effects of dopamine and volume expansion in sick preterm infants. Early Hum Dev 2000;57:157–63.
30. West CR, Groves AM, Williams CE, et al. Early low cardiac output is associated with compromised electroencephalographic activity in very preterm infants. Pediatr Res 2006;59:610–5.
31. Abdel-Hady H, Matter M, Hammad A, et al. Hemodynamic changes during weaning from nasal continuous positive airway pressure. Pediatrics 2008;122: e1086–90.

32. Bouissou A, Rakza T, Klosowski S, et al. Hypotension in preterm infants with significant patent ductus arteriosus: effects of dopamine. J Pediatr 2008;153: 790–4.
33. Paradisis M, Evans N, Kluckow M, et al. Randomized trial of milrinone versus placebo for prevention of low systemic blood flow in very preterm infants. J Pediatr 2009;154:189–95.
34. Kluckow M, Evans N. Superior vena cava flow in newborn infants: a novel marker of systemic blood flow. Arch Dis Child Fetal Neonatal Ed 2000;82: F182–7.
35. Hunt RW, Evans N, Rieger I, et al. Low superior vena cava flow and neurodevelopment at 3 years in very preterm infants. J Pediatr 2004;145:588–92.
36. Kluckow M, Evans N. Low systemic blood flow in the preterm infant. Semin Neonatol 2001;6:75–84.
37. Victor S, Marson AG, Appleton RE, et al. Relationship between blood pressure, cerebral electrical activity, cerebral fractional oxygen extraction, and peripheral blood flow in very low birth weight newborn infants. Pediatr Res 2006;59: 314–9.
38. Victor S, Appleton RE, Beirne M, et al. The relationship between cardiac output, cerebral electrical activity, cerebral fractional oxygen extraction and peripheral blood flow in premature newborn infants. Pediatr Res 2006;60:456–60.
39. Evans N. Functional echocardiography in the neonatal intensive care unit. In: Kleinman CS, Seri I, editors. Hemodynamics and cardiology. Neonatal questions and controversies. Philadelphia: Saunders Elsevier; 2008. p. 83–109.
40. Paradisis M, Evans N, Kluckow M, et al. Pilot study of milrinone for low systemic blood flow in very preterm infants. J Pediatr 2006;148:306–13.
41. Yanowitz TD, Jordan JA, Gilmour CH, et al. Hemodynamic disturbances in premature infants born after chorioamnionitis: association with cord blood cytokine concentrations. Pediatr Res 2002;51:310–6.
42. Yanowitz TD, Baker RW, Roberts JM, et al. Low blood pressure among very-low-birth-weight infants with fetal vessel inflammation. J Perinatol 2004;24: 299–304.
43. Stark MJ, Clifton VL, Wright IM. Microvascular flow, clinical illness severity and cardiovascular function in the preterm infant. Arch Dis Child Fetal Neonatal Ed 2008;93:F271–4.
44. Ashwal S, Dale PS, Longo LD. Regional cerebral blood flow: studies in the fetal lamb during hypoxia, hypercapnia, acidosis, and hypotension. Pediatr Res 1984;18:1309–16.
45. Hernandez MJ, Hawkins RA, Brennan RW. Sympathetic control of regional cerebral blood flow in the asphyxiated newborn dog. In: Heistad DD, Marcus ML, editors. Cerebral blood flow, effects of nerves and neurotransmitters. New York: Elsevier; 1982. p. 359–66.
46. Greisen G. Autoregulation of vital and non-vital organ blood flow in the preterm and term neonate. In: Kleinman CS, Seri I, editors. Hemodynamics and cardiology. Neonatal questions and controversies. Philadelphia: Saunders Elsevier; 2008. p. 19–38.
47. Greisen G. Autoregulation of cerebral blood flow in newborn babies. Early Hum Dev 2005;81:423–8.
48. Seri I, Abbasi S, Wood DC, et al. Regional hemodynamic effects of dopamine in the sick preterm infant. J Pediatr 1998;133:728–34.
49. Helou S, Koehler RC, Gleason CA, et al. Cerebrovascular autoregulation during fetal development in sheep. Am J Physiol 1994;266:H1069–74.

50. Müller T, Löhle M, Schubert H, et al. Developmental changes in cerebral autoregulatory capacity in the fetal sheep parietal cortex. J Physiol 2002;539(3): 957–67.
51. Kotecha N, Hill MA. Myogenic contraction in rat skeletal muscle arterioles: smooth muscle membrane potential and Ca^{2+} signaling. Am J Physiol Heart Circ Physiol 2005;289:H1326–34.
52. Lindauer U, Vogt J, Schuh-Hofer S, et al. Cerebrovascular vasodilation to extraluminal acidosis occurs via combined activation of ATP-sensitive and Ca^{2+}-activated potassium channels. J Cereb Blood Flow Metab 2003;23:1227–38.
53. Wiswell TE, Graziani LJ, Kornhauser MS, et al. Effects of hypocarbia on the development of cystic periventricular leukomalacia in premature infants treated with high-frequency jet ventilation. Pediatrics 1996;98:918–24.
54. Khwaja O, Volpe JJ. Pathogenesis of cerebral white matter injury of prematurity. Arch Dis Child Fetal Neonatal Ed 2008;93:F153–61.
55. Kaiser JR, Gauss CH, Pont MM, et al. Hypercapnia during the first 3 days of life is associated with severe intraventricular hemorrhage in very low birth weight infants. J Perinatol 2006;26:279–85.
56. Fabres J, Carlo WA, Phillips V, et al. Both extremes of arterial carbon dioxide pressure and the magnitude of fluctuations in arterial carbon dioxide pressure are associated with severe intraventricular hemorrhage in preterm infants. Pediatrics 2007;119:299–305.
57. McKee LA, Fabres J, Howard G, et al. P_aCO_2 and neurodevelopment in extremely low birth weight infants. J Pediatr 2009, in press.
58. Bada HS, Korones SB, Perry EH, et al. Mean arterial blood pressure changes in premature infants and those at risk for intraventricular hemorrhage. J Pediatr 1990;117:607–14.
59. Goldstein RF, Thompson RJ, Oehler JM, et al. Influence of acidosis, hypoxaemia, and hypotension on neurodevelopmental outcome in very low birth weight infants. Pediatrics 1995;95:238–43.
60. Watkins AM, West CR, Cooke RW. Blood pressure and cerebral hemorrhage and ischemia in very low birth weight infants. Early Hum Dev 1989;19:103–10.
61. Miall-Allen VM, De Vries LS, Whitelaw AGL. Mean arterial blood pressure and neonatal cerebral lesions. Arch Dis Child 1987;62:1068–9.
62. Seri I. Circulatory support of the sick newborn infant. Semin Neonatol 2001;6: 85–95.
63. Limperopoulos C, Bassan H, Kalish LA, et al. Current definitions of hypotension do not predict abnormal cranial ultrasound findings in preterm infants. Pediatrics 2007;120:966–77.
64. Martens SE, Rijken M, Stoelhorst GM, et al. Leiden Follow-Up Project on Prematurity, The Netherlands. Is hypotension a major risk factor for neurological morbidity at term age in very preterm infants? Early Hum Dev 2003;75: 79–89.
65. Fanaroff JM, Wilson-Costello DE, Newman NS, et al. Treated hypotension is associated with neonatal morbidity and hearing loss in extremely low birth weight infants. Pediatrics 2006;117:1131–5.
66. Dempsey EM, Alhazzani F, Barrington KJ. Permissive hypotension in the extremely low birth weight infant with signs of good perfusion. Arch Dis Child Fetal Neonatal Ed 2009;94:F241–4.
67. Pellicer A, del Carmen Bravo M, Madero R, et al. Early systemic hypotension and vasopressor support in low birth weight infants: impact on neurodevelopment. Pediatrics 2009;123:1369–76.

68. Subhedar NV, Shaw NJ. Dopamine versus dobutamine for hypotensive preterm infants. Cochrane Database Syst Rev 2003;(3):CD001242.
69. Osborn DA, Evans N, Kluckow M, et al. Low superior vena cava flow and effects of inotropes on neurodevelopment to 3 years in preterm infants. Pediatrics 2007; 120:372–80.
70. Meek JH, Tyszczuk L, Elwell CE, et al. Cerebral blood flow increases over the first three days of life in extremely preterm neonates. Arch Dis Child Fetal Neonatal Ed 1998;78:F33–7.
71. Kissack CM, Garr R, Wardle SP, et al. Postnatal changes in cerebral oxygen extraction in the preterm infant are associated with intraventricular hemorrhage and hemorrhagic parenchymal infarction but not periventricular leukomalacia. Pediatr Res 2004;56:111–6.
72. Meek JH, Tyszczuk L, Elwell CE, et al. Low cerebral blood flow is a risk factor for severe intraventricular hemorrhage. Arch Dis Child Fetal Neonatal Ed 1999;81: F15–8.

Intracranial Hemorrhage in the Preterm Infant: Understanding It, Preventing It

Haim Bassan, MD

KEYWORDS

- Prematurity • Germinal matrix • Intraventricular hemorrhage
- Periventricular hemorrhagic infarction
- Posthemorrhagic hydrocephalus • Cerebellar hemorrhage
- Genetic • Terminal vein

Intracranial hemorrhage (ICH) in the premature infant is an acquired lesion with enormous potential impact on morbidity, mortality, and long-term neurodevelopmental outcome. Despite considerably improved neonatal care and increased survival of preterm infants over recent decades, ICH continues to be a significantly worrisome problem. New discoveries in neonatal imaging, cerebral monitoring, and hemodynamics, and greater understanding of inflammatory and genetic mechanisms continue to advance the understanding of ICH in premature infants and to pose new challenges for the creation of early detection and prevention strategies. This article covers the spectrum of ICH in the preterm infant, including germinal matrix intraventricular hemorrhage (GM-IVH), its complications, and associated phenomena, such as the emerging role of cerebellar hemorrhage. The overall aim of this article is to review current knowledge of the mechanisms, diagnosis, outcome, and management of preterm ICH; to revisit the origins from which they emerged; and to discuss future expectations in the enhancement of understanding of ICH with the goal of preventing its occurrence.

GERMINAL MATRIX-INTRAVENTRICULAR HEMORRHAGE

Of all types of cerebral hemorrhages, GM-IVH is the most common and distinctive pathology and cranial ultrasound (CUS) diagnosis in premature infants, with

---

Haim Bassan is supported by the Tel Aviv Sourasky Medical Center Research Fund.
Pediatric Neurology Unit, Neonatal Neurology Service, Dana Children's Hospital, Tel Aviv Sourasky Medical Center, Sackler Faculty of Medicine, Tel Aviv University, 6 Weizman Street, Tel Aviv 64239, Israel
E-mail address: bassan@post.tau.ac.il

Clin Perinatol 36 (2009) 737–762
doi:10.1016/j.clp.2009.07.014
0095-5108/09/$ – see front matter

a consistently high incidence throughout the years.[1] Its complications (periventricular hemorrhagic infarction [PVHI] and posthemorrhagic hydrocephalus [PHH]) and the associated cerebellar hemorrhagic injury (CHI) and periventricular leukomalacia (PVL) are critical determinants of neonatal morbidity, mortality, and long-term neuro-developmental sequelae.[1,2] Although advances in perinatal medicine have led to a significant decrease in the overall incidence of GM-IVH in premature infants (ie, from 50% in the late 1970s to the current 15%–25%),[3–5] GM-IVH continues to be a significant problem in the modern neonatal intensive care unit for several reasons. To begin with, advances in medicine have led to a higher incidence of premature births and a major increase in the survival of premature infants, reaching as high as 85% to 90%.[6,7] Moreover, the incidence of birth and survival of the smallest premature infants who are at the highest risk for developing GM-IVH and its complications have increased during the last decade. Specifically, the incidence of GM-IVH reaches 45% in infants with birth weights less than 750 g, and 35% of these lesions are severe.[8] Finally, it has been suggested that the encouraging decrease in the overall incidence of GM-IVH may have reached a plateau during the last decade.[4,5,9] All of these trends have led to the emergence of a large population of critically ill infants who survive premature birth with the manifestations and complications of GM-IVH and its later neurodevelopmental sequelae.[4,6,10]

CLINICAL DIAGNOSIS OF GERMINAL MATRIX-INTRAVENTRICULAR HEMORRHAGE

GM-IVH in premature infants is typically diagnosed during the first days of life, 50% on the first day and 90% within the first 4 days. Between 20% and 40% of these infants undergo progression of hemorrhage during these first days of life.[1] GM-IVH is usually clinically asymptomatic and diagnosed by routine screening CUS in 25% to 50% of cases, whereas symptoms in the rest of the cases are manifested by either a slow saltatory or acute catastrophic presentation. Deterioration in infants who develop large hemorrhages or PVHI present with various degrees of altered consciousness; cardiorespiratory deterioration; fall in hematocrit; acidosis; blood glucose alterations; inappropriate antidiuretic hormone secretion; bulging fontanel; abnormal neuromotor examination (hypotonia, decreased motility, tight popliteal angle); abnormal eye movement or alignment; abnormal pupillary response; and neonatal seizures.[1,11–13] Clinical neonatal seizures are reported in 17% of infants with GM-IVH and in up to 40% of infants with PVHI,[14] mostly described as generalized tonic seizures or subtle seizures. Several reports suggest that most tonic spells are nonepileptic brainstem release phenomena and that it is difficult to differentiate clinically between these and true epileptic events. In any event, studies on the overall incidence of electro-graphic seizure activity in infants with grade III GM-IVH and PVHI described an inci-dence up to 60% to 75% of cases,[15,16] in which most were subclinical.[16]

IMAGING AND BEDSIDE MONITORING OF GERMINAL MATRIX-INTRAVENTRICULAR HEMORRHAGE

For many years neonatal CUS has been the key diagnostic tool for GM-IVH in prema-ture infants.[17] The severity of GM-IVH has been evaluated by Papile[18] and Volpe's[19] grading systems for the last three decades. Papile[18] grading was originally based on computerized tomography (CT): a grade I hemorrhage is confined to the germinal matrix (the main origin of hemorrhage in the premature infant); a grade II hemorrhage is present in a nondistended lateral ventricle; a grade III hemorrhage has a lateral ventricle distended by blood; and grade IV is a GM-IVH with hemorrhage into the parenchyma. Volpe's classification[19] emphasized two additional important aspects.

First, the severity of GM-IVH depends on the amount of blood in the parasagittal CUS view. In grade II GM-IVH, blood fills less than 50% of the ventricular diameter, whereas it fills greater than 50% of the lateral ventricle in grade III GM-IVH. Secondly, Papile's grade IV has a distinctive mechanism (a venous infarction) and making it a complication of GM-IVH (ie, PVHI) rather than a grade of GM-IVH (see discussion later). Widespread availability, relatively low cost, direct bedside approach, and the high resolution for blood detection have resulted in CUS becoming the first-line imaging for GM-IVH. CT had been used in the original studies of GM-IVH in the preterm brain,[13,18] but concerns over radiation effects on the immature brain have led to its no longer being recommended for diagnostic purposes.

Doppler ultrasound has been used to evaluate the arterial and venous systems of the premature infant, including delineation of normative flow velocity parameters.[20–23] In the context of GM-IVH, Doppler ultrasound is widely used in research studies, and current clinical use is limited to measurements of resistive indices of the periclallosal or middle cerebral arteries as an indirect measure of cerebral vascular resistance that informs treatment decisions in PHH. Doppler ultrasound can also be used for the imaging and flow velocity measurements of the terminal vein that is implicated in PVHI, but the clinical importance of this application remains undetermined.

Although the superiority of MRI over CUS for the detection of associated white matter abnormalities and smaller size petechial hemorrhages is well recognized,[24] its use in the early critical period during the first days of life[25,26] is currently hindered by its limited availability, the logistics of transportation, concerns over sedation, and the high cost. These limitations hamper the clinical use of desirable sequences, such as diffusion, spectroscopy, and MR angiography, for the prediction and early detection of GM-IVH and its complications. Clinically, MRI is more frequently used at later time points (term equivalent or after several months) to follow the evolution and consequences of GM-IVH.[27] Importantly, using such sequences as gradient-echo T2-weighted imaging (T2*, susceptibility) enables the detection of residual blood products for long periods of time following the acute hemorrhagic event.

Finally, the last decade has witnessed intense research in the development of bedside techniques for continuous hemodynamic and electrophysiologic monitoring for prediction and early detection of GM-IVH and its progression during critical postnatal periods. The introduction of near infrared spectroscopy (NIRS), a noninvasive, portable technique utilizing light in the near infrared range (700–1000 nm), provided continuous bedside measurements of changes in cerebral oxygenation and hemodynamics. The summation of changes in cerebral concentration of the basic NIRS parameters, oxyhemoglobin (HbO_2) and deoxyhemoglobin (Hb), yields the changes in total cerebral hemoglobin concentration (HbT); conversely, changes in the difference between the cerebral concentration of these two variables provides the hemoglobin difference (HbD) signal. Newly developed spatially resolved NIRS techniques further allow the absolute measurement of the concentration ratio of oxyhemoglobin to total hemoglobin ([TOI] tissue oxygenation index). Relatively short-term changes in HbT concentration reflect changes in cerebral blood volume. Conversely, results of animal studies have suggested that hemoglobin difference is a reliable surrogate of cerebral blood flow (CBF).[28] The TOI measurement mostly reflects oxygen saturation in the cerebral venous compartment. These measures became even more clinically meaningful when they were used to determine the fractional oxygen extraction,[29] and particularly when time locked to the infants' mean arterial blood pressure measurement, allowing continuous assessment of cerebral pressure autoregulation (see discussion later).[30–32] NIRS was used in research on premature infants at risk for GM-IVH[33] or those who developed GM-IVH[30,31] and PHH[34]; however, adaptation of this technique into clinical practice still requires further development and validation.

Background and epileptiform electroencephalography (EEG) abnormalities are reportedly associated with GM-IVH[14,35,36]; however, there is disagreement over the need for continuous EEG monitoring for the detection of electrographic seizures and the long-term benefits of treating them. Another cerebral monitoring technique, amplitude integrated EEG (aEEG), also allows continuous monitoring of background electrocortical activity and detection of epileptiform patterns.[37] Preliminary reports have suggested that electrocortical aEEG abnormalities and epileptiform activity are common in preterm infants with GM-IVH and may precede CUS abnormalities,[15,16,38] but the usefulness of this technique in the intensive care setting for detection of GM-IVH and its advantages or disadvantages over long-term conventional EEG monitoring are still undetermined.

MECHANISMS OF THE GERMINAL MATRIX-INTRAVENTRICULAR HEMORRHAGE

The mechanism of GM-IVH is multifactorial and involves a combination of vascular-anatomic immaturity and complex hemodynamic factors. The impact of emerging inflammatory and genetic factors is currently being investigated.

Vascular Anatomic Vulnerability of the Premature Infant

The pathogenesis of GM-IVH in premature infants fundamentally involves the unusual vascular vulnerability of the germinal matrix, the origin of intraventricular hemorrhage in the immature brain. In addition, choroid plexus hemorrhage is also present in 50% of postmortem GM-IVH cases.[39] The germinal matrix that surrounds the fetal ventricular system gradually involutes to reside over the body of the caudate between 24 and 28 weeks of gestation and at the level of the head of the caudate in the thalamostriate groove between 28 and 34 weeks, finally involuting towards the 36th week of gestation.[40] This tissue is the source of future neuronal and glial cells and is highly vascularized to fulfill the high metabolic demands of the intensely proliferating cells.[1] The rich capillary network of the germinal matrix is composed of high-caliber, irregular, thin-walled (deficient in the muscularis layer), and immature fragile vessels predisposed to rupture.[41] Furthermore, the germinal matrix lies within an arterial end zone, and it is directly connected to the deep galenic venous system,[40,42] thereby exposing it to insults of arterial ischemia-reperfusion and to venous congestion.[40,43]

As suggested by the seminal contribution of Pape and Wigglesworth,[40] it is noteworthy that the immature cerebral venous system has several vulnerabilities that likely make it a major contributor for the genesis of GM-IVH and its complications. First, the development of the cerebral venous system occurs late in relation to that of the arteries. Second, there is sequential remodeling and considerable individual variation in the pattern and size of the different veins entering the internal cerebral veins. Third, immature veins are of high caliber and thin walled, branching parallel to the ventricular system and therefore, tending to collapse. Fourth, because of the relative paucity of superficial cortical veins between 24 and 28 weeks of gestation, most of the cerebral venous drainage is dependent on the dominant deep galenic system that drains the germinal matrix and most of the white matter. Finally, the major veins of the deep system (particularly the terminal [thalamostriate] vein) pass directly through the germinal matrix and change direction in a U-turn fashion (**Fig. 1**).[40] For all these reasons, the immature deep galenic system is prone to venous congestion and stasis, making it of potentially major importance for the development of GM-IVH and its complications.

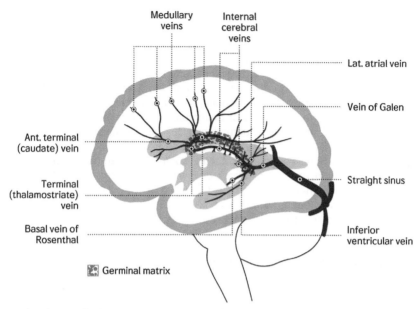

Fig. 1. The deep galenic venous system, sagittal view. The terminal vein is the main vein draining the white matter; it changes its direction, making a U-turn on joining the internal cerebral vein. The periventricular veins, particularly the terminal vein, pass directly through the germinal matrix. Note that the direction of most of the periventricular veins is parallel to that of the ventricular system. (*Adapted from* Volpe JJ. Intracranial hemorrhage. In: Neurology of the newborn. 5th edition. Philadelphia: WB Saunders; 2008. p. 518; with permission.)

Hemodynamic Factors

It is likely that rupture and hemorrhage of the vulnerable germinal matrix requires the coexistence of several intrinsic and extrinsic hemodynamic factors. One intrinsic factor believed to be impaired in sick premature infants is cerebral pressure autoregulation, which is the ability to maintain a relatively constant CBF across a range of cerebral perfusion pressures. Such impairment renders these infants susceptible to both cerebral hypoperfusion and ischemia at the border zone germinal matrix vessels and to bursts of hyperperfusion that can potentially tear the fragile germinal matrix vessels.[44] An association between cerebral pressure passivity and abnormal CO_2 vasoreactivity, as measured by the xenon-133 clearance technique, and the development of GM-IVH was shown in the study of Pryds and colleagues.[45] Tsuji and colleagues[30] used coherence analysis to measure the concordance between mean arterial blood pressure and CBF (as measured by NIRS) to identify pressure passivity. They found that a cerebral pressure passive circulation was significantly associated with GM-IVH and PVL. A subsequent NIRS study by Soul and colleagues[31] demonstrated that periods of cerebral pressure passivity are common in premature infants, and that these were significantly associated with low gestational age and birth weight, and with systemic hypotension. Others have found no association between autoregulation and GM-IVH.[46]

Multisystem immaturity, particularly of the cardiorespiratory system, and the resultant instability of the premature infant can generate various extrinsic factors associated with significant cerebral hemodynamic changes that potentially interfere with the integrity of the vulnerable germinal matrix. Furthermore, some of these factors, specifically hypercarbia, hypoxia, and hypoglycemia, could lead to "paretic" cerebral vasodilatation and cause secondary autoregulatory impairment.[44] The following extrinsic factors have been reported as antecedents of GM-IVH: (1) risk factors for low CBF, including hypotensive events, and frank perinatal asphyxia[47]; (2) risk factors for increased CBF, including hypertension, bolus fluid infusion, pressor treatment, hypercarbia, low hematocrit, pain, and handling[48–50]; (3) risk factors for elevated cerebral venous pressure, including respiratory distress syndrome, positive pressure ventilation, pneumothorax, or pulmonary hemorrhage[9]; and (4) fluctuating CBF.[51,52] The latter observation of fluctuation of CBF (in comparison with stable circulation), as measured by Doppler, was found to be a strong predictor for later development of GM-IVH, and it was suggested that this fluctuating pattern is more common in ventilated infants who are out of synchrony with the ventilator.[51,52] Kissack and colleagues[29] showed that fluctuating fractional oxygen extraction was associated with GM-IVH and PVHI; because fractional oxygen extraction reflects cerebral oxygen delivery and, indirectly, CBF, their data also support the proposition that hemodynamic instability may play a role in the etiology of GM-IVH and PVHI. All the circulatory abnormalities of the cerebral arterial system taken together with those of the venous system could result in net fluctuations of perfusion pressure, important for the genesis of GM-IVH.[53]

Cytokines and Vasoactive, Angiogenic, and Growth Factors

The role of cytokines and of vasoactive, angiogenic, and growth factors in the pathogenesis of GM-IVH is not well understood and their relative contribution is still under investigation. Epidemiologic and experimental studies have suggested an association between infection, inflammatory cytokines, and GM-IVH,[54–56] whereas others did not find such an association.[9,57] Several studies documented an association between GM-IVH and elevated cytokines, particularly interleukin-6, -1, -8, and tumor necrosis factor-α.[56,58,59] Furthermore, preliminary evidence suggested a role for cytokine genes as risk modifiers for GM-IVH and PVL.[60,61] Triggers of cytokine generation in the context of GM-IVH could be maternal and placental infection and inflammation and hypoxic ischemia-reperfusion insult. The mechanisms by which cytokines may be implicated in GM-IVH are by effects on the vascular endothelia causing hemodynamic alterations[62] or frank endothelial damage of the germinal matrix.[56] Cytokines may also activate the coagulation system and induce nitric oxide production.[56] Cytokines can additionally induce cyclooxygenase-2 expression, a major source of prostaglandin production, which in turn produces vasodilatation that may further alter cerebral autoregulation.[44] Prostanoids can also induce the production and release of vascular endothelial growth factor (VEGF), a potent angiogenic factor. Indeed, overexpression of VEGF and a vascular destabilizing factor (angiopoietin 2) was recently described in the germinal matrix of both premature rabbits and premature human infants, suggesting that excessive angiogenesis in the germinal matrix may lead to a propensity to hemorrhage.[63] Furthermore, treatment with celecoxib (cyclooxygenase-2 inhibitor) decreased VEGF and angiopoetin 2 levels, and germinal matrix endothelial proliferation, and substantially decreased the incidence of GM-IVH in the premature rabbit model.[63] Two additional factors, adrenomedullin (a vasoactive peptide) and activin A (a transforming growth factor), were found elevated in blood samples of infants who later developed GM-IVH. It is unknown, however, whether they are merely markers for hypoxic injury or compensatory factors, or whether they provide a mechanistic contribution (eg, alteration of autoregulation) to the development of GM-IVH.[64,65]

Finally, premature infants who died or had severe GM-IVH were found to have diminished levels of thyroid-stimulating hormone and thyroxine, although current belief is that hypothyroxinemia is not implicated in the pathogenesis of GM-IVH but rather serves as a marker of disease severity or a physiologic response to lower the metabolic rate and oxygen consumption as a protective measure.[66,67]

Coagulation and Platelet Abnormalities

The role of coagulation and platelet function in the pathogenesis of GM-IVH is uncertain. Hypothetically, abnormal coagulation could predispose to germinal matrix hemorrhage and hemorrhagic infarction. Prolonged bleeding time, prothrombin time, partial thromboplastin time,[68] low prothrombin activity,[69] lower platelet count,[68,70] and disturbed platelet function (adhesion and aggregation)[68,71] have all been reported in GM-IVH. Because coagulation and platelet disturbances are generally common during the first days of life of sick premature infants,[72–75] it is difficult to define their precise role. Furthermore, the failure of several trials using procoagulant therapies raises even more questions about this association.

Genetic Factors

There are several reasons to suspect that genetic factors may play a part in the pathogenesis of GM-IVH. First, despite their characteristic anatomic and hemodynamic vulnerability, most premature infants do not develop GM-IVH; to the contrary, clinically stable premature infants could still develop GM-IVH, even to a severe degree. Second, despite major advances in perinatal medicine aimed at achieving strict hemodynamic stability (eg, improved ventilatory techniques, control of blood pressure), the incidence of GM-IVH probably reached a plateau during the last decade,[4,5,9] suggesting that additional factors may have a role in the genesis of GM-IVH. Finally, a recent twin study suggested that familial factors contribute to susceptibility for GM-IVH, among other neonatal complications.[76] Because not all infants with GM-IVH develop PVHI and PHH, one can further hypothesize a genetic predisposition for the development of these complications, and several genetic factors have been suggested as potential modulators in GM-IVH and its complications. Thrombophilia may be one of them, presumably by germinal vessel or medullary vein occlusion triggering high-pressure bleeding or hemorrhagic infarction, respectively, but expert opinions are inconsistent. For example, the incidence of being a carrier of the point mutation in the factor V gene (Gln506-FV) was higher among infants with GM-IVH.[77] Prothrombin G20210A mutation was also found in a considerably higher prevalence in a cohort of premature infants with GM-IVH (12%) than in those without (2%), although the difference was not statistically significant.[78] Conversely, carrier state of a factor V Leiden or prothrombin G20210A mutation predicted a low rate of GM-IVH in another study,[79] whereas others were also unable to find an association between thrombophilia and the occurrence or severity of GM-IVH.[80]

Recently it has been proposed that a specific mutation in a collagen gene of the endothelial basement membrane (*Col4a1* mutation)[81] conspires with environmental stress (eg, vaginal delivery, premature birth) in causing severe cerebral hemorrhage. It is reasonable to hypothesize that mutations in collagen genes may predispose to rupture of the germinal matrix vessels and the parenchymal veins. In a mutant mouse model of procollagen type IVα (Col4a1 mutations) all the mice developed perinatal intracerebral hemorrhage and 20% of the survivors developed porencephalic cysts. Importantly, mutations in this gene (mapped to human chromosome 13q34) were also found in human subjects with familial porencephaly[82] and recently in two siblings born preterm with antenatal PVHI followed by porencephaly.[83] Finally, genetic polymorphisms in the promoter region of the gene encoding the proinflammatory cyto-kine interleukin-6 were linked to severe GM-IVH and PVL[60] and to impaired cognitive development.[61] Other investigators were not able to confirm these associations.[84]

Taken together, these new observations suggest that genetic factors could operate on various levels by altering intravascular coagulation, germinal matrix structure, cerebral autoregulation integrity, and inflammatory mechanisms, and therefore could predispose certain vulnerable premature infants to GM-IVH or its complications.

COMPLICATIONS OF GERMINAL MATRIX-INTRAVENTRICULAR HEMORRHAGE
Periventricular Hemorrhagic Infarction

This lesion is a major complication of GM-IVH. It is unilateral in 65% to 75% of cases, it is commonly asymmetric when it occurs bilaterally, and it is associated in 67% to 88% of cases with a large ipsilateral GM-IVH.[85,86] Furthermore, it can be associated with all grades of GM-IVH (grades I–III), and more than one half of the lesions are detected during the second and third postnatal day, suggesting that PVHI is a complication of GM-IVH.[86] PVHI is currently diagnosed in approximately 4% of infants born weigh-ing less than 1500 g, an incidence that can reach 15% to 30% in the smallest (<750 g) premature infants.[9] In earlier CUS studies, it was thought that a large intraventricular hemorrhage could rupture the ependyma and simply extend directly into the adjacent white matter, and hence this lesion was previously classified as grade IV GM-IVH.[18] Pathology studies, however, have demonstrated that the hemorrhagic parenchymal component is a perivascular infarction in the distribution of the fan-shaped periventric-ular medullary veins[43,87,88] and that the ependyma is intact in the acute stages[87] before the appearance of porencephaly. These studies suggested that terminal vein compression by the GM-IVH results in impaired venous drainage and congestion of the medullary veins, which in turn leads to hypoxia-ischemia, infarction, and finally hemorrhagic transformation in the periventricular white matter.[1] Almost a decade later, Taylor[89] found decreased flow velocity and displacement of the ipsilateral terminal vein using Doppler in living infants with PVHI (**Fig. 2**). Perivascular hemor-rhage and presumed intravascular thrombi along the medullary veins were subse-quently demonstrated in an MRI study by Counsell and colleagues,[26] confirming original pathologic studies that suggested intravascular thrombi in the medullary

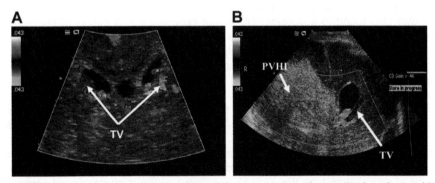

Fig. 2. The terminal vein in relation to PVHI. (A) Normal terminal veins (TVs) as depicted by color Doppler in a premature infant (26 weeks) with a normal cranial ultrasound (angled coronal view). (B) Massive right GM-IVH and PVHI in a premature infant (27 weeks). Note that the right TV is compressed. The left TV is seen traversing a smaller germinal matrix hemorrhage (angled coronal view).

veins.[88] Govaert and colleagues[90] and Dudink and colleagues[91] suggested that the pathogenesis of temporal and parietotemporal (atrial) distribution PVHIs may not stem from terminal vein involvement but rather are secondary to involvement of the inferior ventricular and lateral atrial veins, respectively. The lateral atrial veins make a sharp lateral turn through the periatrial germinal matrix and are prone to compression by a germinal matrix hemorrhage (see **Fig. 1**). Finally, an alternative sequence of a secondary hemorrhage into a PVL lesion is another possible mechanism that is probably less common; it may coexist with the "classic" venous PVHI and be difficult to distinguish by conventional CUS.[1] Doppler and MR venography studies of the terminal vein and other periventricular veins could presumably distinguish between these mechanisms, but data are currently not available.

The consequences of PVHI are primarily destruction of the motor and associative white matter axons and preoligodendrocytes within the evolving porencephalic cyst. In addition, the development of the overlying gray matter may be secondarily impaired, presumably because of interruption of thalamocortical fibers (retrograde maturational neuronal injury); destruction of the dorsal telencephalic subventricular zone; subplate neurons; and interruption of neuronal and glial migration toward their cortical destination.[92]

Progressive Posthemorrhagic Hydrocephalus

Progressive PHH (**Fig. 3**) involves one quarter of infants with GM-IVH who develop progressive ventricular dilatation.[93] Another quarter of infants with GM-IVH develop nonprogressive ventricular dilatation that results from parenchymal loss (ie, PVL or PVHI). It is noteworthy that these two processes commonly coexist (ie, PVHI followed by progression to PHH). Hydrocephalus can develop acutely by direct blood clot obstruction, subacutely, or chronically by secondary obstructive inflammatory changes of the ependyma and/or arachnoid that progress to gliosis, which in turn interferes with CSF flow. These secondary mechanisms are supported by studies that reveal decreased fibrinolytic activity providing clot sustenance in premature infants with GM-IVH,[94] and increased levels of platelet-derived transforming growth factor β_1[95] and procollagen I C-propeptide[96] in the CSF of infants with PHH, triggering collagen fiber formation and fibrosis in CSF spaces. The vulnerable regions for acute

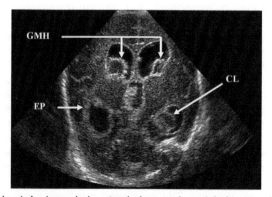

Fig. 3. Posthemorrhagic hydrocephalus. Angled coronal cranial ultrasound view of a premature infant (25 weeks) who developed posthemorrhagic hydrocephalus. Note the dilated frontal and temporal horns of the lateral ventricles, germinal matrix hemorrhage (GMH), intraventricular blood clot (CL), and the hyperechogenic ependyma (EP).

blood clot obstruction and for secondary inflammatory fibrotic changes are the arachnoid villi, aqueduct, fourth ventricle outlet, basilar cisterns, and peritentorial subarachnoid spaces. The resulting types of hydrocephalus are either communicating (considered the most common type); obstructive; or a combination of the two.[97] Based on the findings of animal and clinical studies, it is believed that the deleterious consequences of PHH are primarily related to its injurious effects on the periventricular white matter, leading to cystic or diffuse PVL by three parallel mechanisms: (1) reduction in periventricular CBF and metabolism,[34,98] (2) direct mechanical injury on periventricular axons,[99] and (3) inflammatory injury. The latter is considered a possibility because cytokines[100] and free intraventricular iron[101] measured in the CSF of infants with PHH could be involved in further injurious cascades to cellular elements (particularly preoligodendrocytes and the vascular endothelium) in the periventricular white matter. The importance of this route of injury has not yet been established.

PATHOLOGIES ASSOCIATED WITH GERMINAL MATRIX-INTRAVENTRICULAR HEMORRHAGE
Cerebellar Hemorrhagic Injury

With the advent of the mastoid CUS view, CHI is detected in 3% of infants weighing less than 1500 g, with an almost threefold increase in infants weighing less than 750 g, suggesting a propensity of this type of hemorrhage among preterm infants.[102] Noteworthy, small petechial cerebellar hemorrhages are probably not visible on CUS because pathologic studies revealed an incidence reaching 20% in low-birth-weight infants.[103] The cerebellum undergoes intense growth during this critical period and is therefore vulnerable to injurious processes. Furthermore, prematurity per se seemed to be associated with significantly smaller cerebellar volumes as early as term-corrected age, further emphasizing its specific vulnerability.[104,105] The pathogenesis of CHI in the premature infant is uncertain. Limperopoulos and colleagues[102] reported that 77% of the cases were associated with supratentorial GM-IVH and pathologic studies revealed even a higher association.[106] Furthermore, it seems that the two lesions share the same clinical antecedents and risk factors, suggesting that they may occur concomitantly.[102] The role of cerebellar pressure passivity (ie, unstable hemodynamics) has not yet been studied. The location of CHIs corresponds to the location of the cerebellar germinal matrices in the subependymal and subpial layers. Unilateral hemispheral CHI was seen in 70% of cases, vermian hemorrhage in 20%, and combined bi-hemispheric and vermian hemorrhage in 9%.[102] Taken together, current data suggest that CHI can result from cerebellar germinal matrix hemorrhage (subependymal or subpial); primary hemorrhage; ischemic hemorrhagic transformation of either arterial or venous origin; or their combinations. It was also suggested that CHI could be secondary to dissection of blood through the fourth ventricle or subarachnoid spaces following massive GM-IVH.[107] The injurious hemorrhage to the highly proliferating cerebellar cells eventually results in several types of significant atrophic consequences: unilateral hemispheric, unilateral hemispheric plus vermis, and partial or complete bilateral hemispheric plus vermis atrophy.[108] Severe cerebellar atrophy combined with pontine hypoplasia has been described.[109,110] It was also suggested that CHI could secondarily impair the development of the cerebral hemispheres. In a recent study, unilateral primary CHI resulted in decreased contralateral cerebral brain volume, whereas bilateral CHI was associated with bilateral reductions in cerebral brain volumes. The postulated mechanism responsible for these abnormalities relates to interruption of the cerebellothalamocortical pathway (crossed cerebellocerebral diaschisis), further extending the spectrum of CHI sequelae to additional disruption of supratentorial neural systems.[111]

Extra-Axial Hemorrhage

It is difficult to visualize extra-axial hemorrhage by CUS. As a result, the true incidence of subarachnoid hemorrhage is unknown, but it is estimated to be relatively common in premature infants, whereas subdural hemorrhage is less frequently observed by CUS in this group. Most cases of preterm subarachnoid hemorrhage are associated with GM-IVH, whereas primary subarachnoid hemorrhage is probably less common.[1] In addition to being involved in the evolution of GM-IVH to PHH (obstructive arachnoiditis),[97,112] subarachnoid hemorrhage could be one of the reasons for neonatal seizures in the setting of GM-IVH (irritation of the cerebral convexity), and could also be involved in secondary cerebral gray matter[113] and cerebellar[111] growth impairment that could follow GM-IVH (see later).

Periventricular Leukomalacia

Sonographic studies have suggested a strong association between GM-IVH and echolucencies, echodensities, and nonprogressive ventriculomegaly (ie, the CUS biomarkers of cystic and diffuse PVL).[5,114,115] This association is even stronger in pathology studies, which demonstrate a common occurrence of GM-IVH and PVL in up to 75% of cases.[39] The two pathologies may develop in parallel. For example, preceding ischemia could injure the germinal matrix and the periventricular white matter, leading to both GM-IVH and PVL. Another possibility is that GM-IVH can be followed by PVL through three connector links: (1) iron from red blood cells can induce free radical formation and result in white matter injury; (2) cytokines originating directly from the blood or from the inflamed ependyma could cause direct cellular effects on preoligodendrocytes, vascular endothelia, and astrocytic or neuronal cells[56]; and (3) the hemorrhagic destruction of the germinal matrix may abolish its glial precursors and may impede later development of white matter.[92]

Impaired Cerebellar and Supratentorial Gray Matter Growth

Advanced quantitative MRI techniques allow delineation of decreased volumes of several cerebral topographies in GM-IVH survivors. Limperopoulos and colleagues[111] showed that supratentorial lesions, such as PVHI and PVL, are associated with impaired growth and development of the contralateral cerebellar hemisphere, even in the absence of primary cerebellar injury (**Fig. 4**). The suggested mechanism of this phenomenon is injury to specific supratentorial projection areas that lead to trophic withdrawal (crossed cerebellar diaschisis).[111] A recent study also showed that severe GM-IVH was associated with disrupted cerebellar microstructure, as reflected in abnormal apparent diffusion coefficient and fractional anisotropy.[116] Finally, even uncomplicated GM-IVH (ie, without parenchymal involvement) has been associated with impaired growth of the supratentorial cortical gray matter at term equivalent age.[113] The sequelae of germinal matrix destruction that may prevent neuronal and astrocytic precursor cells from reaching their cortical destination is one proposed explanation.[113] Alternatively, the circulating subarachnoid blood and resultant free radical formation may directly injure the surface of the cerebral cortex.

WHAT DETERMINES THE OUTCOME OF GERMINAL MATRIX-INTRAVENTRICULAR HEMORRHAGE?

The outcome of GM-IVH is primarily determined by the presence of parenchymal lesions: PVHI with its resultant porencephalic cyst; cystic or diffuse PVL (whether in the context of PHH or accompanying "uncomplicated" GM-IVH); CHI; decreased supratentorial gray matter and cerebellar volumes; and associated brainstem and

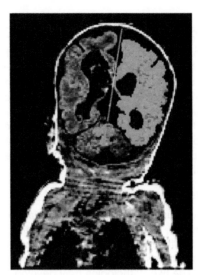

Fig. 4. Coronal SPGR sequence, MRI scan (volumetric analysis), showing a right PVHI associated with decreased volume of the left contralateral cerebellar hemisphere. Yellow demonstrates comparison of a right cerebral hemispheric volume with left cerebellar hemispheric volume; green demonstrates comparison of a left cerebral hemispheric volume with right cerebellar hemispheric volume. (*From* Limperopoulos C, Soul JS, Haidar H, et al. Impaired trophic interactions between the cerebellum and the cerebrum among preterm infants. Pediatrics 2005;116:844–50; with permission.)

hippocampal hypoxic injury (discussed elsewhere[39]). Because most outcome studies rely on initial CUS diagnosis, they may overlook several of these determinants that are below CUS resolution. Furthermore, another underrecognized factor that may contribute to the outcome of GM-IVH is the presence of neonatal seizure activity. Based on animal studies, it was suggested that secondary electrical seizure activity that accompanies neonatal cerebral insults can by itself alter cerebral hemodynamics,[117] neuronal connectivity, receptor expression, and synaptic plasticity, and decrease the threshold for later epilepsy and result in worsening of long-term neurologic outcome.[118,119] It is currently unknown, however, whether neonatal seizures in the context of GM-IVH are merely a marker of severe injury or pose an additional clinical impact on subsequent long-term outcome of GM-IVH survivors, a topic that deserves further research.

Outcome of Germinal Matrix-Intraventricular Hemorrhage and Periventricular Hemorrhagic Infarction

The incidence of major neurodevelopmental sequelae (cerebral palsy and/or mental retardation) in infants with grade I and grade II GM-IVH is generally considered equal to or slightly higher than that for premature infants with a normal CUS.[120,121] The presence of a larger hemorrhage in grade III GM-IVH is associated with an increased risk (35%–50%) for major sequelae. When GM-IVH is complicated by PVHI, the risk of major neurodevelopmental sequelae increases to a staggering 75%.[122,123] This finding is in comparison with a large study carried out three decades ago in which major sequelae affected almost 90% of survivors.[85] Moreover, in a more recent study, Bassan and colleagues[122] suggested that functional outcome, as measured by the Vineland questionnaire, was relatively preserved in 67% of survivors. This trend of improved outcome may be the result of more intensive and widespread early habilitation practices in modern countries. In that study of 30 PVHI survivors, 60% had spastic cerebral palsy, 50% had low cognitive scores, and over 20% were epileptic.[122] Furthermore, one quarter of PVHI survivors had a visual field defect, mostly the inferior, presumably secondary to injury to the optic radiation. Impairment of the visual fields should be taken into consideration for planning developmental strategies. The mortality of PVHI survivors, which reached 60%[85] in earlier reports, continues to decrease and is now approximately 30% to 40%.[9,124]

Grading the severity of PVHI as a predictor of outcome is important for decision-making in patient management and for use as a tool for inclusion in future clinical trials. Bassan and colleagues[86,122] showed that the severity of PVHI could be graded based on three CUS parameters: (1) extent, (2) bilaterality, and (3) the presence of a midline shift (**Fig. 5**). The grouping of three sonographic severity items into a single CUS-based severity system allows improved severity and prognostic assessment of PVHI compared with reliance on separate factors. Based on this score, a unilateral focal

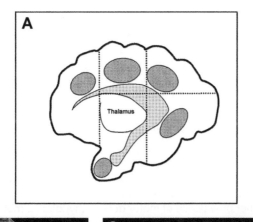

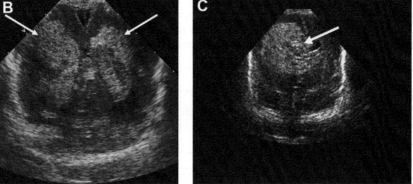

Fig. 5. PVHI severity scoring. The PVHI severity score is derived from the cranial ultrasound study with the maximum PVHI size (maximal size of echogenicity) and is based on three items. (*A*) Lesion extending into greater than or equal two territories. (*B*) Bilateral lesions (*arrows*). (*C*) Midline shift (*arrow*). A study with none of these features is scored 0. A study with all three features is scored 3. (*From* Bassan H, Limperopoulos C, Visconti K, et al. Neurodevelopmental outcome in survivors of periventricular hemorrhagic infarction. Pediatrics 2007;120:785–92; with permission.)

PVHI lesion that involves one territory carries an overall risk profile similar to that of grade III GM-IVH, whereas the risk for major sequelae is above 95% for extensive bilateral PVHI lesions (**Table 1**). Further studies to validate this scoring system are needed.

The evolution of PVHI to multiple cysts (as opposed to a single porencephalic cyst) was also suggested as a predictor for motor sequelae,[122] whereas reports in the literature on the topographic location of PVHI in relation to outcome are inconsistent.[122,125] Finally, asymmetric myelination of the posterior limb of the internal capsule, as seen by MRI at term equivalent, was suggested by De Vries and colleagues[27] as an early predictor of hemiplegia in PVHI.

Outcome of Posthemorrhagic Hydrocephalus

Based on current reports, it is estimated that only 5% to 30% of PHH survivors have a normal long-term neurodevelopmental outcome.[97] A common finding in many PHH outcome studies is the strong correlation between the severity of a preceding cerebral injury and outcome.[126,127] It is also suggested, however, that PHH per se poses an additional risk for neurodevelopmental sequelae, beyond the original risk of the preceding GM-IVH. A recent large-scale study reported that the risk for significant neurodevelopmental sequelae increased significantly, from 55% (grade III GM-IVH) and 63% (PVHI) to 78% and 92%, respectively, when complicated by PHH requiring shunt insertion.[128] Moreover, based on our local data of all disabled PHH survivors, approximately 50% had a profound impairment (ie, severe disabling quadriparetic cerebral palsy and/or profound mental retardation). It seems that progressive PHH, particularly if associated with prior PVHI, is currently the most ominous complication of prematurity.

Outcome of Cerebellar Hemorrhagic Injury

The adverse long-term cognitive and social sequelae of CHI confer a greater importance to its occurrence. In a recent study of 35 premature infants who suffered CHI, Limperopoulos and colleagues[108] showed that over 40% of survivors had cognitive and social communication developmental disabilities and functional limitations in addition to a higher prevalence of motor deficits (hypotonia, motor delay, oculomotor and gait abnormalities). Global developmental and functional deficits, including positive autism screening, were particularly prevalent in cases involving the cerebellar vermis. In that study, cognitive, language, and social outcomes were comparable in infants with isolated CHI and those with combined CHI and supratentorial injury,

Table 1
Percentages of infants with abnormal neuromotor and cognitive outcomes as a function of PVHI severity scoring

Outcome	PVHI Severity Score[a]			
	0	1	2	3
% Abnormal neuromotor examination	0–33	57–66	90	100
% Abnormal cognition	14	50	70	70

[a] See **Fig. 5** for definition.

Adapted from Bassan H, Benson CB, Limperopoulos C, et al. Ultrasonographic features and severity scoring of periventricular hemorrhagic infarction in relation to risk factors and outcome. Pediatrics 2006;117:2111–8; and Bassan H, Limperopoulos C, Visconti K, et al. Neurodevelopmental outcome in survivors of periventricular hemorrhagic infarction. Pediatrics 2007;120:785–92; with permission.

although the latter group had greater motor deficits.[108] Johnsen and colleagues[109,110] described a selected subgroup of ex-preterm infants with an extensive cerebellar injury associated with pontine hypoplasia and supratentorial parenchymal injury. These infants demonstrated a high prevalence of profound neurologic impairment, including microcephaly, spastic quadriplegia, dystonia, ataxia, and seizures.

PREVENTION AND MANAGEMENT OF GERMINAL MATRIX-INTRAVENTRICULAR HEMORRHAGE

Goals are the prevention of GM-IVH when possible, halting its progression, and reducing its complications. Given the peculiar perinatal onset of GM-IVH, prevention issues are addressed by antenatal, intrapartum, and postnatal approaches. Another important feature of GM-IVH is its tendency to progress, with a delay in the appearance of some of the PVHI and virtually all the PHH complications, suggesting a window of opportunity during which preventive interventions may be initiated.

Antenatal and Intrapartum Measures

Modern perinatal medicine is currently characterized by an approach aimed at reducing the incidence of prematurity and, consequently, of GM-IVH. The various measures to be taken include (1) special obstetric care for high-risk pregnancies; (2) treatment of bacterial vaginosis, which may be effective for reducing premature delivery and preventing fetal maternal inflammatory reactions; and (3) prevention of an imminent premature labor using tocolytic agents. Additional measures aimed at reducing the complications of prematurity, such as GM-IVH, include in utero transfer to a tertiary center and cesarean section delivery in selected cases. Cesarean sections have been suggested by some investigators as being beneficial for avoiding the increased cerebral venous pressure during vaginal labor and for preventing GM-IVH,[129] whereas others could not demonstrate such an association.[55]

Several antenatal pharmacologic interventions have been proposed. Antenatal corticosteroids are currently the only modality repeatedly shown in several studies to be associated with a reduction in the incidence of GM-IVH and overall reduction in mortality rates.[130] Another appealing antenatal treatment is magnesium sulfate, commonly used for tocolysis but also with vascular stabilizing, anti-inflammatory, and neuroprotective properties. Magnesium sulfate has been associated with lower risks of cerebral palsy in premature infants. In a recent prospective trial,[131] antenatal administration of magnesium sulfate before anticipated early preterm delivery was associated with decreased rates of moderate and severe cerebral palsy among survivors. Others have suggested a reduction in the incidence of GM-IVH following maternal administration of magnesium sulfate[132]; however, most data do not show any benefit on the incidence of GM-IVH per se, and so its effects on reducing cerebral palsy rates may operate by alternate mechanisms. Other antenatal therapeutics, such as phenobarbital and vitamin K, seemed not to be beneficial for the prevention of GM-IVH.[133]

Postnatal Interventions

Because GM-IVH is strongly associated with both intrinsic and extrinsic hemodynamic effectors, optimal ventilation and strict hemodynamic control of the premature infant are among the cornerstones of preventing GM-IVH and its progression. The neonatal cardiorespiratory management of premature infants is beyond the scope of this article.

Several postnatal *pharmacologic agents* have been proposed for the prevention of GM-IVH:

1. *Pancuronium*, a muscle paralysis agent used in ventilated premature infants, was able to correct the hazardous fluctuating cerebral circulation, prevent pneumothorax and hemodynamic changes during suctioning, and most importantly decrease the overall incidence of GM-IVH. A Cochrane meta-analysis of all relevant reports showed that neuromuscular paralysis with pancuronium seems to have a favorable effect on GM-IVH in ventilated preterm infants with evidence of asynchronous respiratory efforts, although its routine use could not be recommended because of uncertainty about the safety and long-term pulmonary and neurologic effects of its prolonged use.[134]

2. *Phenobarbital* for the prevention of GM-IVH was studied in 10 trials. Results were inconsistent and a meta-analysis showed no significant beneficial effect and raised concerns about increased need for mechanical ventilation.[135]

3. *Vitamin E* is a free radical scavenger intended to protect the germinal matrix from hypoxic damage. Several initial trials showed a decrease in the incidence or severity of GM-IVH[136] but a later study reported a high incidence of GM-IVH in a subgroup of treated infants.[137] A Cochrane meta-analysis of 26 randomized trials revealed that vitamin E supplementation in preterm infants did reduce the risk of GM-IVH but, because of concerns about increasing the risk of sepsis when used intravenously in high doses (serum tocopherol levels >3.5 mg/dL), it was concluded that current evidence does not support its routine intravenous use.[138]

4. Several *procoagulant* and *anticoagulant* prophylaxis treatments were studied for the prevention of GM-IVH, but results were either negative or inconsistent and so they are not currently recommended. Fresh frozen plasma initially showed promise[139] but demonstrated no detectable effects in a later randomized trial.[140] Factor XIII concentrate was studied and found to be effective in only one trial.[141] Ethamsylate, a drug that inhibits prostacyclin production and promotes platelet adhesion and aggregation, was found beneficial in four studies; however, a subsequent large multicenter randomized trial failed to find any beneficial effect.[142,143] Antithrombin III was associated with a reduced incidence and progression of ICH in one study,[144] but incidence was not affected in another study, although the rates of severe GM-IVH cases were reduced.[145] Finally, in a recent pilot study on 10 preterm infants, activated factor VII was initially introduced as a prophylaxis but was not associated with a decrease in GM-IVH rates.[146]

5. Ment and colleagues[147] showed that *indomethacin* prophylaxis significantly decreases the overall incidence and severity of GM-IVH. As a cyclooxygenase-1 and -2 inhibitor, indomethacin can decrease prostaglandin synthesis and therefore decrease CBF. Together with its antioxidative and vascular maturation properties, indomethacin is postulated to protect the fragile germinal matrix vessels, but follow-up studies showed no beneficial effect of indomethacin on the incidence of cerebral palsy and only modest effects on cognition.[148] A large Canadian prospective trial[149] and a meta-analysis of all major indomethacin trials[150] concluded that despite the fact that indomethacin reduces the frequency of patent ductus arteriosus and severe GM-IVH, it does not improve the rate of survival without neurosensory impairment. Several reasons for this puzzling phenomenon have been proposed: gender differences (ie, beneficial effect in males but not females)[151] and genetic differences in the cyclooxygenase-2 gene.[152]

Neonatal individualized developmental care, recently introduced into modern neonatal intensive care units, is associated with improved overall outcome of premature infants and specific reduction in GM-IVH.[153,154] The lack of reduction in GM-IVH in one trial[155] was explained by late onset of initiation of intervention beyond 5 days of age. Reduced manipulation per se could be one of the reasons for its effect on GM-IVH reduction, as demonstrated previously.[156] Given the beneficial effects of this methodology on infants without GM-IVH, however, alternative pathways must play a role in the impact of developmental care on outcome.[157] As such, the importance and relative contribution of GM-IVH reduction to the overall improved outcome in infants subjected to developmental care are not clear.

A short discussion on the *management of PHH* is in order. The main therapeutic dilemma in PHH stems from its unpredictable course, with 60% of the infants undergoing spontaneous arrest or resolution and 40% finally requiring a ventriculoperitoneal shunt, the definitive treatment of progressive PHH.[93] It is also frequently difficult to clearly delineate between a frank hydrocephalic process and an atrophic nonprogressive ventricular dilatation because they often coexist. Moreover, in clinical trials early (before the onset of PHH) serial lumbar punctures were used unsuccessfully to prevent the evolution of GM-IVH to PHH.[158] Early intrathecal fibrinolytic therapy (urokinase, tissue plasminogen activator) also failed to prevent hydrocephalus that required shunting.[133] Once PHH is established, the main therapeutic obstacle stems from a neurosurgical restriction: to reduce the complication rate, shunting needs to be delayed for several weeks while the infant's weight (and presumably the absorptive peritoneal surface area) increases, and the potentially obstructive levels of blood products decreases. Unfortunately, ischemia and inflammation could be deleterious to the developing brain during this critical period of time, particularly in infants who have already sustained other forms of injury, such as PVL or PVHI. Several methods have been proposed for temporary treatment of progressive PHH while awaiting optimal conditions for permanent shunt insertion or spontaneous resolution. Repeated lumbar punctures may temporarily arrest the progression of PHH, but the long-term benefit of this approach remains unknown.[97] One large multicenter trial failed to find any advantage of early and rigorous tapping over conservative, less frequent tapping.[159] Acetazolamide and furosemide are mostly avoided because of concerns over neurotoxicity and nephrocalcinosis.[133] Several invasive policies are used for temporary CSF diversion, including external ventricular drainage (either direct or subcutaneously tunneled) and placement of a subcutaneous ventricular reservoir (ventriculosubgaleal shunt).[160,161] Policy preferences differ from center to center and are generally dictated by local experience and not on evidence-based recommendations. One novel technique involving drainage, irrigation, and fibrinolytic therapy was found not to be beneficial in a multicenter trial.[162] Finally, the potential role of endoscopic coagulation of the choroid plexus in decreasing CSF production has not yet been determined.[163]

FUTURE DIRECTIONS

GM-IVH remains a significant problem of prematurity, with a large number of survivors sustaining neurodevelopmental sequelae. The anatomic and hemodynamic mechanisms of GM-IVH have been the subjects of intense study over the past four decades. These factors were partially addressed by evolving perinatal practices that led to an initial decrease in the incidence of GM-IVH. The last decade has not witnessed any significant change in the incidence of GM-IVH, however, and so the search for means of prevention is ongoing. Advances in imaging, and emerging inflammatory and genetic discoveries, have begun to change the understanding of this multifaceted entity. The formulation of safe and effective management strategies awaits implementation of valid techniques for cerebral hemodynamic measurements, early use of advanced MRI sequences during the first days of life, and genetic assessments for infants at risk, all representing means by which to assist in decision-making for optimal timing of intervention and better selection of patients for clinical trials. Of special note is the urgent need for innovative, safe techniques for the prevention and treatment of PHH, the outcome of which remains grave.

ACKNOWLEDGMENTS

Esther Eshkol and Shaye Moore are thanked for editorial assistance. Sigalit Siso is thanked for graphic assistance. Adré du Plessis is thanked for his critical review.

REFERENCES

1. Volpe JJ. Intracranial hemorrhage: neurology of the newborn. 5th edition. Phila-delphia: W.B. Saunders Co.; 2008. p. 481–588.
2. du Plessis AJ, Volpe JJ. Intracranial hemorrhage in the newborn infant. In: Burg FD, Ingelfinger JR, Wald ER, et al, editors, Gellis & Kagan's current pediatric therapy, vol. 16. Philadelphia: W.B. Saunders Company; 1999. p. 304–8.
3. Philip AG, Allan WC, Tito AM, et al. Intraventricular hemorrhage in preterm infants: declining incidence in the 1980's. Pediatrics 1989;84:797–801.
4. Horbar JD, Badger GJ, Carpenter JH, et al. Trends in mortality and morbidity for very low birth weight infants, 1991–1999. Pediatrics 2002;110(1 Pt 1): 143–51.
5. Hamrick SE, Miller SP, Leonard C, et al. Trends in severe brain injury and neuro-developmental outcome in premature newborn infants: the role of cystic periven-tricular leukomalacia. J Pediatr 2004;145(5):593–9.
6. Hack M, Fanaroff AA. Outcomes of children of extremely low birthweight and gestational age in the 1990's. Early Hum Dev 1999;53(3):193–218.
7. Anthony S, Ouden L, Brand R, et al. Changes in perinatal care and survival in very preterm and extremely preterm infants in The Netherlands between 1983 and 1995. Eur J Obstet Gynecol Reprod Biol 2004;112(2):170–7.
8. Wilson-Costello D, Friedman H, Minich N, et al. Improved survival rates with increased neurodevelopmental disability for extremely low birth weight infants in the 1990s. Pediatrics 2005;115(4):997–1003.
9. Bassan H, Feldman HA, Limperopoulos C, et al. Periventricular hemorrhagic infarction: risk factors and neonatal outcome. Pediatr Neurol 2006;35(2):85–92.
10. O'Shea TM, Klinepeter KL, Goldstein DJ, et al. Survival and developmental disability in infants with birth weights of 501 to 800 grams, born between 1979 and 1994. Pediatrics 1997;100(6):982–6.
11. Dubowitz LM, Levene MI, Morante A, et al. Neurologic signs in neonatal intraven-tricular hemorrhage: a correlation with real-time ultrasound. J Pediatr 1981;99: 127–33.
12. Moylan FM, Herrin JT, Krishnamoorthy K, et al. Inappropriate antidiuretic hormone secretion in premature infants with cerebral injury. Am J Dis Child 1978;132(4):399–402.
13. Krishnamoorthy KS, Fernandez RA, Momose KJ, et al. Evaluation of neonatal intracranial hemorrhage by computerized tomography. Pediatrics 1977;59(2): 165–72.
14. Strober JB, Bienkowski RS, Maytal J. The incidence of acute and remote seizures in children with intraventricular hemorrhage. Clin Pediatr (Phila) 1997; 36(11):643–7.

15. Hellstrom-Westas L, Klette H, Thorngren-Jerneck K, et al. Early prediction of outcome with aEEG in preterm infants with large intraventricular hemorrhages. Neuropediatrics 2001;32(6):319–24.
16. Hellstrom-Westas L, Rosen I, Svenningsen NW. Cerebral function monitoring during the first week of life in extremely small low birthweight (ESLBW) infants. Neuropediatrics 1991;22(1):27–32.
17. Pape KE, Blackwell RJ, Cusick G, et al. Ultrasound detection of brain damage in preterm infants. Lancet 1979;1(8129):1261–4.
18. Papile LA, Burstein J, Burstein R, et al. Incidence and evolution of subependymal and intraventricular hemorrhage: a study of infants with birth weights less than 1,500 gm. J Pediatr 1978;92:529–34.
19. Volpe JJ. Intracranial hemorrhage: germinal matrix-intraventricular hemorrhage of the premature infant: neurology of the newborn. Philadelphia: W.B. Saunders; 1995. p. 403–62.
20. Dean LM, Taylor GA. The intracranial venous system in infants: normal and abnormal findings on duplex and color Doppler sonography. AJR Am J Roentgenol 1995;164(1):151–6.
21. Quinn M, Ando Y, Levene M. Cerebral arterial and venous flow-velocity measurements in post-hemorrhagic ventricular dilation and hydrocephalus. Dev Med Child Neurol 1992;34:863–9.
22. Horgan JG, Rumack CM, Hay T, et al. Absolute intracranial blood-flow velocities evaluated by duplex Doppler sonography in asymptomatic preterm and term neonates. AJR Am J Roentgenol 1989;152(5):1059–64.
23. Taylor GA, Madsen JR. Neonatal hydrocephalus: hemodynamic response to fontanelle compression: correlation with intracranial pressure and need for shunt placement. Radiology 1996;201(3):685–9.
24. Maalouf EF, Duggan PJ, Counsell SJ, et al. Comparison of findings on cranial ultrasound and magnetic resonance imaging in preterm infants. Pediatrics 2001;107(4):719–27.
25. Maalouf EF, Duggan PJ, Rutherford MA, et al. Magnetic resonance imaging of the brain in a cohort of extremely preterm infants. J Pediatr 1999;135(3):351–7.
26. Counsell SJ, Maalouf EF, Rutherford MA, et al. Periventricular haemorrhagic infarct in a preterm neonate. Europ J Paediatr Neurol 1999;3(1):25–7.
27. de Vries LS, Groenendaal F, van Haastert IC, et al. Asymmetrical myelination of the posterior limb of the internal capsule in infants with periventricular haemorrhagic infarction: an early predictor of hemiplegia. Neuropediatrics 1999;30(6):314–9.
28. Tsuji M, duPlessis A, Taylor G, et al. Near infrared spectroscopy detects cerebral ischemia during hypotension in piglets. Pediatr Res 1998;44:591–5.
29. Kissack CM, Garr R, Wardle SP, et al. Postnatal changes in cerebral oxygen extraction in the preterm infant are associated with intraventricular hemorrhage and hemorrhagic parenchymal infarction but not periventricular leukomalacia. Pediatr Res 2004;56(1):111–6.
30. Tsuji M, Saul JP, du Plessis AJ, et al. Cerebral intravascular oxygenation correlates with mean arterial pressure in critically ill premature infants. Pediatrics 2000;106(4):625–32.
31. Soul JS, Hammer PE, Tsuji M, et al. Fluctuating pressure-passivity is common in the cerebral circulation of sick premature infants. Pediatr Res 2007;61(4): 467–73.
32. Wong FY, Leung TS, Austin T, et al. Impaired autoregulation in preterm infants identified by using spatially resolved spectroscopy. Pediatrics 2008;121(3): e604–11.

33. Munro MJ, Walker AM, Barfield CP. Hypotensive extremely low birth weight infants have reduced cerebral blood flow. Pediatrics 2004;114(6):1591–6.
34. Soul JS, Eichenwald E, Walter G, et al. CSF removal in infantile posthemorrhagic hydrocephalus results in significant improvement in cerebral hemodynamics. Pediatr Res 2004;55(5):872–6.
35. Aso K, Abdab-Barmada M, Scher MS. EEG and the neuropathology in premature neonates with intraventricular hemorrhage. J Clin Neurophysiol 1993; 10(3):304–13.
36. Clancy RR, Tharp BR, Enzman D. EEG in premature infants with intraventricular hemorrhage. Neurology 1984;34(5):583–90.
37. Hellstrom-Westas L, Rosen I. Continuous brain-function monitoring: state of the art in clinical practice. Semin Fetal Neonatal Med 2006;11(6):503–11.
38. Olischar M, Klebermass K, Waldhoer T, et al. Background patterns and sleep-wake cycles on amplitude-integrated electroencephalography in preterms younger than 30 weeks gestational age with peri-/intraventricular haemorrhage. Acta Paediatr 2007;96(12):1743–50.
39. Armstrong DL, Sauls CD, Goddard-Finegold J. Neuropathologic findings in short-term survivors of intraventricular hemorrhage. Am J Dis Child 1987;141: 617–21.
40. Pape KE, Wigglesworth JS. Haemorrhage, ischaemia and the perinatal brain. Philadelphia: J.B. Lippincott; 1979.
41. Hambleton G, Wigglesworth JS. Origin of intraventricular haemorrhage in the preterm infant. Arch Dis Child 1976;51(9):651–9.
42. Nakamura Y, Okudera T, Fukuda S, et al. Germinal matrix hemorrhage of venous origin in preterm neonates. Hum Pathol 1990;21(10):1059–62.
43. Takashima S, Tanaka K. Microangiography and vascular permeability of the subependymal matrix in the premature infant. Can J Neurol Sci 1978;5(1):45–50.
44. du Plessis AJ. Cerebrovascular injury in premature infants: current understanding and challenges for future prevention. Clin Perinatol 2008;35(4): 609–41, v.
45. Pryds O, Greisen G, Lou H, et al. Heterogeneity of cerebral vasoreactivity in preterm infants supported by mechanical ventilation. J Pediatr 1989;115:638–45.
46. Tyszczuk L, Meek J, Elwell C, et al. Cerebral blood flow is independent of mean arterial blood pressure in preterm infants undergoing intensive care. Pediatrics 1998;102:337–41.
47. Low J, Froese A, Galbraith R, et al. The association between preterm newborn hypotension and hypoxemia and outcome during the first year. Acta Paediatr 1993;82:433–7.
48. Kohlhauser C, Bernert G, Hermon M, et al. Effects of endotracheal suctioning in high-frequency oscillatory and conventionally ventilated low birth weight neonates on cerebral hemodynamics observed by near infrared spectroscopy (NIRS). Pediatr Pulmonol 2000;29(4):270–5.
49. Limperopoulos C, Gauvreau KK, O'Leary H, et al. Cerebral hemodynamic changes during intensive care of preterm infants. Pediatrics 2008;122(5): e1006–13.
50. Perry EH, Bada HS, Ray JD, et al. Blood pressure increases, birth weight-dependent stability boundary, and intraventricular hemorrhage. Pediatrics 1990;85(5):727–32.
51. Perlman JM, McMenamin JB, Volpe JJ. Fluctuating cerebral blood-flow velocity in respiratory-distress syndrome: relation to the development of intraventricular hemorrhage. N Engl J Med 1983;309:204–9.

52. van Bel F, Van de Bor M, Stijnen T, et al. Aetiological role of cerebral blood-flow alterations in development and extension of peri-intraventricular haemorrhage. Dev Med Child Neurol 1987;29(5):601–14.
53. Perlman JM, Volpe JJ. Are venous circulatory abnormalities important in the pathogenesis of hemorrhagic and/or ischemic cerebral injury? Pediatrics 1987;80(5):705–11.
54. Hansen A, Leviton A. Labor and delivery characteristics and risks of cranial ultrasonographic abnormalities among very-low-birth-weight infants. Am J Obstet Gynecol 1999;181:997–1006.
55. Linder N, Haskin O, Levit O, et al. Risk factors for intraventricular hemorrhage in very low birth weight premature infants: a retrospective case-control study. Pediatrics 2003;111(5 Pt 1):e590–5.
56. Dammann O, Leviton A. Maternal intrauterine infection, cytokines, and brain damage in the preterm newborn. Pediatr Res 1997;42(1):1–8.
57. Sarkar S, Kaplan C, Wiswell TE, et al. Histological chorioamnionitis and the risk of early intraventricular hemorrhage in infants born < or =28 weeks gestation. J Perinatol 2005;25(12):749–52.
58. Yanowitz TD, Jordan JA, Gilmour CH, et al. Hemodynamic disturbances in premature infants born after chorioamnionitis: association with cord blood cytokine concentrations. Pediatr Res 2002;51(3):310–6.
59. Tauscher MK, Berg D, Brockmann M, et al. Association of histologic chorioamnionitis, increased levels of cord blood cytokines, and intracerebral hemorrhage in preterm neonates. Biol Neonate 2003;83(3):166–70.
60. Harding DR, Dhamrait S, Whitelaw A, et al. Does interleukin-6 genotype influence cerebral injury or developmental progress after preterm birth? Pediatrics 2004;114(4):941–7.
61. Harding D, Brull D, Humphries SE, et al. Variation in the interleukin-6 gene is associated with impaired cognitive development in children born prematurely: a preliminary study. Pediatr Res 2005;58(1):117–20.
62. Yanowitz TD, Potter DM, Bowen A, et al. Variability in cerebral oxygen delivery is reduced in premature neonates exposed to chorioamnionitis. Pediatr Res 2006; 59(2):299–304.
63. Ballabh P, Xu H, Hu F, et al. Angiogenic inhibition reduces germinal matrix hemorrhage. Nat Med 2007;13(4):477–85.
64. Gazzolo D, Marinoni E, Giovannini L, et al. Circulating adrenomedullin is increased in preterm newborns developing intraventricular hemorrhage. Pediatr Res 2001;50(4):544–7.
65. Florio P, Perrone S, Luisi S, et al. Increased plasma concentrations of activin a predict intraventricular hemorrhage in preterm newborns. Clin Chem 2006; 52(8):1516–21.
66. Paul DA, Leef KH, Stefano JL, et al. Low serum thyroxine on initial newborn screening is associated with intraventricular hemorrhage and death in very low birth weight infants. Pediatrics 1998;101(5):903–7.
67. Kantor MJ, Leef KH, Bartoshesky L, et al. Admission thyroid evaluation in very-low-birth-weight infants: association with death and severe intraventricular hemorrhage. Thyroid 2003;13(10):965–9.
68. Setzer ES, Webb IB, Wassenaar JW, et al. Platelet dysfunction and coagulopathy in intraventricular hemorrhage in the premature infant. J Pediatr 1982;100(4):599–605.
69. Salonvaara M, Riikonen P, Kekomaki R, et al. Intraventricular haemorrhage in very-low-birthweight preterm infants: association with low prothrombin activity at birth. Acta Paediatr 2005;94(6):807–11.

70. Andrew M, Castle V, Saigal S, et al. Clinical impact of neonatal thrombocytopenia. J Pediatr 1987;110(3):457–64.
71. Rennie JM, Doyle J, Cooke RW. Elevated levels of immunoreactive prostacyclin metabolite in babies who develop intraventricular haemorrhage. Acta Paediatr Scand 1987;76(1):19–23.
72. Lupton BA, Hill A, Whitfield MF, et al. Reduced platelet count as a risk factor for intraventricular hemorrhage. Am J Dis Child 1988;142(11):1222–4.
73. Linder N, Shenkman B, Levin E, et al. Deposition of whole blood platelets on extracellular matrix under flow conditions in preterm infants. Arch Dis Child Fetal Neonatal Ed 2002;86(2):F127–30.
74. Levy-Shraga Y, Maayan-Metzger A, Lubetsky A, et al. Platelet function of newborns as tested by cone and plate(let) analyzer correlates with gestational age. Acta Haematol 2006;115(3–4):152–6.
75. Rajasekhar D, Barnard MR, Bednarek FJ, et al. Platelet hyporeactivity in very low birth weight neonates. Thromb Haemost 1997;77(5):1002–7.
76. Bhandari V, Bizzarro MJ, Shetty A, et al. Familial and genetic susceptibility to major neonatal morbidities in preterm twins. Pediatrics 2006;117(6):1901–6.
77. Petaja J, Hiltunen L, Fellman V. Increased risk of intraventricular hemorrhage in preterm infants with thrombophilia. Pediatr Res 2001;49(5):643–6.
78. Aronis S, Bouza H, Pergantou H, et al. Prothrombotic factors in neonates with cerebral thrombosis and intraventricular hemorrhage. Acta Paediatr Suppl 2002;91(438):87–91.
79. Gopel W, Gortner L, Kohlmann T, et al. Low prevalence of large intraventricular haemorrhage in very low birthweight infants carrying the factor V Leiden or prothrombin G20210A mutation. Acta Paediatr 2001;90(9):1021–4.
80. Kenet G, Maayan-Metzger A, Rosenberg N, et al. Thrombophilia does not increase risk for neonatal complications in preterm infants. Thromb Haemost 2003;90(5):823–8.
81. Gould DB, Phalan FC, Breedveld GJ, et al. Mutations in Col4a1 cause perinatal cerebral hemorrhage and porencephaly. Science 2005;308(5725):1167–71.
82. Breedveld G, de Coo IF, Lequin MH, et al. Novel mutations in three families confirm a major role of COL4A1 in hereditary porencephaly. J Med Genet 2006;43(6):490–5.
83. de Vries LS, Koopman C, Groenendaal F, et al. COL4A1 mutation in two preterm siblings with antenatal onset of parenchymal hemorrhage. Ann Neurol 2009; 65(1):12–8.
84. Gopel W, Hartel C, Ahrens P, et al. Interleukin-6-174-genotype, sepsis and cerebral injury in very low birth weight infants. Genes Immun 2006;7(1):65–8.
85. Guzzetta F, Shackelford G, Volpe S, et al. Periventricular intraparenchymal echodensities in the premature newborn: critical determinant of neurologic outcome. Pediatrics 1986;78(6):995–1006.
86. Bassan H, Benson CB, Limperopoulos C, et al. Ultrasonographic features and severity scoring of periventricular hemorrhagic infarction in relation to risk factors and outcome. Pediatrics 2006;117(6):2111–8.
87. Gould SJ, Howard S, Hope PL, et al. Periventricular intraparenchymal cerebral haemorrhage in preterm infants: the role of venous infarction. J Pathol 1987; 151:197–202.
88. Takashima S, Mito T, Ando Y. Pathogenesis of periventricular white matter hemorrhages in preterm infants. Brain Dev 1986;8:25–30.
89. Taylor GA. Effect of germinal matrix hemorrhage on terminal vein position and patency. Pediatr Radiol 1995;25:1S37–1S40.

90. Govaert P, Smets K, Matthys E, et al. Neonatal focal temporal lobe or atrial wall haemorrhagic infarction. Arch Dis Child Fetal Neonatal Ed 1999;81(3):F211–6.
91. Dudink J, Lequin M, Weisglas-Kuperus N, et al. Venous subtypes of preterm periventricular haemorrhagic infarction. Arch Dis Child Fetal Neonatal Ed 2008;93:F201–6.
92. Volpe JJ. Brain injury in premature infants: a complex amalgam of destructive and developmental disturbances. Lancet Neurol 2009;8(1):110–24.
93. Murphy BP, Inder TE, Rooks V, et al. Posthaemorrhagic ventricular dilatation in the premature infant: natural history and predictors of outcome. Arch Dis Child Fetal Neonatal Ed 2002;87(1):F37–41.
94. Whitelaw A, Mowinckel M, Abildgaard U. Low levels of plasminogen in cerebrospinal fluid after intraventricular haemorrhage a limiting factor for clot lysis? Acta Paediatr 1995;84:933–6.
95. Whitelaw A, Christie S, Pople I. Transforming growth factor-beta1: a possible signal molecule for posthemorrhagic hydrocephalus? Pediatr Res 1999;46(5): 576–80.
96. Heep A, Stoffel-Wagner B, Soditt V, et al. Procollagen I C-propeptide in the cerebrospinal fluid of neonates with posthaemorrhagic hydrocephalus. Arch Dis Child Fetal Neonatal Ed 2002;87(1):F34–6.
97. du Plessis AJ. Posthemorrhagic hydrocephalus and brain injury in the preterm infant: dilemmas in diagnosis and management. Semin Pediatr Neurol 1998; 5(3):161–79.
98. Soul JS, Taylor GA, Wypij D, et al. Noninvasive detection of changes in cerebral blood flow by near-infrared spectroscopy in a piglet model of hydrocephalus. Pediatr Res 2000;48(4):445–9.
99. Del Bigio MR. Neuropathological changes caused by hydrocephalus. Acta Neuropathol 1993;85(6):573–85.
100. White RP, Leffler CW, Bada HS. Eicosanoid levels in CSF of premature infants with posthemorrhagic hydrocephalus. Am J Med Sci 1990;299(4): 230–5.
101. Savman K, Nilsson UA, Blennow M, et al. Non-protein-bound iron is elevated in cerebrospinal fluid from preterm infants with posthemorrhagic ventricular dilatation. Pediatr Res 2001;49(2):208–12.
102. Limperopoulos C, Benson CB, Bassan H, et al. Cerebellar hemorrhage in the preterm infant: ultrasonographic findings and risk factors. Pediatrics 2005; 116(3):717–24.
103. Flodmark O, Becker LE, Harwood-Nash DC, et al. Correlation between computed tomography and autopsy in premature and full-term neonates that have suffered perinatal asphyxia. Radiology 1980;137:93–103.
104. Limperopoulos C, Soul JS, Gauvreau K, et al. Late gestation cerebellar growth is rapid and impeded by premature birth. Pediatrics 2005;115(3):688–95.
105. Allin M, Matsumoto H, Santhouse AM, et al. Cognitive and motor function and the size of the cerebellum in adolescents born very pre-term. Brain 2001; 124(Pt 1):60–6.
106. Grunnet ML, Shields WD. Cerebellar hemorrhage in the premature infant. J Pediatr 1976;88(4 Pt 1):605–8.
107. Donat JF, Okazaki H, Kleinberg F. Cerebellar hemorrhages in newborn infants. Am J Dis Child 1979;133(4):441.
108. Limperopoulos C, Bassan H, Gauvreau K, et al. Does cerebellar injury in premature infants contribute to the high prevalence of long-term cognitive, learning, and behavioral disability in survivors? Pediatrics 2007;120(3):584–93.

109. Johnsen SD, Tarby TJ, Lewis KS, et al. Cerebellar infarction: an unrecognized complication of very low birthweight. J Child Neurol 2002;17(5):320–4.

110. Johnsen SD, Bodensteiner JB, Lotze TE. Frequency and nature of cerebellar injury in the extremely premature survivor with cerebral palsy. J Child Neurol 2005;20(1):60–4.

111. Limperopoulos C, Soul JS, Haidar H, et al. Impaired trophic interactions between the cerebellum and the cerebrum among preterm infants. Pediatrics 2005;116(4):844–50.

112. Hansen AR, DiSalvo D, Kazam E, et al. Sonographically detected subarachnoid hemorrhage: an independent predictor of neonatal posthemorrhagic hydrocephalus? Clin Imaging 2000;24(3):121–9.

113. Vasileiadis GT, Gelman N, Han VK, et al. Uncomplicated intraventricular hemorrhage is followed by reduced cortical volume at near-term age. Pediatrics 2004; 114(3):e367–72.

114. de Vries LS, Van Haastert IL, Rademaker KJ, et al. Ultrasound abnormalities preceding cerebral palsy in high-risk preterm infants. J Pediatr 2004;144(6): 815–20.

115. Kuban K, Sanocka U, Leviton A, et al. White matter disorders of prematurity: association with intraventricular hemorrhage and ventriculomegaly. The Developmental Epidemiology Network. J Pediatr 1999;134(5):539–46 [see comments].

116. Tam EW, Ferriero DM, Xu D, et al. Cerebellar development in the preterm neonate: effect of supratentorial brain injury. Pediatr Res 2009;66:102–6.

117. Perlman J, Volpe J. Seizures in the preterm infant: effects on cerebral blood flow velocity, intracranial pressure, and arterial blood pressure. J Pediatr 1983;102: 288–93.

118. Cornejo BJ, Mesches MH, Coultrap S, et al. A single episode of neonatal seizures permanently alters glutamatergic synapses. Ann Neurol 2007;61(5): 411–26.

119. Lombroso CT. Neonatal seizures: gaps between the laboratory and the clinic. Epilepsia 2007;48(Suppl 2):83–106.

120. Kuban KC, Allred EN, O'Shea TM, et al. Cranial ultrasound lesions in the NICU predict cerebral palsy at age 2 years in children born at extremely low gestational age. J Child Neurol 2009;24(1):63–72.

121. Laptook AR, O'Shea TM, Shankaran S, et al. Adverse neurodevelopmental outcomes among extremely low birth weight infants with a normal head ultrasound: prevalence and antecedents. Pediatrics 2005;115(3):673–80.

122. Bassan H, Limperopoulos C, Visconti K, et al. Neurodevelopmental outcome in survivors of periventricular hemorrhagic infarction. Pediatrics 2007;120(4): 785–92.

123. Broitman E, Ambalavanan N, Higgins RD, et al. Clinical data predict neurodevelopmental outcome better than head ultrasound in extremely low birth weight infants. J Pediatr 2007;151(5):500–5, 505.e1–2.

124. Roze E, Kerstjens JM, Maathuis CG, et al. Risk factors for adverse outcome in preterm infants with periventricular hemorrhagic infarction. Pediatrics 2008; 122(1):e46–52.

125. Rademaker KJ, Groenendaal F, Jansen GH, et al. Unilateral haemorrhagic parenchymal lesions in the preterm infant: shape, site and prognosis. Acta Paediatr 1994;83(6):602–8.

126. Hanigan WC, Morgan AM, Anderson RJ, et al. Incidence and neurodevelopmental outcome of periventricular hemorrhage and hydrocephalus in a regional population of very low birth weight infants. Neurosurgery 1991;29(5):701–6.

127. Futagi Y, Suzuki Y, Toribe Y, et al. Neurodevelopmental outcome in children with posthemorrhagic hydrocephalus. Pediatr Neurol 2005;33(1):26–32.
128. Adams-Chapman I, Hansen NI, Stoll BJ, et al. Neurodevelopmental outcome of extremely low birth weight infants with posthemorrhagic hydrocephalus requiring shunt insertion. Pediatrics 2008;121(5):e1167–77.
129. Leviton A, Fenton T, Kuban KC, et al. Labor and delivery characteristics and the risk of germinal matrix hemorrhage in low birth weight infants. J Child Neurol 1991;6(1):35–40.
130. Crowley P. WITHDRAWN: prophylactic corticosteroids for preterm birth. Cochrane Database Syst Rev 2006;(3):CD000065.
131. Rouse DJ, Hirtz DG, Thom E, et al. A randomized, controlled trial of magnesium sulfate for the prevention of cerebral palsy. N Engl J Med 2008;359(9): 895–905.
132. Di Renzo GC, Mignosa M, Gerli S, et al. The combined maternal administration of magnesium sulfate and aminophylline reduces intraventricular hemorrhage in very preterm neonates. Am J Obstet Gynecol 2005;192(2):433–8.
133. Whitelaw A. Intraventricular haemorrhage and posthaemorrhagic hydrocephalus: pathogenesis, prevention and future interventions. Semin Neonatol 2001; 6(2):135–46.
134. Cools F, Offringa M. Neuromuscular paralysis for newborn infants receiving mechanical ventilation. Cochrane Database Syst Rev 2000;(4):CD002773.
135. Whitelaw A, Odd D. Postnatal phenobarbital for the prevention of intraventricular hemorrhage in preterm infants. Cochrane Database Syst Rev 2007;(4): CD001691.
136. Chiswick ML, Johnson M, Woodhall C, et al. Protective effect of vitamin E (DL-alpha-tocopherol) against intraventricular haemorrhage in premature babies. Br Med J (Clin Res Ed) 1983;287(6385):81–4.
137. Phelps DL, Rosenbaum AL, Isenberg SJ, et al. Tocopherol efficacy and safety for preventing retinopathy of prematurity: a randomized, controlled, double-masked trial. Pediatrics 1987;79(4):489–500.
138. Brion LP, Bell EF, Raghuveer TS. Vitamin E supplementation for prevention of morbidity and mortality in preterm infants. Cochrane Database Syst Rev 2003;(4):CD003665.
139. Beverley DW, Pitts-Tucker TJ, Congdon PJ, et al. Prevention of intraventricular haemorrhage by fresh frozen plasma. Arch Dis Child 1985;60(8):710–3.
140. The Northern Neonatal Nursing Initiative [NNNI] Trial Group. A randomized trial comparing the effect of prophylactic intravenous fresh frozen plasma, gelatin or glucose on early mortality and morbidity in preterm babies. Eur J Pediatr 1996; 155(7):580–8.
141. Shirahata A, Nakamura T, Shimono M, et al. Blood coagulation findings and the efficacy of factor XIII concentrate in premature infants with intracranial hemorrhages. Thromb Res 1990;57(5):755–63.
142. The EC Ethamsylate Trial Group. The EC randomised controlled trial of prophylactic ethamsylate for very preterm neonates: early mortality and morbidity. Arch Dis Child 1994;70(3 Suppl):F201–5.
143. Elbourne D, Ayers S, Dellagrammaticas H, et al. Randomised controlled trial of prophylactic etamsylate: follow up at 2 years of age. Arch Dis Child Fetal Neonatal Ed 2001;84(3):F183–7.
144. Brangenberg R, Bodensohn M, Burger U. Antithrombin-III substitution in preterm infants: effect on intracranial hemorrhage and coagulation parameters. Biol Neonate 1997;72(2):76–83.

145. Fulia F, Cordaro S, Meo P, et al. Can the administration of antithrombin III decrease the risk of cerebral hemorrhage in premature infants? Biol Neonate 2003;83(1):1–5.

146. Veldman A, Josef J, Fischer D, et al. A prospective pilot study of prophylactic treatment of preterm neonates with recombinant activated factor VII during the first 72 hours of life. Pediatr Crit Care Med 2006;7(1):34–9.

147. Ment LR, Oh W, Ehrenkranz RA, et al. Low-dose indomethacin and prevention of intraventricular hemorrhage: a multicenter randomized trial. Pediatrics 1994; 93(4):543–50.

148. Ment LR, Vohr B, Allan W, et al. Outcome of children in the indomethacin intra-ventricular hemorrhage prevention trial. Pediatrics 2000;105(3 Pt 1):485–91.

149. Schmidt B, Davis P, Moddemann D, et al. Long-term effects of indomethacin prophylaxis in extremely-low-birth-weight infants. N Engl J Med 2001;344(26): 1966–72.

150. Fowlie PW, Davis PG. Prophylactic indomethacin for preterm infants: a system-atic review and meta-analysis. Arch Dis Child Fetal Neonatal Ed 2003;88(6): F464–6.

151. Ohlsson A, Roberts RS, Schmidt B, et al. Male/female differences in indometh-acin effects in preterm infants. J Pediatr 2005;147(6):860–2.

152. Harding DR, Humphries SE, Whitelaw A, et al. Cognitive outcome and cyclo-oxygenase-2 gene (-765 G/C) variation in the preterm infant. Arch Dis Child Fetal Neonatal Ed 2007;92(2):F108–12.

153. Als H, Lawhon G, Duffy FH, et al. Individualized developmental care for the very low-birth-weight preterm infant. JAMA 1994;272:853–8.

154. Wielenga JM, Smit BJ, Merkus MP, et al. Individualized developmental care in a Dutch NICU: short-term clinical outcome. Acta Paediatr 2007;96(10):1409–15.

155. Als H, Gilkerson L, Duffy FH, et al. A three-center, randomized, controlled trial of individualized developmental care for very low birth weight preterm infants: medical, neurodevelopmental, parenting, and caregiving effects. J Dev Behav Pediatr 2003;24(6):399–408.

156. Szymonowicz W, Yu VY, Walker A, et al. Reduction in periventricular haemor-rhage in preterm infants. Arch Dis Child 1986;61(7):661–5.

157. Als H, Duffy FH, McAnulty GB, et al. Early experience alters brain function and structure. Pediatrics 2004;113(4):846–57.

158. Mantovani JF, Pasternak JF, Mathew OP, et al. Failure of daily lumbar punctures to prevent the development of hydrocephalus following intraventricular hemor-rhage. J Pediatr 1980;97(2):278–81.

159. Ventriculomegaly Trial Group. Randomised trial of early tapping in neonatal posthaemorrhagic ventricular dilatation. Arch Dis Child 1990;65(1):3–10.

160. Weninger M, Salzer H, Pollak A, et al. External ventricular drainage for treatment of rapidly progressive posthemorrhagic hydrocephalus. Neurosurgery 1992;31: 52–8.

161. Rahman S, Teo C, Morris W, et al. Ventriculosubgaleal shunt: a treatment option for progressive posthemorrhagic hydrocephalus. Childs Nerv Syst 1995;11(11): 650–4.

162. Whitelaw A, Evans D, Carter M, et al. Randomized clinical trial of prevention of hydrocephalus after intraventricular hemorrhage in preterm infants: brain-washing versus tapping fluid. Pediatrics 2007;119(5):e1071–8.

163. Pople IK, Ettles D. The role of endoscopic choroid plexus coagulation in the management of hydrocephalus. Neurosurgery 1995;36(4):698–701 [discussion: 2].

The Role of Toll-like Receptors in Perinatal Brain Injury

Carina Mallard, PhD[a], Xiaoyang Wang, MD, PhD[a,b],
Henrik Hagberg, MD, PhD[c,d],*

KEYWORDS

- TLRs • Injury • Neonatal • Innate immunity • Immature brain
- Lipopolysaccharide

The innate immune response is the first line of defense to protect the host from invading microbes. It is now well recognized that innate reactions are also activated in the central nervous system (CNS), an organ that once was believed to be immune privileged. The ability to mount an effective innate immune response in the CNS is likely to be critical for pathogen elimination and vital to host survival. However, it is also evident that chronic or acute dysregulated inflammation in the CNS can cause tissue damage and neurodegeneration. Microglia, which are the resident phagocytes of the CNS, and astrocytes are strongly activated in association with brain injury. Both cell types participate in the initiation of neuroinflammation through the production of cytokines and chemokines and also in the recruitment and activation of peripheral immune cells into the CNS, functions likely to be at least partially mediated via innate reactions.

This article focuses on the innate immune system in the CNS and how it may play a role in brain injury, with particular emphasis on the developing brain.

The work was supported by the Swedish Medical Research Council (VR 2006-2783, Carina Mallard [CM]; VR 2006-3396, Henrik Hagberg [HH]), the Wilhelm and Martina Lundgren Foundation (CM, Xiaoyang Wang [XW]), the Åhlén Foundation (CM), the Frimurare Barnhus Foundation (CM), Governmental Grants to University Hospitals in Sweden (ALFGBG-11101, HH, CM) and MRC United Kingdom (award DSRR P19381, HH).

[a] Department of Neuroscience and Physiology, Perinatal Center, Sahlgrenska Academy at the University of Gothenburg, Medicinaregatan 11, 41390 Gothenburg, Sweden
[b] Department of Pediatrics, The Third Affiliated Hospital of Zhengzhou University, Kanfu Qian Street 7, 450052, Zhengzhou, China
[c] Department of Obstetrics and Gynecology, Perinatal Center, Sahlgrenska Academy at the University of Gothenburg, Östra Sjukhuset, 416 85 Gothenberg, Sweden
[d] Department of Obstetrics, Institute of Reproductive and Developmental Biology, Imperial College London, Du Cane Road, London W12 0NN, UK
* Corresponding author.
E-mail address: h.hagberg@imperial.ac.uk (H. Hagberg).

Clin Perinatol 36 (2009) 763–772
doi:10.1016/j.clp.2009.07.009
0095-5108/09/$ – see front matter

TOLL-LIKE RECEPTORS

Innate immunity depends on inflammatory host cells, such as macrophages, neutrophils, dendritic cells, and natural killer cells, that express pattern recognition receptors (PRRs). The PRRs sense pathogen-associated molecular patterns (PAMPs) from various microorganisms, which results in initiation of intracellular signaling pathways and production of inflammatory mediators including cytokines, chemokines and interferons (IFNs). In turn these mediators can modulate the immune response, including the subsequent adaptive immune responses. A recently discovered family of PRRs, the so-called toll-like receptors (TLRs) are transmembrane receptors, recognizing PAMPs from various microbes.

To date, 11 human TLRs and 13 mouse TLRs have been identified. Different TLRs recognize specific PAMPs from various pathogens, ranging from lipids, lipoproteins, and proteins to nucleic acids. TLR4, which was the first receptor to be identified, together with its extracellular components myeloid differentiation 2 (MD2) and cluster of differentiation 14 (CD14), recognizes lipopolysaccharide (LPS) from gram-negative bacteria. TLR2 forms heterodimers with TLR1 and TLR6, and these receptor complexes recognize molecules expressed on gram-positive bacteria, such as peptidoglycan, lipopeptides, and lipoproteins. TLR5 binds mainly bacterial flagellin. The group of TLR3, 7, 8 and 9 is present on intracellular vesicles, such as endosomes and lysosomes, where they detect nucleic acids from bacteria and viruses.

Signaling through TLRs depends on recruitment of intracellular toll-interleukin-1 receptor (TIR)-domain–containing adaptors. So far 5 adaptors have been identified. Four are stimulatory, namely (1) myeloid differentiation primary response gene 88 (MyD88), (2) MyD88-adaptorlike (Mal), (3) TIR-domain–containing adaptor protein inducing IFNβ (TRIF), and (4) TRIF-related adaptor molecule (TRAM); in contrast, sterile α- and armadillo-motif containing protein (SARM) is inhibitory via interference with TRIF functions. TLR4 activates the MyD88-dependent and TRIF-dependent pathways, whereas TLR3 signals only through the TRIF adaptor protein, and the rest of the TLRs use the MyD88-dependent pathway only. Several excellent articles further discuss the intracellular signaling pathway.[1,2]

TOLL-LIKE RECEPTOR EXPRESSION IN CNS

The mRNA expression of TLR2 and TLR4 in the adult rodent brain was first described by Laflamme and Rivest.[3] Using in situ hybridization, they found TLR2 and TLR4 mRNA expression under basal conditions, mainly in the leptomeninges, choroid plexus, and circum-ventricular organs. TLRs have also been detected in human cerebral tissue.[4] Less is known about TLR expression in the developing brain. TLR4 gene transcripts were demonstrated in the newborn rat brain by reverse transcription-polymerase chain reaction (RT-PCR),[5] and protein expression of TLR3 and TLR8 has been identified particularly during embryonic development.[6,7] TLR2 expression is low before birth and increases during the first 2 weeks of life.[7] Brain expression of TLRs is generally low in fetal and adult tissue samples, when compared with other tissues.[8]

The cellular localization of TLRs has predominantly been studied in cell culture systems. In vitro studies generally demonstrate that microglia cells express mRNA encoding for a wide range of different TLR family members, whereas astrocytes are more restricted and they primarily express only TLR2 and TLR3. There are, however, substantial inconsistencies among different studies and also between gene expression and identification of the proteins. Despite most TLRs being detected by RT-PCR, when using immunohistochemistry under basal conditions, only TLR2 expression was detected at low level in microglia, neurons, ependymal cells, and astrocytes,[9] and TLR13 in neurons[10] in the murine brain. In rodent cell cultures, TLR2, 3 and 4 proteins have been demonstrated in neurons,[11] although neuronal TLR expression has not been replicated in vivo by in situ hybridization.[12] Recently, TLR2 and TLR4 immunopositive cells were found in neural progenitor cells in the hippocampus.[13] In the developing brain, TLR8 immunohistochemical staining has been localized to cortical neurons and axons.[6] Collectively, data show that TLRs are widely expressed in the brain, and evidence suggests that some TLRs are developmentally regulated.

FUNCTIONS OF TOLL-LIKE RECEPTORS IN CNS

In a study using TLR4 chimeric mice, Chakravarty and Herkenham[12] showed that TLR4 expression in the CNS is necessary to mount an appropriate cytokine response in the brain in response to systemic LPS exposure. Mice that are specifically lacking TLR4 in peripheral immune cells had defective cytokine production in the serum after peripheral LPS injection, but cytokine production in the CNS was relatively intact. In contrast, mice with peripheral TLR4-expressing cells, but lacking specific CNS TLR4, were unable to mount a CNS cytokine response, suggesting specific functions for TLRs in the brain.

Further studies indicate that TLRs may play important roles in cerebral cell proliferation and brain development. Inflammation has a strong effect on progenitor cells and reduces adult hippocampal neurogenesis.[14,15] TLR2 and TLR4 are expressed on adult neural progenitor cells but appear to have opposite effects on neurogenesis. TLR2 deficiency in mice resulted in impaired hippocampal neurogenesis, whereas the absence of TLR4 enhanced proliferation and neuronal differentiation.[13] The detrimental effects of TLR4 on progenitor cells was shown to be dependent on prostaglandin E2 receptors,[16] which is further supported by the protective effect on hippocampal neurogenesis by cyclooxygenase inhibitors.[17]

Also during normal brain development, TLRs appear to play a role in neural progenitor cell proliferation. TLR3 is expressed at high levels in the embryonic brain in mice and TLR3 deficiency increases proliferation of neural progenitor cells, suggesting that TLR3 is a negative regulator of neurogenesis in the developing brain.[7] TLR8 is also expressed at high levels during brain development, and in cultured cortical neurons, TLR8 stimulation inhibits neurite outgrowth.[6] Taken together, these studies strongly suggest that TLRs have specific functions in the adult and the developing brain, which are distinct from classical immune responses.

PATHOPHYSIOLOGIC ROLE OF TOLL-LIKE RECEPTORS
TLRs and Adult Brain Injury

Increasing evidence indicates that TLRs play an important role in several CNS pathologies in the human. For example, a rare genetic single nucleotide polymorphism in TLR4 has been associated with increased susceptibility to meningococcal infection,[18] and one study has shown that the TLR4 gene C119A polymorphism is associated with ischemic stroke among ethnic Chinese in Taiwan.[19] TLRs are also believed to be important in autoimmune disease, as reviewed elsewhere[20]; for example, expression of TLR3 and TLR4 is enhanced in the brain and spinal cord of patients with multiple sclerosis.[4] Furthermore, it has been suggested that TLRs play a fundamental role in Alzheimer disease.[21] Stimulation of the innate immune system, via TLR9, reduced the amyloid burden up to 80% in mice.[22] Activation of TLR4 has been proposed to induce Parkinson diseaselike injury, where the following was shown: exposure of pregnant rats to LPS resulted in long-term loss of dopaminergic neurons in the

Table 1
The role of TLRs in acute adult brain damage

Reference	Model	Effect
25	• Denervation of hippocampus • TLR2 KO mice • C3H/HeJ and C3H/HeN mice	• Denervation-induced TLR2 upregulation in hippocampus • TLR2 KO mice showed transient reductions of cytokine and chemokine expression and delayed T-cell recruitment • TLR2 deficiency conferred a decrease in microglia expansion up to 5d postdenervation • Denervation did not induce TLR2 upregulation in astrocytes • TLR4 deficiency did not affect the neuroinflammatory response
26	• TLR4 deficient C57BL/10ScCr mice and WT control C57BL/10ScSn • C3H/HeJ and C3H/HeN MCAO model	• Two strains of TLR4-deficient mice (C3H/HeJ and C57BL/10ScNJ) showed reduced infarction at 24h after permanent MCAO • iNOS, COX-2, MMP-9 were reduced in mutants, but not IL-1β or TNF-α at 24h after MCAO • Neurologic and behavioral status were improved in mutants at 1wk after MCAO. • Observed expression of TLR4 after MCAO in astrocytes, microglia, and blood vessels
11	• TLR2 KO • C3HeJ and C3H/HeN • focal MCAO model	• TLR2 KO and TLR4 mutant mice showed reduced brain damage and improved functional outcome after MCAO • Cultured neurons from TLR2 KO and TLR4 mutant mice were protected against energy-deprivation–induced cell death and showed reduced expression of pJNK, AP-1, and caspase-3. • MCAO resulted in rapid increases in TLR2 and 4 immunoreactivity in neurons (1h) in cerebral cortex and delayed (36h) TLR2 in microglia
27	• MCAO model • C3H/HeJ and C3H/HeN	• TLR4-deficient mice (C3H/HeJ) had reduced cerebral infarct size and brain edema and less neurologic impairment after MCAO. • C3H/HeJ mice had lower serum level of TNF-α and IL-6
28	• Spinal cord injury female C3H/HeJ & HeOuJ • TLR2 KO mice	• mRNAs for TLR1, 2, 4, 5, and 7 were increased after sterile SCI • TLR2 was expressed on astrocytes and CNS macrophages, whereas TLR4 was predominantly expressed on CNS macrophages following SCI. • TLR2 KO and TLR4 mutant mice showed impaired locomotor recovery after SCI that was associated with unusual patterns of demyelination, neuroinflammation, and gliosis
29	• Transient MCAO model • TLR2 KO mice	• TLR2, 4, 9 mRNAs and genes, related to TLR2 signal pathway, were induced in the ipsilateral mouse brain hemispheres after transient MCAO • TLR2-protein was expressed mainly on microglia in the postischemic brain tissue but also on selected endothelial cells, neurons, and astrocytes • TLR2 KO mice showed decreased infarct volume at 2d after MCAO

30	• TLR2 KO mice • MCAO model	• TLR2 mRNA was upregulated in WT mice after MCAO • TLR2 KO mice developed smaller brain infarctions compared with WT mice • In ischemic brains, TLR2 protein was expressed in lesion-associated microglia
31	• TLR4 deficient C57BL/10ScCr mice and WT control C57BL/10ScSn • Global cerebral ischemia/reperfusion	• TLR4-deficient C57BL/10ScCr mice displayed decreased neuronal damage and reduced neuronal apoptosis, following global cerebral ischemia/reperfusion • TLR4 immunoreactivity was increased in the HF and caudate-putamen at 72h, following ischemia in WT mice • Ischemia/reperfusion stimulated NFκB p65 nuclear translocation in the HF of WT mice. • TLR4 deficiency prevented upregulation of IL-6, TNF-α, Fas-L, and HMGB1 in the HF in response to ischemia • Phosphorylation of Akt and GSK3β was increased in the HF of TLR4 deficiency mice after the insult
32	• C3H/HeJ and C3h/HeN • Transient MCAO model	• TLR4 mutant C3H/HeJ mice showed reduced brain injury and reduced number of TUNEL- and caspase-3-positive cells after MCAO. • TLR4 mutation promoted the survival of axotomized retinal ganglion cells • The TLR4 mutants had reduced pERK-2, pJNK-1, pJNK-2, and p38 following MCAO • The number of iNOS positive cells was reduced but the number of neutrophils (MPO+) and microglia (Iba1+) were increased in TLR-4 mutants following MCAO
33	• TLR2 gene knockout mice (TLR2 KO, B6.129-TLR2tm1kir/J) • TLR4 deficient C57BL/10ScCr mice and WT control C57BL/10ScSn deficient • MCAO model	• In TLR4 deficient mice (C57BL/10ScCr), brain infarct size was decreased and neurologic function was improved as compared with WT mice following MCAO • TLR2 KO mice showed higher mortality, decreased neurologic function, and increased brain infarct size • NFκB DNA binding activity was decreased in TLR4 mice but increased in TLR2 KO mice following MCAO • The phosphorylation of Akt and ERK1/2 that was evoked by cerebral ischemia was attenuated in TLR2 KO compared with TLR4 mice

Abbreviations: AP-1, activator protein-1; COX-2, cyclooxygenase 2; ERK, extracellular signal-regulated kinase; Fas-L, Fas ligand; HF, hippocampal formation; GSK3β, glycogen synthase kinase 3 beta; HMGB1, high mobility group box 1; Iba1, ionized calcium binding adaptor molecule 1; IL, interleukin; iNOS, inducible nitric oxide synthase; KO, knock out; MCAO, medial cerebral artery occlusion; MMP-9, matrix metallopeptidase 9; MPO, myeloperoxidase; mRNA, messenger RNA; NFκB, NF-kappa-B–inducing kinase; pERK, phosphorylated ERK; pJNK, phosphorylated Jun N-terminal kinase; SCI, spinal cord injury; TUNEL, terminal-deoxynucleotidyl-transferase–mediated dUTP nick end labeling; WT, wild-type.

substantia nigra and increased tumor necrosis factor (TNF)-α levels in the striatum in the offspring.[23] However, there are conflicting observations in fetal sheep, where intra-uterine LPS exposure did not affect dopaminergic neurons.[24]

It is now well recognized that injured tissue can release endogenous PAMPs that stimulate the innate immune system. Numerous articles have been published that show the involvement of TLRs in experimental acute adult brain injury, following ischemia or trauma, as summarized in **Table 1**. These studies suggest that the activation of TLR2 or TLR4 may be detrimental in acute CNS injury and that these receptors may be novel neuroprotective targets.

TLRs and Perinatal Brain Injury

Very little is known about the direct role of TLRs in neonatal brain injury in humans, and most data are incidental to other inflammatory parameters, such as associations of cytokines with preterm birth and cerebral palsy. However, emerging data suggest a role for TLRs in preterm birth. Human placenta and fetal membranes express TLRs, and the expression of TLR2 and TLR4 is enhanced in preterm delivery with histologic chorioamnionitis.[34–36] Several studies have shown an association between preterm birth and TLR polymorphisms.[37–39]

Animal studies have demonstrated a strong link between the TLR4 agonist LPS and brain injury, in fetal and newborn animals.[40] The direct involvement of TLRs has been examined in newborn animals. LPS, injected directly into the developing brain of mice and rats, induces white matter injury[41,42]; deletion of the TLR4 gene prevented LPS-induced oligodendrocyte death in vitro.[41] Systemic administration of LPS has also

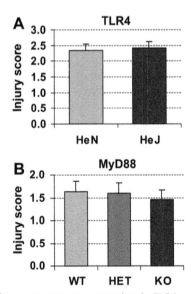

Fig. 1. (A) C3H mice that have spontaneous mutation in TLR4 gene (C3H/HeJ, n = 54) and respective controls (C3H/HeN, n = 44) were subjected to hypoxia-ischemia at postnatal day (PND) 9. Brain injury was evaluated by macroscopic scoring at 3 days after hypoxia-ischemia; $P > .05$. (B) Littermates of C57BL/6 mice lacking the gene for MyD88 (MyD88 KO, n = 22), C57BL/6 wild type (WT, n = 28), and heterozygotes (HET, n = 34) were subjected to hypoxia-ischemia at PND 9; brain injury was evaluated by macroscopic scoring at 3 days after hypoxia-ischemia; $P > .05$.

been shown to induce white matter lesions in fetal sheep[43] and newborn kittens.[44] The investigators have previously shown that LPS sensitizes the developing rat and mouse brain to subsequent hypoxia-ischemia,[5,45–47] if it is administered systemically[5,45,47] between the amniotic and chorionic membranes[46] or directly into the brain.[48] Data suggest that these effects are mediated through the TLR adaptor protein MyD88.[49] However, in contrast to the adult, TLR4 or MyD88 deficiency does not confer protection from hypoxia-ischemia in neonatal mice (**Fig. 1**, Wang and colleagues, 2007, unpublished data); this fact suggests that the inflammatory mechanisms, following a "sterile" inflammatory insult, differ with development.

There are few studies on TLR2 in immature brain injury, but its involvement has been proposed in neurodegeneration that is induced by group B streptococci.[50] However, the TLR2 agonist, lipoteichoic acid, does not affect vulnerability to hypoxia-ischemia in immature rats[51]; MyD88 gene deletion not affecting the extent of hypoxic-ischemic brain injury (see **Fig. 1**) suggests that TLR2 may not be critical in response to sterile insults in the newborn.

TLR3 may be important because it inhibits axonal growth and could be anticipated to negatively influence the regenerative response after injury.[52] Furthermore, prenatal administration of the TLR3 agonist polyI:C to pregnant rodents impairs subcortical dopaminergic activity and cognitive function.[53] Hypothetically, activation of TLR3 receptors, by virus or other exogenous or endogenous agonists, may have adverse effects on the developing CNS; this possibility requires further investigation.

SUMMARY

The discovery of the presence of TLRs in the CNS has initiated a new intense area of research, to understand their role in the brain. Emerging evidence suggests that CNS TLRs may serve other functions than the classic immune responses known in peripheral tissue. During normal brain development and adult neurogenesis, TLRs appear to regulate cell proliferation, differentiation, and neurite outgrowth. Furthermore, TLRs have been implicated in acute ischemic brain injury in the adult. TLR microbial agonists can clearly injure the developing brain; however, the role of TLRs in "sterile" hypoxia-ischemia–induced inflammation in the developing brain remains unclear and seems to differ from that in the adult. Further studies need to determine whether different TLRs are important at different developmental stages and which TLRs are regulated in acute perinatal brain injury.

REFERENCES

1. O'Neill LA, Bowie AG. The family of five: TIR-domain-containing adaptors in Toll-like receptor signalling. Nat Rev Immunol 2007;7(5):353–64.
2. Kawai T, Akira S. The roles of TLRs, RLRs and NLRs in pathogen recognition. Int Immunol 2009;21(4):317–37.
3. Laflamme N, Rivest S. Toll-like receptor 4: the missing link of the cerebral innate immune response triggered by circulating gram-negative bacterial cell wall components. FASEB J 2001;15(1):155–63.
4. Bsibsi M, Ravid R, Gveric D, et al. Broad expression of Toll-like receptors in the human central nervous system. J Neuropathol Exp Neurol 2002;61(11):1013–21.
5. Eklind S, Mallard C, Leverin AL, et al. Bacterial endotoxin sensitizes the immature brain to hypoxic–ischaemic injury. Eur J Neurosci 2001;13(6):1101–6.
6. Ma Y, Li J, Chiu I, et al. Toll-like receptor 8 functions as a negative regulator of neurite outgrowth and inducer of neuronal apoptosis. J Cell Biol 2006;175(2):209–15.

7. Lathia JD, Okun E, Tang SC, et al. Toll-like receptor 3 is a negative regulator of embryonic neural progenitor cell proliferation. J Neurosci 2008;28(51):13978–84.

8. Nishimura M, Naito S. Tissue-specific mRNA expression profiles of human toll-like receptors and related genes. Biol Pharm Bull 2005;28(5):886–92.

9. Mishra BB, Mishra PK, Teale JM. Expression and distribution of Toll-like receptors in the brain during murine neurocysticercosis. J Neuroimmunol 2006;181(1–2):46–56.

10. Mishra BB, Gundra UM, Teale JM. Expression and distribution of Toll-like receptors 11–13 in the brain during murine neurocysticercosis. J Neuroinflammation 2008;5:53.

11. Tang SC, Arumugam TV, Xu X, et al. Pivotal role for neuronal Toll-like receptors in ischemic brain injury and functional deficits. Proc Natl Acad Sci U S A 2007; 104(34):13798–803.

12. Chakravarty S, Herkenham M. Toll-like receptor 4 on nonhematopoietic cells sustains CNS inflammation during endotoxemia, independent of systemic cytokines. J Neurosci 2005;25(7):1788–96.

13. Rolls A, Shechter R, London A, et al. Toll-like receptors modulate adult hippocampal neurogenesis. Nat Cell Biol 2007;9(9):1081–8.

14. Ekdahl CT, Claasen JH, Bonde S, et al. Inflammation is detrimental for neurogenesis in adult brain. Proc Natl Acad Sci U S A 2003;100(23):13632–7.

15. Monje ML, Toda H, Palmer TD. Inflammatory blockade restores adult hippocampal neurogenesis. Science 2003;302(5651):1760–5.

16. Keene CD, Chang R, Stephen C, et al. Protection of hippocampal neurogenesis from toll-like receptor 4-dependent innate immune activation by ablation of prostaglandin E2 receptor subtype EP1 or EP2. Am J Pathol 2009;174(6):2300–9.

17. Bastos GN, Moriya T, Inui F, et al. Involvement of cyclooxygenase-2 in lipopolysaccharide-induced impairment of the newborn cell survival in the adult mouse dentate gyrus. Neuroscience 2008;155(2):454–62.

18. Emonts M, Hazelzet JA, de Groot R, et al. Host genetic determinants of Neisseria meningitidis infections. Lancet Infect Dis 2003;3(9):565–77.

19. Lin YC, Chang YM, Yu JM, et al. Toll-like receptor 4 gene C119A but not Asp299Gly polymorphism is associated with ischemic stroke among ethnic Chinese in Taiwan. Atherosclerosis 2005;180(2):305–9.

20. Fischer M, Ehlers M. Toll-like receptors in autoimmunity. Ann N Y Acad Sci 2008; 1143:21–34.

21. Salminen A, Ojala J, Kauppinen A, et al. Inflammation in Alzheimer's disease: amyloid-beta oligomers trigger innate immunity defence via pattern recognition receptors. Prog Neurobiol 2009;87(3):181–94.

22. Scholtzova H, Kascsak RJ, Bates KA, et al. Induction of toll-like receptor 9 signaling as a method for ameliorating Alzheimer's disease-related pathology. J Neurosci 2009;29(6):1846–54.

23. Ling Z, Gayle DA, Ma SY, et al. In utero bacterial endotoxin exposure causes loss of tyrosine hydroxylase neurons in the postnatal rat midbrain. Mov Disord 2002; 17(1):116–24.

24. Dean JM, Farrag D, Zahkouk SA, et al. Cerebellar white matter injury following systemic endotoxemia in preterm fetal sheep. Neuroscience 2009;160(3):606–15.

25. Babcock AA, Wirenfeldt M, Holm T, et al. Toll-like receptor 2 signaling in response to brain injury: an innate bridge to neuroinflammation. J Neurosci 2006;26(49): 12826–37.

26. Caso JR, Pradillo JM, Hurtado O, et al. Toll-like receptor 4 is involved in brain damage and inflammation after experimental stroke. Circulation 2007;115(12): 1599–608.

27. Cao CX, Yang QW, Lv FL, et al. Reduced cerebral ischemia-reperfusion injury in Toll-like receptor 4 deficient mice. Biochem Biophys Res Commun 2007;353(2): 509–14.

28. Kigerl KA, Lai W, Rivest S, et al. Toll-like receptor (TLR)-2 and TLR-4 regulate inflammation, gliosis, and myelin sparing after spinal cord injury. J Neurochem 2007;102(1):37–50.

29. Ziegler G, Harhausen D, Schepers C, et al. TLR2 has a detrimental role in mouse transient focal cerebral ischemia. Biochem Biophys Res Commun 2007;359(3):574–9.

30. Lehnardt S, Lehmann S, Kaul D, et al. Toll-like receptor 2 mediates CNS injury in focal cerebral ischemia. J Neuroimmunol 2007;190(1–2):28–33.

31. Hua F, Ma J, Ha T, et al. Activation of Toll-like receptor 4 signaling contributes to hippocampal neuronal death following global cerebral ischemia/reperfusion. J Neuroimmunol 2007;190(1–2):101–11.

32. Kilic U, Kilic E, Matter CM, et al. TLR-4 deficiency protects against focal cerebral ischemia and axotomy-induced neurodegeneration. Neurobiol Dis 2008;31(1): 33–40.

33. Hua F, Ma J, Ha T, et al. Differential roles of TLR2 and TLR4 in acute focal cerebral ischemia/reperfusion injury in mice. Brain Res 2009;1262:100–8.

34. Kim YM, Romero R, Chaiworapongsa T, et al. Toll-like receptor-2 and -4 in the chorioamniotic membranes in spontaneous labor at term and in preterm parturition that are associated with chorioamnionitis. Am J Obstet Gynecol 2004;191(4): 1346–55.

35. Beijar EC, Mallard C, Powell TL. Expression and subcellular localization of TLR-4 in term and first trimester human placenta. Placenta 2006;27(2–3):322–6.

36. Koga K, Cardenas I, Aldo P, et al. Activation of TLR3 in the trophoblast is associated with preterm delivery. Am J Reprod Immunol 2009;61(3):196–212.

37. Krediet TG, Wiertsema SP, Vossers MJ, et al. Toll-like receptor 2 polymorphism is associated with preterm birth. Pediatr Res 2007;62(4):474–6.

38. Heinzmann A, Mailaparambil B, Mingirulli N, et al. Association of interleukin-13/-4 and Toll-like receptor 10 with preterm births. Neonatology 2009;96(3):175–81.

39. Koga K, Aldo PB, Mor G. Toll-like receptors and pregnancy: trophoblast as modulators of the immune response. J Obstet Gynaecol Res 2009;35(2):191–202.

40. Hagberg H, Peebles D, Mallard C. Models of white matter injury: comparison of infectious, hypoxic-ischemic, and excitotoxic insults. Ment Retard Dev Disabil Res Rev 2002;8(1):30–8.

41. Lehnardt S, Lachance C, Patrizi S, et al. The toll-like receptor TLR4 is necessary for lipopolysaccharide-induced oligodendrocyte injury in the CNS. J Neurosci 2002;22(7):2478–86.

42. Pang Y, Cai Z, Rhodes PG. Disturbance of oligodendrocyte development, hypomyelination and white matter injury in the neonatal rat brain after intracerebral injection of lipopolysaccharide. Brain Res Dev Brain Res 2003;140(2):205–14.

43. Mallard C, Welin AK, Peebles D, et al. White matter injury following systemic endotoxemia or asphyxia in the fetal sheep. Neurochem Res 2003;28(2):215–23.

44. Gilles FH, Averill DR Jr, Kerr CS. Neonatal endotoxin encephalopathy. Ann Neurol 1977;2(1):49–56.

45. Eklind S, Mallard C, Arvidsson P, et al. Lipopolysaccharide induces both a primary and a secondary phase of sensitization in the developing rat brain. Pediatr Res 2005;58(1):112–6.

46. Wang X, Hagberg H, Nie C, et al. Dual role of intrauterine immune challenge on neonatal and adult brain vulnerability to hypoxia-ischemia. J Neuropathol Exp Neurol 2007;66(6):552–61.

47. Wang X, Svedin P, Nie C, et al. N-acetylcysteine reduces lipopolysaccharide-sensitized hypoxic-ischemic brain injury. Ann Neurol 2007;61(3):263–71.
48. Coumans AB, Middelanis JS, Garnier Y, et al. Intracisternal application of endotoxin enhances the susceptibility to subsequent hypoxic-ischemic brain damage in neonatal rats. Pediatr Res 2003;53(5):770–5.
49. Wang X, Stridh L, Li W, et al. Lipopolysaccharide sensitizes neonatal hypoxic-ischemic brain injury in a MyD88 dependent manner. J Immunol 2009, in press.
50. Lehnardt S, Henneke P, Lien E, et al. A mechanism for neurodegeneration induced by group B Streptococci through activation of the TLR2/MyD88 pathway in microglia. J Immunol 2006;177(1):583–92.
51. Eklind S, Arvidsson P, Hagberg H, et al. The role of glucose in brain injury following the combination of lipopolysaccharide or lipoteichoic acid and hypoxia-ischemia in neonatal rats. Dev Neurosci 2004;26(1):61–7.
52. Cameron JS, Alexopoulou L, Sloane JA, et al. Toll-like receptor 3 is a potent negative regulator of axonal growth in mammals. J Neurosci 2007;27(47):13033–41.
53. Ozawa K, Hashimoto K, Kishimoto T, et al. Immune activation during pregnancy in mice leads to dopaminergic hyperfunction and cognitive impairment in the offspring: a neurodevelopmental animal model of schizophrenia. Biol Psychiatry 2006;59(6):546–54.

Long-term Outcome of Preterm Infants and the Role of Neuroimaging

Eliza Myers, MD, Laura R. Ment, MD*

KEYWORDS

- Prematurity • Outcome • Follow-up
- Neuroimaging • Plasticity

A recent report of the Institute of Medicine defines preterm birth as one of the major public health problems of this decade.[1] With preterm birth come preterm survivors—more every year—and as survival rates increase, the next great imperative for perinatal medicine is to understand and prevent the serious adverse neurodevelopmental outcomes of preterm birth. Neonatology as a field of medicine is recently organized, with the first Neonatal Intensive Care Unit in the United States opening in 1965 at Yale University School of Medicine and with the American Academy of Pediatrics recognizing Neonatology as a subspecialty field in 1975. Exogenous surfactant was first described as a therapy for Respiratory Distress Syndrome in 1980,[2] and surfactant replacement therapy was first recognized in a policy statement by the American Academy of Pediatrics in 1999.[3] Antenatal steroid use was formalized in a National Institutes of Health consensus statement in 1994, and recognized by the American College of Obstetricians and Gynecologists shortly thereafter.[4] These therapies have revolutionized survival rates for very preterm neonates, but many have questioned the neurodevelopmental cost. An understanding of both changing patterns of survival and emerging long-term neurodevelopmental disability is necessary to address outcome in the prematurely born.

TRENDS IN PREVALENCE, MORTALITY, AND MORBIDITY

From 1965 through the early 1990s, survival statistics improved annually, with steadily decreasing mortality at every gestational age (GA) and birth weight (BW) point.[1] Progress since the 1990s to the present is less clear. A review for the National Institute of

This work was supported by NS 27116 and NICHD T32 07094 from the National Institutes of Health.

Department of Pediatrics, Yale University School of Medicine, P.O. Box 208064, New Haven, CT 06520-8064, USA

* Corresponding author.

E-mail address: laura.ment@yale.edu (L.R. Ment).

Child Health and Human Development (NICHD) Neonatal Research Network in 2007 found that the infant mortality rate rose between 2001 and 2002, from 6.8 per 1000 live births to 7.0 per 1000 live births, for the first time in 4 decades, whereas the survival of very low birth weight (VLBW) infants changed "almost imperceptibly" between 1997 and 2002.[5] At the same time, the overall incidence for premature birth is slowly increasing, mostly in the late preterm infant but also in the very and extremely low birth weight (ELBW) infant: from 1.2% in 1980 to 1.5% in 2006.[6] These data are particularly useful because they consolidate standardized information across multiple level-III perinatal centers.

That the incidence of neurodevelopmental disability in preterm populations has been reported to change little over time is a phenomenon documented in several reviews.[1] Taken together, then, the coincidence of increasing incidence of VLBW and ELBW infants (501–1500 g)—the same infants at highest risk for neurodevelopmental impairment—with the lack of progress in overall morbidity of these infants suggests that increasing numbers of impaired infants are surviving every year. In 2005, Wilson-Costello and colleagues[7] concluded just that; in their single perinatal center, whereas overall survival increased in the 1990s compared with the 1980s, the risk for significant neurodevelopmental impairment also increased. This study concludes that the absolute numbers of ELBW (500–999 g) survivors is increasing in both the unimpaired and impaired groups.

These and other epidemiologic studies are difficult to compare because of differences between institutional practices, definitions (particularly comparing BW categories with weeks of gestation when describing prematurity), patient populations, and follow-up parameters, but the overall trend in the United States seems to be toward an increasing number of premature births, with increasing survival rates that perhaps outpace improvements in morbidity, such that increasing numbers of both impaired and intact premature infants are surviving every year. It is therefore possible that overall survival is increasing at the expense of intact survival, although this, too, is impossible to know until the most current generation of survivors reaches follow-up age.

Whether or not increasing incidence of impaired survival is the case, the next imperative in neonatology is to better understand the pathophysiology of preterm birth, the role of neurologic injury on neurodevelopmental impairment, and the potential for recovery in the injured preterm brain. This review attempts to report the current understanding of neurodevelopmental outcome of premature infants in the postsurfactant/antenatal steroid era, and to describe current practices of monitoring the developing brain.

PRESENT STATUS OF OUTCOME DATA

Outcome for surviving infants is defined by various neurodevelopmental impairments and by general measures of health, including chronic respiratory diseases, growth parameters, and recurrent infections. This review focuses on the neurodevelopmental dysfunctions. These disabilities, including cerebral palsy, mental retardation, and visual and hearing deficits, exist on a spectrum ranging from mild involvement (including learning disability, language disability, attention deficit-hyperactivity disorder and coordination, behavior, and social-emotional disorders) to profound impairment.[1] This spectrum of deficits represents the sequelae of that injury to the developing brain associated with preterm birth.

The group of premature infants born since 1995, the postsurfactant/antenatal steroid era, is just now reaching adolescence. Little data yet exist describing this cohort's neurodevelopmental outcome at adolescence and beyond. Until studies are published describing this post-1995 cohort, the next best options for understanding the present state of neonatal outcomes are (1) to examine data that describe late outcomes (adolescence and adulthood) of earlier cohorts of infants, and (2) to evaluate data that describe early outcomes (toddler and childhood) of more contemporary cohorts. Both options are potentially flawed.

When looking at much earlier cohorts of infants, those born before the 1980s, the outcome data must be considered in light of multiple confounding variables: these studies likely represent the hardiest of preterms who survived in an era when the norm included less aggressive resuscitations and fewer aggressive postnatal interventions (thereby selecting for the most robust of preterms), and probably represent a large percentage of small for GA but near-term or term infants, thereby skewing results toward the favorable spectrum. Indeed, studies that describe premature infants born before 1950 report none to minimal neurodevelopmental impairment in adulthood; however, these survivors of prematurity likely represent the healthiest of preterms.[8,9]

Although comparing details of outcome data from multiple institutions and eras is difficult, certain themes emerge. The smallest and most premature infants always are at greatest risk for poor neurodevelopmental outcome, and usually, male infants are at increased risk compared with female neonates. In 2000, Saigal and colleagues reported that 72% of adolescents less than 750 g BW and 53% of those with BW of 750 to 1000 g had significant deficits at school age; these deficits were present even in children without neurosensory impairments and in those with normal intelligence quotients (IQs).[10] More recently, Larroque and colleagues reported from a nationwide study in France that 42% of children born at 24 to 28 weeks and 31% born at 29 to 32 weeks needed special health care support due to neurologic sequelae, compared with only 16% of those born at 39 to 40 weeks.[11] Both of these groups noted that, in addition to those children with the lowest GAs, male neonates were most vulnerable to adverse neurodevelopmental outcomes. Being female and having singleton gestation, normal intrauterine growth with increased BW, and a complete course of antenatal steroids are all factors associated with higher survival rates.[12]

Early Prognosticating is Unreliable

Outcome data describing more recent cohorts of infants at younger follow-up ages are limited by the testing instruments employed and the timing of the follow-up. "Long-term" studies often extend follow-up to only 2 or 3 years of age, which may be too early to predict prognosis at school age or beyond. One review by Voss and colleagues of literature describing prognostic data suggests that follow-up must be at least to age 6 years to make a reliable cognitive diagnosis. These investigators tracked 129 preterms (median BW 794 g and 27 weeks GA) for 6 to 10 years and found that cognitive developmental prognosis at term corrected age was only 49% correct, with almost 40% "false favorable overrating." Not until age 3 and 4 years was the developmental diagnosis 70% right, and this age group still had almost 15% false favorable overrating.[13] In this study the "too bad prognosis" (or overly negative diagnosis) remained stable at about 10% to 15% for all time points. Whereas this study describes an unreliable testing experience with an emphasis on false favorable overrating, other studies describe similar poor predictive validity with an emphasis on false negative scoring. Hack and colleagues describe 330 preterms (mean BW 811 g and 26.4 weeks corrected GA) in whom a subnormal Mental Developmental Index score at corrected age 20 months is poorly predictive of cognitive function at age 8 years.

An exception is children with significant neurosensory impairment or severe abnormalities on cranial ultrasound, in whom early scores are predictive of adverse outcome at school age.[14] Both Voss and Hack describe that early testing is generally unreliable for later outcome, with the exception of the most severely and obviously affected children. As will be described later, the potential for predicting the trajectory of a child's development may be better realized with advances in neuroimaging.

Preterms at Adolescence and Young Adulthood

Recent studies describing adolescent and young adult outcome measures of premature infants report on births that occurred in the late 1970s, a time when overall survival was markedly less than it is now, and when perinatal interventions did not include such interventions as antenatal steroids and surfactant.[15] The survivors described in these studies may therefore represent the most vigorous of premature infants, such that the outcomes described are perhaps skewed toward a positive outlook. An example of this situation is the recent population-based study from Norway describing nearly 1 million babies born between 1967 and 1983; in this study, whereas survival of infants at less than 28 weeks GA was only 17.8%, when these survivors were assessed at ages 20 to 36 years, they had rates of cerebral palsy of 9.7%, and of mental retardation (MR) of only 4.4%.[16] In contrast, current status of babies born at less than 28 weeks can be extrapolated from the most recent report from the NICHD Neonatal Research Network, in which survival of babies 501 to 1000 g ranges from a mean of 55% to 88%.[5] Current status about incidence of cerebral palsy (CP) and cognitive deficit in babies less than 28 weeks is less reassuring, with incidence of CP in babies less than 28 weeks ranging from 7% to 17% and MR ranging from 10% to 12%.[1] Nevertheless, this and other studies are heartening in the overall picture they paint of adolescent and young adult survivors. Hack and colleagues[17] describe a cohort of young adults born between 1977 and 1979 at a mean BW of 1200 g and a mean GA of 29 weeks; this cohort was found to have decreased school performance at 20 years of age but also decreased risk-taking behaviors, including substance use and abuse, contact with the police, and sexual activity. Similarly reassuring is a report by Saigal and colleagues that ELBW survivors in adolescence, while recognizing and self-reporting more functional disability than term comparisons, place as high a value on health-related *quality* of life as term comparisons. This group of ELBW survivors had good self-reported quality of life despite having, as a group, 27% neurosensory impairment (compared with 2% for term comparisons) and 17% self-reported cognitive impairment (compared with 3% for terms).[18] The findings of Hack and Saigal suggest that many of the outcome measures used to define success of neonatal intervention may not always contribute to the final quality of life of the survivor. Saigal and colleagues also report on a cohort of ELBW survivors in whom, even among those deemed impaired at childhood, many make a successful transition from childhood and adolescence to adulthood. Saigal and colleagues describe this as a "lifetime perspective" in which, over the course of a survivor's lifetime, subtle deficits are slowly repaired, suggesting a potential recovery of function over time.[19]

Contemporary Preterms at Childhood

Recent studies describing school-age outcome measures of premature infants report on infants born up to the mid-1990s. These studies report outcomes that reflect the current state of neonatology, in particular the use of antenatal steroids and surfactants. Marlow and colleagues describe a geographic cohort of extremely preterm infants (less than or equal to 25 weeks) born in 1995; at 6 years of age, this group was compared with both normative data (equivalent to a 1970s cohort) and a contemporary cohort. When compared with normative data, the preterms were found to be as impaired as would be expected from past studies; 21% had IQ scores 2 SD below the normative mean. When compared with their peers, twice as many preterms had an IQ more than 2 SD below the contemporary mean. This finding demonstrates the potential for underestimating the impairment of preterm children. This study also reports the percentage of live births surviving without severe to moderate disability: less than 1% of 22-week gestations, 3% of 23-week gestations, 9% of 24-week gestations, and 20% of 25-week gestations.[20] A geographic cohort study by Anderson and colleagues describes a group of children of less than 28 weeks or BW less than 1000 g born in 1991 to 1992. The preterm children were compared at age 8 years with term controls in measures of cognitive ability, behavioral outcome, and educational progress, and were found to be at significantly increased risk for impairment in all 3 measures. The smallest infants in the preterm group (BW less than 749 g) had significantly lower cognitive and academic scores than larger preterm infants.[21] These and other recent outcome studies at school age provide a sobering reminder that the smallest, most immature infants are particularly vulnerable to injury.

Cerebral Palsy as a Marker of Outcome

Because CP is a motor disorder of central origin, and because its incidence is inversely related to GA, CP is often used as a marker of neonatal outcome.[22] Follow-up results from the Swedish national prospective study suggested that, for children born in 1990 to 1992, the incidence of CP was 14% for infants born at 23 to 24 weeks GA, 19% for those of 25 to 26 weeks GA, and 3% for infants born after 27 weeks of gestation.[23] Furthermore, analysis of 2 large cohort studies suggests no change in CP rates over time for infants born at 32 weeks GA or less, staying at an overall rate of 7% to 10%.

COGNITIVE DEFICITS

Preterm children have IQ scores ranging from within normal range to below range, but even when the scores are within 1 SD of normal they are significantly lower than those of their term peers. The youngest, most immature preterms are the most affected, and Johnson reports a decrease of 1.5 to 2.5 points per decreasing week of GA.[24] Of note, many studies report parental IQ or parental educational attainment as a significant variable in favorable cognitive outcome, suggesting the potential for environmental influence and biologic recovery.[25,26]

NEUROSENSORY DEFICITS

As with other neurodevelopmental impairments, the smallest and most immature preterms are at greatest risk for neurosensory deficits compared with term infants. Since 1970, the incidence of blindness has decreased from up to 10% to less than 3% with current cryotherapies and laser therapies for retinopathy of prematurity and with attention to supplemental oxygen delivery.[27] Even with these techniques, blindness affects up to 8% of the smallest survivors (less than 25 weeks GA), and corrective lenses are worn by almost 25% of school-age children born at less than 26 weeks GA compared with only 4% of term controls.[20] Hearing deficits are similarly prevalent, with up to 7% of babies born at less than 1000 g having severe hearing loss with unilateral or bilateral deafness. Wilson-Costello and colleagues report a significant increase in severe hearing deficits from 3% in 1982 to 1989 to 6% in 1990 to 1998 in these smallest survivors.[7] This effect was likely due to postnatal steroid use, as the same group reported a significant decrease in deafness in a subsequent era (2000–2002), from 6% to 1%, when postnatal steroid use decreased.[28] Another longitudinal review of preterms born at less than 28 weeks and followed until age 3 years demonstrated an incidence of permanent hearing loss at 3.1%, with no significant change from 1974 to 2003.[29]

LONGITUDINAL OUTCOME STUDIES

The longitudinal outcome studies presented in **Table 1** represent a critical body of work regarding the long-term cognitive and motor impairment outcome of prematurely born infants. Taken together, these data from 1977 to 1995, bridging multiple generations of neonatal care and dramatically improved survival rates, imply that cognitive scores are not improving over time in preterm children as they enter adolescence and adulthood, and that the neurodevelopmental sequelae present in childhood are persisting into later life. These data highlight the need for improved understanding of the neurologic injury of preterm birth, such that neurodevelopmental outcomes are ameliorated.

CURRENT PERSPECTIVE ON NEUROIMAGING

In this review thus far the neurodevelopmental disabilities of the prematurely born have been extensively described, yet the underlying alterations in brain development responsible for these changes and the time at which these changes become predictive of later outcome remain poorly understood. New magnetic resonance image (MRI) modalities and analysis tools, including diffusion tensor imaging (DTI) and voxel-based morphometry (VBM), are contributing to the understanding of neurologic sequelae of preterm birth by providing microstructural evidence of injury sustained by the preterm brain. DTI, by assessing water diffusion in cerebral tissues, reveals important information at a microstructural level about both maturational processes and the impact of injury on the developing preterm brain. Likewise, VBM offers automated structural analysis of cerebral images to detect regional microstructural morphologic differences. These techniques document changes both in major white matter tracts, including the corpus callosum and internal capsule, and in those subcortical regions serving language and executive function in the prematurely born. Multiple factors, including degree of prematurity, alterations in axonal microcircuitry, and vulnerability in oligodendroglial precursors, may contribute to these microstructural findings. Taken together, these imaging methods demonstrate alterations in neural connectivity and cortical maturation that perhaps predict long-term outcome in the prematurely born. Given that current testing strategies are poorly predictive of later outcome, and that the markers used to define later outcome are themselves poor indicators of later quality of life, these neuroimaging techniques will likely play a critical role in predicting, understanding, and managing neurodevelopmental injury for future premature infants.

CLINICAL AND VOLUMETRIC MRI STUDIES

Numerous MRI studies have documented the macrostructural sequelae of premature birth in the newborn period and beyond.[30–33] One major finding is that of decreased white matter volumes, even in relatively healthy preterm infants with no evidence of perinatal brain injury at term equivalent age, and the presumptive secondary changes in neural connectivity.[34–38] A second important finding is that of regional vulnerability. There are regional differences in development in the human brain; these include not only the timing of maximal brain growth but also patterns of synaptogenesis and cerebral myelination.[39,40] These events occur earliest in the primary sensory and motor areas, and latest in the prefrontal cortex.[41–43] Of significance for the preterm

Table 1
Cohorts with longitudinal follow-up

Years Cohort Born	Birth Weight or Gestational Age	N born	N Survived	Age at Follow-up	N evaluated	Full-Scale IQ[a]	Cerebral Palsy
Hack et al[14,73]							
1992–1995	<1000 g	330	238	20 mo	200	MDI 75.6 ± 16	29 (15%)
				8 y	200	MPC 87.8 ± 19	31 (16%)
Hack et al[17,74]							
1977–1979	<1500 g	490	312	8 y	249	VIQ 95.7 ± 18 PIQ 94.2 ± 17.7	Not reported
				20 y	242	87 ± 15	15 (6.2%)
O'Brien et al[75]							
1979–1982	<33 wk	320	224	8 y	207	104 ± 18	8 (5%) n = 150
				14–15 y	151	95 ± 18	6 (4%) n = 149
Hack et al[76,77]							
1982–1986	<750 g	243	73	7 y	68	MPC 87 ± 15	9 (13%)
				11–14 y	59	Not reported	6 (10%)
Pinto-Martin et al, Whitaker et al[78–81]							
1984–1987	<2000 g	1105	901	2 y	611	MDI 105.6 ± 19.7	113 (14.6%)
				6 y	538	SB:FE 103.4 ± 11.9	Not reported
			868	9 y	488	98.7 ± 14.3	Not reported
				16 y	474 nondisabled only	97.27 ± 14.57	Not reported
Vohr et al[82–84]							
1989–1992	600–1250 g	505	384	4.5 y	337	86.0 ± 15.8 to 88.9 ± 17.8	23 (7%)
				8 y	328	85 ± 24 to 95.7 ± 18	26 (7.9%)
				12 y	375	87.9 ± 18.3	Not reported
Saigal et al[10,85]							
1977–1982	501–1000 g		169	8 y	113 (only 1977–1981 evaluated)	91 ± 16	Not reported
				12–16 y	150 (full cohort evaluated)	89 ± 19	Not reported

Abbreviations: MDI, Mental Developmental Index of the Bayley Scales of Infant Development; MPC, Mental Processing Composite; PIQ, performance IQ; SB:FE, Composite Index of the Stanford Binet, Fourth Edition; VIQ, verbal IQ.
[a] If not otherwise noted, IQ is full-scale IQ from the Wechsler Intelligence Scales for Children.

population is the prominent maturation of the central white matter and the temporal auditory cortex during the third trimester of gestation, suggesting that those regions might be most susceptible to the injury of preterm birth.[44]

Studying 8-year-old ex-preterm subjects and term control children, Reiss and colleagues reported decreased white matter in the central sensory motor regions as well as in the temporal lobes of the preterm group.[35] Similarly, serial studies by Mewes and colleagues of preterm neonates with no evidence for perinatal brain injury demonstrated moderately decreased white matter volumes when compared with matched control infants at term equivalent age.[38] White matter of the precentral and central region developed more slowly than that of other regions in the preterm infants, and the data suggested alterations in the course of myelination for preterms.

DIFFUSION TENSOR IMAGING

DTI, a recent MR modality that assesses the diffusion of water across the axes of white matter bundles, is a powerful technique to explore the structural basis of white matter and cortical development, and has been used to evaluate brain injury in preterms.[45,46] Water diffusion is impeded by large white matter bundles that themselves delineate functional connectivity, such that the patterns of diffusion in multiple planes suggest the connectivity of anatomically remote areas. Fractional anisotropy (FA) values are a measure of fiber tract organization, and for multiple central white matter regions FA values have been noted to be significantly lower in the preterm group. Those infants with the lowest GAs (<28 weeks GA) had additional reductions in FA in the external capsule, the posterior limb of the internal capsule (PLIC), and the isthmus and mid-body of the corpus callosum[47] and, studying preterm neonates of 26 to 32 weeks GA, Dudink and colleagues reported a significant correlation between GA and FA of the PLIC bilaterally.[48] Taken together, these data suggest that the central white matter is the region of increased vulnerability in the developing preterm brain during the third trimester of gestation, and that this vulnerability is inversely related to GA.[49,50]

DTI parameters may provide useful neurodevelopmental outcome prognostic data. Gross motor function and CP are attributed to alterations in central white matter development in the preterm population. These changes have been demonstrated in a DTI study of 137 neonates by Arzoumanian and colleagues, in which FA values at term equivalent age in the right PLIC were significantly lower for preterm children with CP than those with normal motor examinations.[51] Drobyshevsky and colleagues similarly demonstrated that, for preterm neonates of less than 32 weeks GA, the Bayley Psychomotor Developmental Index at 18 to 24 months correlated with FA values in the internal capsule at 30 weeks GA.[52] Also using DTI in 24 preterm infants at term equivalent age, Rose and colleagues noted highly significant negative correlations between the left and right PLIC and the Gross Motor Functional scale when examined at age 4 years.[53]

Differences in DTI parameters between preterm and term equivalents persist into adolescence. When DTI is used to evaluate VLBW preterms at adolescence, regional differences in FA are associated with neurodevelopmental impairments. Skranes showed that low FA values in the internal capsule were correlated with visual motor and visual perceptual deficits in the preterm group at age 15 years. Low FA values in the external capsule and inferior and middle superior fasciculus were correlated with low IQ. This study offers the first preliminary data indicating that abnormalities in the neonatal period persist into adolescence, and that these abnormalities correlate with clinically significant injury (**Figs. 1** and **2**).[54]

Other DTI regions not yet explored in the newborn period may also be predictive of adverse long-term outcome. Constable and colleagues showed significant changes in

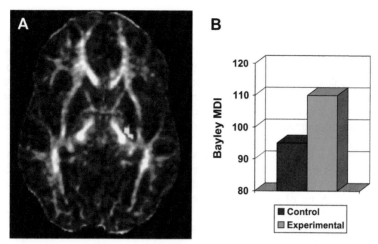

Fig. 1. Skranes and colleagues have shown that the left posterior limb of the internal capsule (PLIC) is associated with visual motor and visual perceptual outcome of preterm infants at adolescence.[54] In the newborn period, the left PLIC has been shown to correlate with Bayley Mental Developmental Index (MDI) scores in infants exposed to the Newborn Individualized Developmental Care and Assessment Program.[86] (A) Axial image of the left PLIC in preterm subjects scanned at age 12 years. (B) Bayley scores for control and experimental groups at 9 months.[86] (Panel A: *Courtesy of* C. Lacadie, Magnetic Resonance Research Center, Yale University.)

FA in preterms compared with term controls at age 12 years, and these changes were significantly correlated with cognitive testing scores. Constable and colleagues also noted gender effects; one notable finding was that of reduced FA in the uncinate fasciculus, a critical language pathway, in preterm males, associated with poor cognitive and language scores.[55]

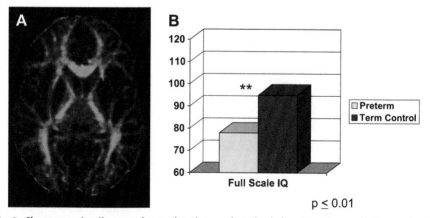

Fig. 2. Skranes and colleagues have also shown that the left external capsule is associated with lower IQ scores in preterm infants at adolescence.[54] (A) Axial image of the left external capsule in preterm infants scanned at age 12 years. (B) Total IQ scores for preterm versus term control 12-year-olds evaluated by Skranes and colleagues.[54] (Panel A: *Courtesy of* C. Lacadie, Magnetic Resonance Research Center, Yale University.)

VOXEL-BASED MORPHOMETRY

VBM is a neuroimaging analysis technique that allows detailed anatomic investigation of the white matter microstructure. Only a few VBM studies have been performed on preterm subjects during the newborn period, but many more have examined preterm subjects at adolescence and early adulthood. In one newborn period study, Srinivasan and colleagues noted reduced thalamic and lentiform volumes in deep gray matter in preterm-born infants at term equivalent age, when compared with term-born infants. These reduced volumes were most marked in subjects with supratentorial white matter injury.[56]

Studying ex-preterm infants at age 14 years, Gimenez and colleagues noted significant differences in thalamic nuclei volume between preterms and term controls; preterm thalamic volumes were significantly decreased, and these volume differences correlated with tests of verbal fluency for the ex-preterm group (**Fig. 3**).[57] Taken together, these studies suggest that injury to deep gray matter structures is persistent into adolescence and clinically relevant, and might provide a focus for future neuroimaging follow-up studies.

Other VBM studies on ex-preterm infants at adolescence demonstrate clinically significant volume reductions, but there are as yet no neonatal studies with which to compare this work. Isaacs and colleagues conducted a neuroimaging study of ex-preterm subjects at adolescence who had been born at less than 30 weeks' gestation and demonstrated that absolute IQ scores were related to areas in both the parietal and temporal lobes, suggesting that emerging neonatal VBM studies in preterm subjects may also provide data with important predictive possibilities.[58] Future studies will most certainly interrogate these regions of interest in the prematurely born at term equivalent (**Table 2**).

FUNCTIONAL MAGNETIC RESONANCE IMAGING

Functional MRI (fMRI) is an emerging MRI modality that uses the different magnetic properties of oxygenated and deoxygenated blood to track hemodynamic activity. This map of hemodynamic activity, termed blood oxygenation level dependent

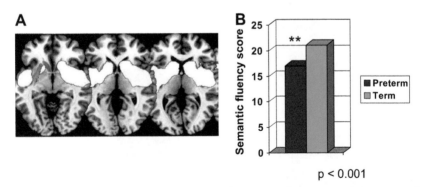

Fig. 3. Gimenez and colleagues employed voxel-based morphometry to demonstrate that prematurely born subjects have less thalamic gray at age 14 years than term control subjects. These data correlate with verbal fluency scores in the preterm group.[57] (*A*) VBM image of the thalamus of prematurely born subjects scanned at age 12 years. (*B*) Verbal fluency scores for preterms versus term controls as evaluated by Gimenez and colleagues. (Panel A: *Courtesy of* S. Kesler, Ph.D, Stanford University School of Medicine.)

Table 2
MRI markers of outcome

Author	Number	Gestational Age, Birth Weight	MRI Age	Age at Follow-up	MRI Change	Clinical Correlate
DTI						
Als[86]	30 PT	28–33 wk	2 wk CGA	18–24 mo	Higher RA; left IC in early intervention group	Improved behavioral function at 9 mo correlated with DTI changes
Arzoumanian[51]	63 PT	<33 wk, <1800 g	Term	18–24 mo CGA	Reduced FA in right posterior IC	Abnormal neuroexam, ±CP, correlated with DTI changes
Skranes[54]	34 PT, 47 T	<1500 g	15 y	15 y	Reduced FA in IC, EC, CC, and sup, mid sup and inf fasciculus	Low FA in EC and inf and mid sup fasciculus correlated with low IQ
VBM						
Srinivasan[56]	40 PT, 8 T	<34 wk	Term		Thal/lentiform nucleus volumes significantly smaller than term controls	
Gimenez[57]	30 PT, 30 T	<33 wk	14 y	14 y	Several thalamic nuclei significantly smaller than term controls	Poor semantic fluency correlated with decreased thalamic volumes

Abbreviations: CC, corpus callosum; CGA, corrected gestational age; DTI, diffusion tensor imaging; EC, external capsule; FA, fractional anisotropy; IC, internal capsule; PT, preterm; RA, relative anisotropy; T, term; VBM, voxel-based morphometry.

(BOLD) contrast, allows assessment of resting state cerebral activity and also neural processing in response to cerebral tasks.[59] Although no cognitive correlations are yet described, fMRI will likely play an important role in evaluating the microstructural mechanisms that support brain development.[60,61] Most recently, functional neuroimaging data have been used to examine interactions between spatially distinct regions, or "functional connectivity," in typically developing children and adolescents.[62,63]

fMRI has been used with reliability in ex-preterm and term-born neonates in infancy.[64–66] Seghier and colleagues[67] employed DTI and fMRI to appreciate recovery from injury in the developing brain; a neonate who suffered left-sided visual cortex injury after a perinatal stroke was followed through 20 months of age, at which time there was emergence of BOLD activation in the left optical pathways where previously there had been none. This report highlights 2 important themes: first, that the developing brain is resilient, and second, that DTI and fMRI may be used to demonstrate structure-function correlation in preterm subjects.

Evidence for alterations in neural connectivity

Multiple fMRI studies have identified functionally distinct pathways in the preterm developing brain, particularly in the realms of language and memory, and functional connectivity analyses provide additional support for these findings.[68–70] The significance of functionally distinct pathways in the preterm brain is that such pathways might represent either compensatory paths or unpruned neonatal systems that allow the preterm to recover from the injury associated with preterm birth. A recent publication demonstrates alterations in functional connectivity for preterms at adolescence. Schafer and colleagues show that whereas preterms and terms at adolescence do similarly well on a simple language task, and activate similar semantic processing areas, the preterms employ different neural pathways for semantic processing.[61] In an auditory task conducted by Santhouse and colleagues, preterms with corpus callosum (CC) thinning exhibited greater right-sided activation than the preterms without CC thinning and the term controls, suggesting that this group of preterms had developed an alternative neural pathway, presumably to compensate for the perinatal injury that resulted in CC thinning. This same group also exhibited increased right-sided activation in a visual stimulation task that required working memory, also suggesting an alternative neural pathway.[71]

SUMMARY

Preterm neonates are at high risk for neurodevelopmental disabilities. Longitudinal data from at least 7 different cohorts born between 1977 and 1995 demonstrate several important points: assessment during early childhood may not be predictive of outcome at school and beyond, and, although lower than term controls, testing scores for preterm subjects are stable from school entry through adolescence.

The challenge for neonatologists and neurologists alike is identifying early markers of outcome in the prematurely born. The authors suggest that the role of neuroimaging in the future will be to identify the babies most at risk. It is already known that DTI abnormalities present at term equivalent age and at adolescence are associated with clinically significant deficits, suggesting that the injuries present at term equivalent age might predict impairment in adolescence. Similarly, VBM changes present in term equivalent neonates are also present in adolescents, and correlate with clinically significant cognitive deficits. The next generation of neonatal outcome studies will need to evaluate a large, perhaps multicenter cohort of at-risk infants, employing multiple modalities of serial imaging and retaining the cohort for long-term follow-up.

In her review of outcome measures of neonatal intensive care survivors, Hack describes that to best qualify and quantify disability, neonatologists need "specific measures of impairments and their residual disability" rather than subjective assessments.[72] Neuroimaging will provide those specific measures.

REFERENCES

1. Behrman RE, Stith Butler A. Institute of medicine committee on understanding premature birth and assuring healthy outcomes board on health sciences outcomes: preterm birth: causes, consequences, and prevention. Washington, DC: The National Academies Press; 2007.
2. Fujiwara T, Adams FH. Surfactant for hyaline membrane disease. Pediatrics 1980; 66(5):795–8.
3. Surfactant replacement therapy for respiratory distress syndrome. American academy of pediatrics. Committee on fetus and newborn. Pediatrics 1999; 103(3):684–5.
4. Effect of corticosteroids for fetal maturation on perinatal outcomes. NIH Consensus Statement 1994;12(2):1–24.
5. Fanaroff AA, Stoll BJ, Wright LL, et al. Trends in neonatal morbidity and mortality for very low birthweight infants. Am J Ostet Gynecol. 2007;196:147 e141–7.e148.
6. Martin JA, Kung HC, Mathews TJ, et al. Annual summary of vital statistics: 2006. Pediatrics 2008;121(4):788–801.
7. Wilson-Costello D, Friedman H, Minich NM, et al. Improved survival rates with increased neurodevelopmental disability for extremely low birth weight infants in the 1990's. Pediatrics 2005;115:997–1003.
8. Douglas JW, Gear R. Children of low birthweight in the 1946 national cohort. Behaviour and educational achievement in adolescence. Arch Dis Child 1976; 51(11):820–7.
9. Hess JH. Experiences gained in a thirty year study of prematurely born infants. Pediatrics 1953;11(5):425–34.
10. Saigal S, Hoult LA, Streiner DL, et al. School difficulties at adolescence in a regional cohort of children who were extremely low birth weight. Pediatrics 2000;105(2):325–31.
11. Larroque B, Ancel PY, Marret S, et al. Neurodevelopmental disabilities and special care of 5-year-old children born before 33 weeks of gestation (the EPI-PAGE study): a longitudinal cohort study. Lancet 2008;371:813–20.
12. Tyson JE, Parikh NA, Langer J, et al. Intensive care for extreme prematurity—moving beyond gestational age. N Engl J Med 2008;358:1672–81.
13. Voss W, Neubauer A-P, Wachtendorf M, et al. Neurodevelopmental outcome in extremely low birth weight infants: what is the minimum age for reliable developmental prognosis? Acta Pediatr 2007;96:342–7.
14. Hack M, Taylor HG, Drotar D, et al. Poor predictive validity of the Bayley Scales of Infant Development for cognitive function of extremely low birth weight children at school age. Pediatrics 2005;116:333–41.
15. Lorenz JM, Wooliever DE, Jetton JR, et al. A quantitative review of mortality and developmental disability in extremely premature newborns. Arch Pediatr Adolesc Med 1998;152(5):425–35.
16. Moster D, Lie RT, Markestad T. Long-term medical and social consequences of preterm birth. N Engl J Med 2008;359(3):262–73.
17. Hack MB, Flannery DJ, Schluchter M, et al. Outcomes in young adulthood for very-low-birth-weight infants. N Engl J Med 2002;346:149–57.

18. Saigal S, Feeny D, Rosenbaum P, et al. Self-perceived health status and health-related quality of life of extremely low birth weight infants at adolescence. JAMA 1996;276:453–9.
19. Saigal S, Stoskopf B, Streiner DL, et al. Transition of extremely low-birth-weight infants from adolescence to young adulthood. JAMA 2006;295:667–75.
20. Marlow N, Wolke D, Bracewell MA, et al. Neurologic and developmental disability at six years of age after extremely preterm birth. N Engl J Med 2005;352:9–19.
21. Anderson P, Doyle LW, Victorian ICSG. Neurobehavioral outcomes of school-age children born extremely low birth weight or very preterm in the 1990s. JAMA 2003;289:3264–72.
22. Saigal S, Doyle LW. An overview of mortality and sequelae of preterm birth from infancy to adulthood. Lancet 2008;371:261–9.
23. Hagberg B, Hagberg G, Olow I, et al. The changing panorama of cerebral palsy in Sweden: VII. Prevalence and origin in the birth year period 1987–1990. Acta Paediatr 1996;85:954–60.
24. Johnson S. Cognitive and behavioural outcomes following very preterm birth. Semin Fetal Neonatal Med 2007;12(5):363–73.
25. Weisglas-Kuperus N, Hille ET, Duivenvoorden HJ, et al. Intelligence of very preterm or very low birthweight infants in young adulthood. Arch Dis Child Fetal Neonatal Ed 2009;94(3):F196–200.
26. Ment LR, Vohr BR, Allan WA, et al. Change in cognitive function over time in very low-birth-weight infants. JAMA 2003;289:705–11.
27. Doyle LW, Anderson PJ. Improved neurosensory outcome at 8 years of age of extremely low birthweight children born in Victoria over three distinct eras. Arch Dis Child Fetal Neonatal Ed 2005;90(6):F484–8.
28. Wilson-Costello D, Friedman H, Minich N, et al. Improved neurodevelopmental outcomes for extremely low birth weight infants in 2000–2002. Pediatrics 2007; 119:37–45.
29. Robertson CM, Howarth TM, Bork DL, et al. Permanent bilateral sensory and neural hearing loss of children after neonatal intensive care because of extreme prematurity: a thirty-year study. Pediatrics 2009;123(5):e797–807.
30. Huppi PS, Warfield S, Kikinis R, et al. Quantitative magnetic resonance imaging of brain development in premature and mature newborns. Ann Neurol 1998;43: 224–35.
31. Boardman JP, Counsell SJ, Rueckert D, et al. Early growth in brain volume is preserved in the majority of preterm infants. Ann Neurol 2007;62:185–92.
32. Peterson BS, Vohr B, Cannistraci CJ, et al. Regional brain volume abnormalities and long-term cognitive outcome in preterm infants. JAMA 2000;284:1939–47.
33. Allin M, Henderson M, Suckling J, et al. Effects of very low birthweight on brain structure in adulthood. Dev Med Child Neurol 2004;46:46–53.
34. Nosarti C, Al-Asady MH, Frangou S, et al. Adolescents who were born very preterm have decreased brain volumes. Brain 2002;125:1616–23.
35. Reiss AL, Kesler SR, Vohr BR, et al. Sex differences in cerebral volumes of 8-year-olds born preterm. J Pediatr 2004;145:242–9.
36. Dyet LE, Kennea NL, Counsell SJ, et al. Natural history of brain lesions in extremely preterm infants studied with serial magnetic resonance imaging from birth and neurodevelopmental assessment. Pediatrics 2006;118:536–48.
37. Woodward LJ, Anderson PJ, Austin NC, et al. Neonatal MRI to predict neurodevelopmental outcomes in preterm infants. New Engl J Med 2006;355:685–94.
38. Mewes AUJ, Huppi PS, Als H, et al. Regional brain development in serial magnetic resonance imaging of low-risk preterm infants. Pediatrics 2006;118:23–33.

39. Bystron I, Blakemore C, Rakic P. Development of the human cerebral cortex: Boulder Committee revisited. Nature Reviews Neuroscience 2008;9:110–22.
40. Kostovic I, Jovanov-Milosevic N. The development of cerebral connections during the first 20–45 weeks' gestation. Sem Fet Neo Med 2006;11:415–22.
41. Huttenlocher PR. Synaptic density in human frontal cortex—developmental changes and effects of aging. Brain Res 1979;163:195–205.
42. Huttenlocher PR, de Courten C, Garey LJ, et al. Synaptogenesis in human visual cortex-evidence for synapse elimination during normal development. Neuroscience Lett 1982;33:247–52.
43. Huttenlocher PR, deCourten C. The development of synapses in striate cortex of man. Hum Neurobiol 1987;6:1–9.
44. Huttenlocher P, Dabholkar A. Regional differences in synaptogenesis in human cerebral cortex. J Comp Neurol 1997;387:167–78.
45. Mukherjee P, McKinstry RC. Diffusion tensor imaging and tractography of human brain development. Neuroimag Clin N Am 2006;16:19–43.
46. Huppi PS, Dubois J. Diffusion tensor imaging of brain development. Sem Fet Neo Med 2006;11:489–97.
47. Anjari M, Srinivasan L, Allsop JM, et al. Diffusion tensor imaging with tract-based spatial statistics reveals local white matter abnormalities in preterm infants. NeuroImage 2007;35:1021–7.
48. Dudink J, Lequin M, van Pul C, et al. Fractional anisotropy in white matter tracts of very-low-birth-weight infants. Pediatr Radiol 2007;37:1216–23.
49. Berman JI, Mukherjee P, Partridge SC, et al. Quantitative diffusion tensor MRI fiber tractography of sensorimotor white matter development in premature infants. Neuroimage 2005;27:862–71.
50. Miller SP, Vigneron DB, Henry RG, et al. Serial quantitative diffusion tensor MRI of the premature brain: development in new-borns with and without injury. J Magn Reson Imaging 2002;16:621–32.
51. Arzoumanian Y, Mirmiran M, Barnes PD, et al. Diffusion tensor brain imaging findings at term-equivalent age may predict neurologic abnormalities in low birth weight preterm infants. AJNR Am J Neurorad 2003;24:1646–53.
52. Drobyshevsky A, Bregman J, Storey P, et al. Serial diffusion tensor imaging detects white matter changes that correlate with motor outcome in premature infants. Dev Neurosci 2007;29:289–301.
53. Rose J, Mirmiran J, Butler EE, et al. Neonatal microstructural development of the internal capsule on diffusion tensor imaging correlations with severity of gait and motor deficits. Devel Med Child Neurol 2007;49:745–50.
54. Skranes JS, Vangberg TR, Kulseng S, et al. Clinical findings and white matter abnormalities seen on diffusion tensor imaging in adolescents with very low birth weight. Brain 2007;130:654–66.
55. Constable RT, Ment LR, Vohr BR, et al. Prematurely born children demonstrate white matter microstructural differences at age 12 years relative to term controls: an investigation of group and gender effects. Pediatrics 2008;121:306–16.
56. Srinivasan L, Dutta R, Counsell S, et al. Quantification of deep gray matter in preterm infants at term-equivalent age using manual volumetry of 3-tesla magnetic resonance images. Pediatrics 2007;119:759–65.
57. Gimenez M, Junque C, Narberhaus A, et al. Correlations of thalamic reductions with verbal fluency impairment in those born prematurely. Neuroreport 2006;17: 463–6.
58. Isaacs EB, Edmonds CJ, Chong WK, et al. Brain morphometry and IQ measurement in preterm children. Brain 2004;127:2595–607.

59. Ment LR, Constable RT. Injury and recovery in the developing brain: evidence from functional MRI studies of prematurely-born children. Nat Clin Prac Neurol 2007;3:558–71.
60. Fransson P, Skiold B, Horsch S, et al. Resting-state networks in the infant brain. PNAS 2007;104:15531–6.
61. Schafer RJ, Lacadie C, Vohr B, et al. Alterations in functional connectivity for language in prematurely-born adolescents. Brain 2009;132(Pt 3):661–70.
62. Fair DA, Cohen AL, Dosenbach NUF, et al. The maturing architecture of the brain's default network. PNAS 2008;105:4028–32.
63. Fair DA, Dosenbach NUF, Church JA, et al. Development of distinct control networks through segregation and integration. PNAS 2007;104:13507–12.
64. Anderson AW, Marois R, Colson ER, et al. Neonatal auditory activation detected by functional magnetic resonance imaging. Magn Reson Imaging 2001;19:1–5.
65. Born P, Leth H, Miranda MJ, et al. Visual activation in infants and young children studied by functional magnetic resonance imaging. Pediatr Res 1998; 44:578–83.
66. Born AP, Miranda MJ, Rostrup E, et al. Functional magnetic resonance imaging of the normal and abnormal visual system in early life. Neuropediatrics 2000;31: 24–32.
67. Seghier ML, Lazeyras F, Zimine S, et al. Visual recovery after perinatal stroke evidenced by functional and diffusion MRI: case report. BMC Neurol 2005;26:17.
68. Rushe TM, Temple CM, Rifkin L, et al. Lateralisation of language function in young adults born very preterm. Arch Dis Child Fetal Neonatal Ed 2004;89:F112–8.
69. Ment LR, Peterson BS, Vohr B, et al. Cortical recruitment patterns in children born prematurely compared with control children during a passive listening functional magnetic resonance imaging task. J Pediatr 2006;149:490–8.
70. Gimenez M, Junque C, Vendrell P, et al. Hippocampal functional magnetic resonance imaging during a face-name learning task in adolescents with antecedents of prematurity. Neuroimage 2005;25:561–9.
71. Santhouse AM, ffytche DH, Howard RJ, et al. The functional significance of perinatal corpus callosum damage: an fMRI study in young adults. Brain 2002;125: 1782–92.
72. Hack M. Consideration of the use of health status, functional outcome, and quality-of-life to monitor neonatal intensive care practice. Pediatrics 1999; 103(1 Suppl E):319–28.
73. Hack M, Wilson-Costello D, Friedman H, et al. Neurodevelopment and predictors of outcomes of children with birth weights of less than 1000 g. Arch Pediatr Adolesc Med 2000;154:725–31.
74. Hack M, Breslau N, Aram D, et al. The effect of very low birth weight and social risk on neurocognitive abilities at school age. J Dev Behav Pediatr 1992;13(6):412–20.
75. O'Brien F, Roth S, Stewart A, et al. The neurodevelopmental progress of infants less than 33 weeks into adolescence. Arch Dis Child 2004;89(3):207–11.
76. Hack M, Taylor HG, Kelin N, et al. School-age outcomes in children with birth weights under 750 g. New Engl J Med 1994;331:753–9.
77. Hack M, Taylor HG, Klein N, et al. Functional limitations and special health care needs of 10- to 14-year-old children weighing less than 750 grams at birth. Pediatrics 2000;106(3):554–60.
78. Pinto-Martin JA, Riolo S, Chaan A, et al. Cranial ultrasound prediction of disabling and nondisabling cerebral palsy at age two in a low birth weight population. Pediatrics 1995;95:249–55.

79. Whitaker AG, Feldman JF, Rossem RV, et al. Neonatal cranial ultrasound abnormalities in low birth weight infants: relation to cognitive outcomes at six years of age. Pediatrics 1996;98:719–29.

80. Pinto-Martin JA, Whitaker AH, Feldman J, et al. Relation of cranial ultrasound abnormalities in low-birthweight infants to motor or cognitive performance at ages 2, 6 and 9 years. Devel Med Child Neurol 1999;41:826–33.

81. Whitaker AH, Feldman JF, Lorenz JM, et al. Motor and cognitive outcomes in nondisabled low-birth-weight adolescents: early determinants. Arch Pediatr Adolesc Med 2006;160(10):1040–6.

82. Vohr BR, Allan WC, Westerveld M, et al. School-age outcomes of very low birth weight infants in the indomethacin intraventricular hemorrhage prevention trial. Pediatrics 2003;111(4 Pt 1):e340–6.

83. Ment LR, Vohr B, Allan W, et al. Outcome of children in the indomethacin intraventricular hemorrhage prevention trial. Pediatrics 2000;105(3 Pt 1):485–91.

84. Luu TM, Ment LR, Schneider KC, et al. Lasting effects of preterm birth and neonatal brain hemorrhage at 12 years of age. Pediatrics 2009;123:1037–44.

85. Saigal S, Szatmari P, Rosenbaum P, et al. Cognitive abilities and school performance of extremely low birth weight children and matched term control children at age 8 years; a regional study. J Pediatr 1991;118:751–60.

86. Als H, Duffy FH, McAnulty GB, et al. Early experience alters brain function and structure. Pediatrics 2004;114:1738–9.

Autism Spectrum Disorders in Survivors of Extreme Prematurity

Catherine Limperopoulos, PhD[a,b,c,d],*

KEYWORDS

- Prematurity • Autism spectrum disorders • Brain
- MRI • Outcome

The impact of extreme prematurity on the neurodevelopmental outcome in survivors is enormous.[1–6] Advances in perinatal and neonatal care have resulted in dramatic increases in survival of premature infants, most strikingly among the smallest and sickest.[2,3,7,8] Unfortunately, this decrease in mortality has not been accompanied by a similar decrease in long-term neurodevelopmental morbidity among survivors.[3,5,9] Ex-premature infants are at substantial risk for significant and costly lifelong disabilities.[10,11] Of particular concern is the risk for significant higher-order neurodevelopmental impairment in ex-premature children reaching school age. In some studies, up to 50% of ex-preterm infants experience difficulties in executive functioning, learning, and behavior, often requiring special educational support.[12–14] These children are at increased risk for attentional difficulties, hyperactivity,[15] social-behavioral, and communication dysfunction,[16] and for psychiatric disorders in adolescence[16] and adulthood.[14,17–22] Failure to cope with the demands of adulthood is more prevalent among survivors of prematurity, with lower educational and income attainment, and difficulties establishing a family.[11]

Converging lines of evidence point to a significantly increased risk among extremely premature infants for subsequent development of cognitive, learning, behavioral, and

Dr. Limperopoulos is supported by the Canada Research Chairs Program, Canada Research Chair in Brain and Development. This work was supported in part by the LifeBridge Fund and the Trust Family Foundation.

[a] Department of Neurology and Neurosurgery, School of Physical and Occupational Therapy, McGill University, 2300 Tupper Street, Montreal, Quebec, H3H 1P3, Canada

[b] Department of Pediatrics, School of Physical and Occupational Therapy, McGill University, 2300 Tupper Street, Montreal, Quebec, H3H 1P3, Canada

[c] Fetal-Neonatal Neurology Research Group, Department of Neurology, Children's Hospital Boston, Harvard Medical School, 300 Longwood Avenue, Boston, MA 02115, USA

[d] Pediatric Neurology, Montreal Children's Hospital, 2300 Tupper Street A-334, Montreal, Quebec H3H 1P3, Canada

* Pediatric Neurology, Montreal Children's Hospital, 2300 Tupper Street A-334, Montreal, Quebec H3H 1P3, Canada.

E-mail address: catherine.limperopoulos@mcgill.ca

psychoaffective disturbances. Recent reports also suggest an increase in atypical social-behavioral functioning in this population that is strongly suggestive of autism spectrum disorders (ASD). These recent data have triggered a vigorous and highly charged debate, given the potential implications for this growing population of prematurity survivors, their caretakers, and society at large. This article reviews available evidence for prematurity and ASD, examines the potential role of early life neuroanatomic antecedents for these behavior patterns in survivors of extreme preterm birth, and explores future directions in this emerging area of research.

AUTISM SPECTRUM DISORDERS

ASD are a heterogeneous group of behaviorally defined, neurodevelopmental disorders characterized by impaired development in communication, social interaction, and behavior.[23] There are three broad categories (ie, autism, Asperger syndrome, and pervasive developmental disorder not otherwise specified), each with a wide range of effects but shared core symptoms. At the lower-functioning end of the autism spectrum, individuals have impaired reciprocal social interaction, abnormal development and use of language, and repetitive and ritualized behaviors. Conversely, those with Asperger syndrome are higher-functioning with normal intelligence but abnormalities in social interaction. When a child has autistic symptoms that do not fit another ASD diagnosis, pervasive developmental disorder not otherwise specified may be diagnosed.[23]

The earliest behavioral signs of ASD emerge between 1 and 2 years of age, and include impaired social attention, language development, and emotional reactivity.[23] Given the importance of early detection and intervention for children with ASD, the American Academy of Pediatrics has recently published guidelines endorsing autism-specific screening for all children at age 18 months.[24] Early screening tools for ASD, such as the Modified Checklist for Autism in Toddlers (M-CHAT), incorporate items that capture these early signs of ASD. These screening tests identify children who warrant formal testing for the diagnosis of ASD, which is usually made between 2 and 4 years of age.

ASDs are increasingly recognized as a major public health issue in childhood and beyond.[25,26] Although ASD was once considered a rare disorder, the Centers for Disease Control and Prevention recently estimated its prevalence at around 1 in 150.[25] The personal and familial impact of these conditions is often catastrophic. Likewise, the economic cost of ASD to society is enormous, with an estimated annual cost as high as $35 billion per year and an individual lifetime cost of $3.2 million.[27] The potential contribution from increasing survivors of extreme prematurity to this growing population of children with ASD is explored herein.

Etiology of ASD

Although a broad range of etiologies has been implicated in the development of ASD, prevailing consensus favors a multifactorial pathogenesis. A growing body of evidence supports the presence of abnormal fetal brain development in ASD. Many researchers adhere to a triple-hit hypothesis for the development of ASD.[28] In this paradigm, ASD develops in individuals with (1) an underlying biologic vulnerability who experience (2) varying degrees of exogenous stressors (3) during a critical period of brain development.[28–31] The notion that the underlying predisposition to ASD is caused by a single gene defect has been refuted, and current understanding is that the risk of developing ASD is modified by multiple susceptibility and protective genes.[28] The putative genetic factors implicated in ASD form part of a vast and complex area of research that is beyond the scope of this article. Rather, this article explores the other two arms of this triple-hit paradigm, namely the potential role of insults to the immature brain during a critical period of brain development in prematurely born infants. Early life insults may play a role in the development of ASD. Clinical data support the notion of a vulnerability period during the second and third trimester of gestation for subsequent development of ASD and are summarized later.[32,33]

WHAT IS THE RELATIONSHIP BETWEEN PREMATURITY AND ASD?
Prematurity-related Risk Factors and ASD

To date, population-based studies have consistently identified prematurity and low birth weight[34–38] as important perinatal risk factors for the development of ASD. A recent large population-based study of adults born at very low gestational age compared with term-born adults described a significant increased risk for ASD, with a relative risk of 7.3 among those born at 28 to 30 weeks gestation, increasing to nearly 10 in those born at 23 to 27 weeks gestational age.[11] These data suggest that the incidence of ASD among survivors of preterm birth is inversely related to gestational age.

Obstetric complications and intrapartum hypoxia (eg, bleeding during pregnancy, maternal hypotension, cesarean delivery, fetal distress, low Apgar score)[29,35,39,40] and a history of neonatal intensive care[33] have also been reported to increase the risk of autism. Parental infertility and advanced maternal and paternal age at birth are additional risk factors that have been associated with ASD.[39,41,42] Interestingly, a higher prevalence of ASD has recently been linked with in vitro fertilization compared with the general population.[43]

Available evidence suggests that pregnancy, delivery, and neonatal complications increase the risk for ASD through independent etiologic pathways that likely interact with a genetic predisposition, thereby interfering with brain maturation at critical points in development.[29,30,44,45] It is important to note that, to date, population-based studies generally reflect a population born preterm over two decades ago, and the prevalence of ASD among ex-premature infants born in the modern era remains unknown. Given that the greatest advances in survival are among the most premature and critically ill infants, the need to better define the risk of ASD in these new survivors of extreme preterm birth is of unquestionable importance. Moreover, given the established risk of preterm birth associated with in vitro fertilization,[46,47] the complex relationship between in vitro fertilization, prematurity, and ASD needs further definition. Taken together, large population-based studies are needed to allow for a more precise and detailed assessment of exposures and potential confounders for a more conclusive investigation of prematurity-related risk factors and ASD.

Prematurity and Evidence for Social-behavioral Dysfunction

Current understanding of the behavioral and psychosocial health of survivors of very preterm birth indicates that these children are at increased risk for social-behavioral dysfunction. Most notably, low birth weight and gestational age have been identified as important perinatal risk factors for disturbances in social interaction, communication, and behavior[48] and later psychoaffective disorders in adulthood.[18,19,49] During childhood and adolescence, very low birth weight children exhibit greater internalizing and externalizing behavior problems than their peers, and attentional difficulties and hyperactivity.[15,16,50,51] A high prevalence of difficulties with social integration, such as excessive shyness, withdrawn behavior, and more difficulties in establishing social contacts, and antisocial behaviors has also been described.[21,52,53] Noteworthy is the fact that preterm adolescents are far more likely to experience psychiatric symptoms

(46%) than controls (13%), particularly attention deficit, anxiety symptoms, and relational problems.[54,55]

More recent literature has underscored significant concerns about the ability of these children to cope with the demands of adulthood, including lower levels of educational attainment and income, and difficulties with establishing a family.[22] From a social-behavioral perspective, extremely low birth weight adults are reported to have an overall lower level of social competence characterized by significantly higher shyness, behavioral inhibition, lower extraversion and higher neuroticism, impaired interpersonal relationships, and overall lower sociability and emotional well-being than their normal birth weight counterparts.[14,20,22] The personality profile of adults born very preterm is increasingly characterized by behavioral inhibition and negative affectivity, and decreased positive affectivity, collectively, placing them at risk for mental health problems, such as anxiety and depression.[16,21,22] Interestingly, despite increased recognition of psychosocial impairments among prematurity survivors, to date these problems remain clinically underdiagnosed.[56]

Converging evidence points to an increased risk among extremely premature infants for significant future psychiatric and emotional problems. Despite increasing reports of atypical social-behavioral functioning among survivors of extreme preterm birth, little is currently known about the true prevalence of ASD in this vulnerable population.

Prematurity and ASD: What is the Evidence?

The potential role of ASD in the spectrum of social-behavioral dysfunction described in this population has been underexplored. Anecdotal experience in the clinical follow-up of ex-preterm infants in recent years has suggested that a subgroup of infants born very preterm exhibit noticeably atypical social behavioral characteristics, many of which are similar to those typically documented in young children with ASD. Until recently, however, studies linking very low birth weight and ASD have been few and limited largely to small subgroups of higher functioning adolescents and young adults with Asperger disorder,[55,57] or those with severe retinopathy of prematurity.[58] Studies that have reported an association between ASD and prematurity are summarized in **Table 1**. Msall[58] using a parental questionnaire reported a higher prevalence of autism in a cohort of extremely preterm infants (<1251 g) with unfavorable vision status (ie, severe retinopathy of prematurity) (8.5%) versus those with favorable vision status (0.8%) at 8 years of age. Indredavik and colleagues[16,55] have reported increased scores on the Autism Spectrum Screening Questionnaire and an increased prevalence of Asperger syndrome–like symptoms (assessed by interview) in very low birth weight adolescents. The authors speculated that very low birth weight adolescents exhibit a milder form of ASD, and experience particular deficits with encoding and interpreting subtle cues of social relations,[59] which likely implicates cognitive and emotional mechanisms and impaired brain connectivity (described later).

The recent availability of validated screening instruments for detection of early signs of ASD[60] has facilitated the early screening of infants to prompt appropriate referrals for specialized autism diagnostic testing.[61] Stimulated by observations of autism-like behavioral profiles in clinical follow-up of very premature infants, together with the greater availability of ASD screening tools for toddlers, the author and others have recently begun to explore the potential relationship of ADS and survivors of extreme preterm birth. The author's group published the first study that examined the relationship between early signs of autism in young toddlers with a history of extreme prematurity.[62] They performed initial screening for early autistic features using the M-CHAT in a consecutive series of 91 ex-preterm infants born less than

Table 1
Rates of ASD in follow-up studies of infants born preterm

Author	Year	Sample Size	Birth Weight GA	Sample Characteristics	ASD Measure	Age at Follow-up	Rates of ASD
Msall et al[58]	2004	24	<1250 g	Preterm and severe ROP	Parental questionnaire	14–15 y	7 (8.5%) severe ROP 1 (0.8%) favorable vision status
Indredavic et al[55]	2005	104	<1500 g	Preterm and SGA	ASSQ	14–15 y	4 symptoms of Asperger's 1 ASD (2%)
Limperopoulos et al[64]	2007	86	<32 wk GA	Preterm with CBH Preterm with SPI Preterm controls	M-CHAT SCQ (subset)	1–5 years	13 (37%) M-CHAT 5 (33%) SCQ
Limperopoulos et al[62]	2008	91	<1500 g <31 wk GA	Preterm	M-CHAT	18–24 mo	23 (25%)
Kuban et al[63]	2009	988	<28 wk GA	Preterm	M-CHAT	24 mo	212 (22%)
Limperopoulos et al (Limperopoulos, 2009)	2009	42	<32 wk GA	Preterm with CBH	ADOS DSM-IV	6–9 y	12 (28%)

Abbreviations: ADOS, autism diagnostic observation schedule; ASSQ, autism spectrum screening questionnaire; CBH, cerebellar hemorrhagic injury; DSM-IV, *Diagnostic and Statistical Manual of Mental Disorders*, 4th edition; GA, gestational age; M-CHAT, Modified Checklist for Autism in Toddlers; ROP, retinopathy of prematurity; SCQ, Social Communication Questionnaire; SGA, small for gestational age; SPI, supratentorial parenchymal injury.

or equal to 1500 g prospectively recruited at birth. They reported that an alarming 25% of ex-preterm infants (mean of 21 months corrected age) tested positive on these autism screening instruments. Abnormal M-CHAT scores correlated highly with internalizing behavioral problems on the Child Behavior Checklist and socialization and communication deficits on the Vineland Adaptive Behavior Scale. Importantly, with the exception of three children, the cohort was otherwise not affected by significant visual, auditory, and motor (eg, cerebral palsy) impairments. Perinatal risk factors associated with a positive autism screening included lower birth weight, chorioamnionitis, acute intrapartum hemorrhage, male gender, and illness severity on admission.

Kuban and colleagues[63] in a subsequent study also examined the prevalence of a positive screen for ASD using the M-CHAT in a large multicenter study of preterm infants born less than 28 weeks of gestation, and reported more than 21% screened positive for ASD. The authors also examined the impact of sensorimotor and cognitive impairments on a false-positive screening. Major motor (eg, cerebral palsy), cognitive (eg, mental retardation), and significant visual and hearing impairments accounted for more than 50% of the positive M-CHAT screens in their cohort. For example, children with major visual or hearing impairments were eight times more likely to screen positive. Among the subgroup of children who were free of motor, cognitive, visual, and hearing impairments, 10% screened positive, nearly double the expected rate. Noteworthy is the fact that cognitive impairment is frequently present in children with ASD; adjusting for this variable likely underestimates the true prevalence.

A third study to report an association between prematurity and ASD by the author's group examined the developmental consequences in a subgroup of ex-preterm infants with cerebellar hemorrhagic injury,[64] a form of brain injury increasingly recognized among survivors of extreme preterm birth.[65–69] Children underwent formal neurologic examinations and a battery of standardized developmental, functional, and behavioral evaluations, and autism screening questionnaires at a mean age 32 months. Results indicated that children with isolated cerebellar injury versus preterm age-matched controls demonstrated significantly greater motor disabilities, language delays, and cognitive deficits. Notably, 37% of infants with cerebellar injury tested positive for early signs of autism using the M-CHAT. The author speculates that cerebellar hemorrhagic injury in preterm infants was associated with a high prevalence of pervasive neurodevelopmental disabilities and may play a critical and underrecognized role in social, affective, and behavioral dysfunction (discussed later).

Collectively, these initial data strongly suggested that early autistic behaviors seem to be an underappreciated feature in survivors of extreme prematurity, and that these behaviors might be increased by injury and growth failure (see later) to the premature cerebellum. These provocative preliminary findings clearly require confirmation using definitive autism diagnostic tests. One important limitation of the studies summarized previously is that the cut-off scores of screening measures are typically designed to maximize the identification of children at greatest risk, and consequently may compromise both false-positive and false-negative results. Furthermore, the extent to which these initial positive screen rates are transient or indicative of a milder form of ASD that is specific to extreme preterm survivors or merely reflective of future social-emotional impairments is unclear. Long-term studies are urgently needed to examine the sensitivity and specificity of the M-CHAT, and determine the true prevalence of ADS in infants born preterm.

To date, formal follow-up evaluations using the Autism Diagnostic Observation Schedule and *Diagnostic and Statistical Manual of Mental Disorders, 4th edition* criteria in the author's cohort of ex-preterm children with isolated cerebellar hemorrhagic injury who tested positive on initial screening using the M-CHAT (described previously) are revealing that approximately 30% of children meet diagnostic criteria for ASD (Limperopoulos, 2009). The relationship between perinatal risk factors and topography of cerebellar injury is currently under investigation. Ongoing research is needed to better elucidate the prevalence, mechanisms, and neural basis of autism spectrum features in ex-preterm children.

NEUORANATOMIC SUBSTRATES FOR ASD AND PREMATURITY

Neuroimaging and neuropathologic studies in ASD have shown a heterogeneous array of anatomic findings in the cerebrum and cerebellum.[70,71] Although a comprehensive review of this literature is beyond the scope of this article, the potential relationship between altered brain development in ASD and the role of prematurity itself and prematurity-related brain injury is explored.

One of the most striking observations in autism research to date is the lack of neuro-imaging studies that have focused on early neuroanatomic development at the age of clinical onset of autism.[71] Conversely, studies have focused largely on subjects a decade or more after the onset of the disorder, and primarily on higher-functioning autistic individuals. Consequently, there is a glaring lack of early neuroimaging data from around the time of autism diagnosis (ie, between 2 and 4 years of age).[71] More-over, because ASDs are typically diagnosed around age 2 or later, no studies have reported the pre-existing neuroimaging findings in children subsequently diagnosed with ASD. Existing data largely reflect neuroanatomic changes years after the onset of autism, delineating the end result of the pathology of autism rather than the struc-tural changes taking place before or during the emergence of ASD symptoms.[71,72] The neuroanatomic antecedents of ASD remain essentially unknown at the present time. Longitudinal neural anatomic studies before the emergence of ASD features are urgently needed.

Neuroimaging, Prematurity, and ASD

Evidence for neuroimaging abnormalities and ASD in survivors of preterm birth is currently limited to a handful of reports, which are summarized next.

Impaired connectivity

Skranes and colleagues[73] demonstrated that very low birth weight adolescents with symptoms of Asperger disorder all had white matter reduction and ventricular enlarge-ment on MRI. Moreover, higher scores on the Autism Spectrum Screening Question-naire were significantly correlated with impaired connectivity characterized by reduced fractional anisotropy values on diffusion tensor imaging in the external capsule and superior fascicle on the left side. The authors speculate that the low frac-tional anisotropy values may be associated with damage to the immature developing white matter that has long-term consequences on microstructure and connectivity. This damage in turn leads to poor connectivity in commissural and association tracts and impairs the abilities that demand cooperation between different brain regions. Specifically, the external capsule contains fibers that connect the temporal and fontal lobes.[74] These findings corroborate neuroimaging studies reporting white matter abnormalities in the frontal, superior temporal cortex, and temporoparietal junction,[75] and neuropathology reports of smaller frontal and temporal cortical minicolumns in individuals with autism.[76,77]

Impaired cerebellar growth and development

Using advanced three-dimensional volumetric MRI studies in premature infants, the author's group has demonstrated a particularly rapid growth period for the immature cerebellum during the third trimester of gestation, a growth rate that far exceeds that of the cerebral hemispheres.[78] In late gestation, proliferation and migration of the cerebellar granule cells are particularly prominent events,[79] and such insults as hemorrhage and hypoxia-ischemia may injure these immature granule cells, with secondary effects on other cell populations[80] ultimately impairing cerebellar growth and development.[81]

Impaired growth and development of the cerebellum in premature infants may be grouped into two broad categories, based on early neonatal MRI studies.

The first category of cerebellar growth impairment observed in preterm infants is evidence of direct cerebellar injury during the neonatal period. Cerebrovascular (often hemorrhagic) injury is an important and previously underrecognized form of injury to the immature cerebellum, particularly in the extremely low gestational age infant. Although the pathogenesis for this type of injury remains unknown, it is likely related to impaired cerebral autoregulation and vascular fragility of the cerebellar germinal matrices.[82] The author's group has shown that ex-preterm infants with isolated cerebellar hemorrhagic injury were significantly more likely to score positive on initial autism screening compared with those infants without cerebellar injury.[64] Moreover, the presence of associated supratentorial injury (eg, periventricular leukomalacia, periventricular hemorrhagic infarction) did not further increase the risk for testing positive on early autism screening in these infants. It is noteworthy that socialization difficulties and a positive autism screening were almost exclusively associated with injury to the vermis (**Fig. 1**). Recent findings also suggest that unilateral cerebellar hemorrhagic injury is associated with region-specific contralateral cerebral gray and white matter volume reductions in the sensorimotor, premotor, dorsolateral prefrontal, and mid-temporal cortices, suggesting trophic withdrawal (ie, cerebellocerebral crossed diaschisis [Limperopoulos, 2009]). The potential role of such remote contralateral cerebellocerebral growth failure in the subsequent development of cognitive, affective, and behavioral impairment, including ASD, remains unknown.

The second category of cerebellar growth impairment is present in the absence of direct injury to the cerebellum detected by MRI. Using quantitative MRI studies, the author and others[78,83,84] have also shown an increased risk for impaired cerebellar growth in ex-premature infants. Such cerebellar growth impairment is already detectable by quantitative MRI as early as term gestational age equivalent.[78] Whether this growth impairment is caused by cellular injury below the current resolution of MRI, loss of maternal-placental growth factors, or environmental factors injurious to the immature cerebellum remains unknown.[82] Importantly, decreased total cerebellar volume at term equivalent in the absence of direct cerebellar injury is associated with higher M-CHAT scores in toddlers born preterm, controlling for total brain volume and gestational age (Limperopoulos, 2009) (**Fig. 2**). These data support the notion that impaired development of the cerebellum (in the absence of direct cerebellar injury) in the preterm infant may be associated with long-term atypical socioaffective development in this vulnerable population. Taken together, these data suggest that both direct and indirect mechanisms of cerebellar injury seem to stunt cerebellar growth and development in the preterm infant. Likewise, these findings provide important insights into the highly integrated anatomic and functional interactions between the immature cerebrum and cerebellum, and suggest significant remote trophic effects between these structures during development. It is also reasonable to suggest that early life impairment of cerebellar growth plays a central but previously underrecognized role in the long-term cognitive, behavioral, and social deficits associated with brain injury among premature infants.[64] The full extent of the role of cerebellar injury, however, in

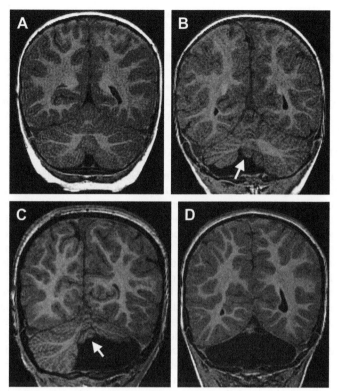

Fig. 1. Relationship between cerebellar injury topography and early signs of ASD. (*A*) Example of a normal cerebellum. (*B*) Unilateral right cerebellar injury without injury to the vermis. (*C*) Unilateral cerebellar and vermis hemorrhagic injury. (*D*) Extensive (near complete) bilateral cerebellar-vermis injury.

the genesis of social behavioral deficits among premature infants remains to be determined.

Neuropathology and Autism

Neuropathologic studies have highlighted evidence of cellular abnormalities and processes that may underlie the neuropathologic substrates of autism. Although

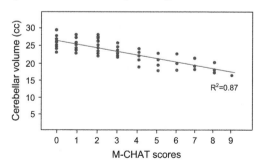

Fig. 2. Relationship between cerebellar volume at term equivalent and M-CHAT scores at follow-up testing between 18 and 24 months corrected age. Higher M-CHAT scores were associated with lower total cerebellar volume at term.

neuroanatomic descriptions from cases of autism are limited, a variety of findings has been described in autopsy studies[28,71,72,85] supporting these cellular and growth abnormalities in the cerebellar, frontal, and temporal cortices. Noteworthy is the fact that 80% of these have demonstrated well-defined cerebellar anatomic abnormalities.[85-89] Importantly, there are no autopsy reports from autistic children around the typical age at diagnosis (ie, 2–4 years). The most commonly described neuropathologic findings in the cerebellum of autistic individuals include glial activation with gliosis, and neuronal degeneration most prominently among the Purkinje neurons.[87]

THE CEREBELLUM: CHANGING CONCEPTS OF ITS FUNCTIONAL ROLES

Available data on the role of the cerebellum and ASD in preterm infants are in harmony with an accumulating experience in older subjects reflecting the relationship between the cerebellum and socioaffective development. Although traditional understanding of the cerebellum's role has been that of a center for motor control,[90] in recent years this traditional view has been challenged by increasing recognition that the cerebellum has an important role in "higher functions," such as cognition, learning, affect, and behavior. Central to this development has been the description of a distinct "cerebellar cognitive affective disorder"[91] in older children[92-94] and adults[91] following cerebellar injury, particularly to the posterior lobe. The cerebellar cognitive affective syndrome is characterized by a constellation of impairments in executive, visual spatial, linguistic, and affective function. Relevant to survivors of extreme preterm birth is an earlier description of an apparent "developmental" form of cerebellar cognitive affective syndrome.[64] Central to the cerebellar cognitive affective disorder is emotional dysregulation, which is usually evident with impaired behavioral modulation and flattening or disinhibition of affect.[95] In addition, obsessive-compulsive traits may be prominent, and behavioral stereotypies and disturbed interpersonal relations that meet criteria for autism.[90] In studies, the features of this developmental cerebellar cognitive affective syndrome show clear overlap with the features of early autism. Of particular note is the fact that these behavioral changes in the cerebellar cognitive affective syndrome are most prominent when the vermis and paravermian regions of the cerebellum are injured, as is the case in a cohort of ex-premature children in which injury to the vermis is strongly associated with early signs of ASD.[64] The relationship between regional cerebellar volumes and ADS in ex-preterm children with cerebellar injury diagnosed with ASD at school age is currently underway.

SUMMARY AND FUTURE DIRECTIONS

Clearly, the most pervasive long-term neurodevelopmental sequelae among survivors of extreme prematurity are those in the areas of cognitive, behavioral, and affective function. Although clinical experience and initial screening tests point to a significant prevalence of autistic-like behaviors in these children, the true nature and severity of these behaviors need further definition. Likewise, the precise mechanisms underlying the development of these autism-like behaviors among ex-premature children are unclear. The precise structure-function relationships between these observations are not yet known. Ongoing research is needed to provide new insight into the true prevalence of diagnosed ASD, and the association between prematurity itself, and the effects of prematurity-related brain injury, and the development of ASD among survivors of extreme prematurity. Importantly, delineation of these relationships provides clinicians with the understanding needed for informed prognostic counseling of future parents of premature infants and for anticipatory guidance, and for the development of more timely and cost-effective models for early intervention and better allocation of resources.

REFERENCES

1. Hagberg B, Hagberg G, Beckung E, et al. Changing panorama of cerebral palsy in Sweden. VIII. Prevalence and origin in the birth year period 1991–94. Acta Paediatr 2001;90(3):271–7.
2. Larroque B, Breart G, Kaminski M, et al. Survival of very preterm infants: epipage, a population based cohort study. Arch Dis Child Fetal Neonatal Ed 2004;89(2): F139–44.
3. Anthony S, Ouden L, Brand R, et al. Changes in perinatal care and survival in very preterm and extremely preterm infants in The Netherlands between 1983 and 1995. Eur J Obstet Gynecol Reprod Biol 2004;112(2):170–7.
4. Vincer MJ, Allen AC, Joseph KS, et al. Increasing prevalence of cerebral palsy among very preterm infants: a population-based study. Pediatrics 2006;118(6):e1621–6.
5. Winter S, Autry A, Boyle C, et al. Trends in the prevalence of cerebral palsy in a population-based study. Pediatrics 2002;110(6):1220–5.
6. Johnson S, Hennessy E, Smith R, et al. Academic attainment and special educational needs in extremely preterm children at 11 years of age: the EPICure study. Arch Dis Child Fetal Neonatal Ed 2009;94(4):F283–9.
7. Darlow BA, Cust AE, Donoghue DA. Improved outcomes for very low birthweight infants: evidence from New Zealand national population based data. Arch Dis Child Fetal Neonatal Ed 2003;88(1):F23–8.
8. Marlow N, Wolke D, Bracewell MA, et al. Neurologic and developmental disability at six years of age after extremely preterm birth. N Engl J Med 2005;352(1):9–19.
9. Tommiska V, Heinonen K, Lehtonen L, et al. No improvement in outcome of nationwide extremely low birth weight infant populations between 1996–1997 and 1999–2000. Pediatrics 2007;119(1):29–36.
10. Rushing S, Ment LR. Preterm birth: a cost benefit analysis. Semin Perinatol 2004; 28(6):444–50.
11. Moster D, Lie RT, Markestad T. Long-term medical and social consequences of preterm birth. N Engl J Med 2008;359(3):262–73.
12. Dahl LB, Kaaresen PI, Tunby J, et al. Emotional, behavioral, social, and academic outcomes in adolescents born with very low birth weight. Pediatrics 2006;118(2): e449–59.
13. Anderson PJ, Doyle LW. Executive functioning in school-aged children who were born very preterm or with extremely low birth weight in the 1990s. Pediatrics 2004;114(1):50–7.
14. Schmidt LA, Miskovic V, Boyle MH, et al. Shyness and timidity in young adults who were born at extremely low birth weight. Pediatrics 2008;122(1):e181–7.
15. Saigal S, Pinelli J, Hoult L, et al. Psychopathology and social competencies of adolescents who were extremely low birth weight. Pediatrics 2003;111(5 Pt 1):969–75.
16. Indredavik MS, Vik T, Heyerdahl S, et al. Psychiatric symptoms and disorders in adolescents with low birth weight. Arch Dis Child Fetal Neonatal Ed 2004;89(5): F445–50.
17. Hack M, Flannery DJ, Schluchter M, et al. Outcomes in young adulthood for very-low-birth-weight infants. N Engl J Med 2002;346(3):149–57.
18. Buka SL, Fan AP. Association of prenatal and perinatal complications with subsequent bipolar disorder and schizophrenia. Schizophr Res 1999;39(2):113–9 [discussion: 60–1].

19. Wahlbeck K, Osmond C, Forsen T, et al. Associations between childhood living circumstances and schizophrenia: a population-based cohort study. Acta Psychiatr Scand 2001;104(5):356–60.
20. Kajantie E. Early-life events: effects on aging. Hormones (Athens) 2008;7(2): 101–13.
21. Elgen I, Sommerfelt K, Markestad T. Population based, controlled study of behavioural problems and psychiatric disorders in low birthweight children at 11 years of age. Arch Dis Child Fetal Neonatal Ed 2002;87(2):F128–32.
22. Allin M, Rooney M, Cuddy M, et al. Personality in young adults who are born preterm. Pediatrics 2006;117(2):309–16.
23. Wetherby AM, Woods J, Allen L, et al. Early indicators of autism spectrum disorders in the second year of life. J Autism Dev Disord 2004;34(5):473–93.
24. Council on Children With Disabilities, Section on Developmental Behavioral Pediatrics, Bright Futures Steering Committee, et al. Identifying infants and young children with developmental disorders in the medical home: an algorithm for developmental surveillance and screening. Pediatrics 2006;118(1):405–20.
25. Kuehn BM. CDC: autism spectrum disorders common. JAMA 2007;297(9):940.
26. Leslie DL, Martin A. Health care expenditures associated with autism spectrum disorders. Arch Pediatr Adolesc Med 2007;161(4):350–5.
27. Ganz ML. The lifetime distribution of the incremental societal costs of autism. Arch Pediatr Adolesc Med 2007;161(4):343–9.
28. Casanova MF. The neuropathology of autism. Brain Pathol 2007;17(4):422–33.
29. Bolton PF, Murphy M, Macdonald H, et al. Obstetric complications in autism: consequences or causes of the condition? J Am Acad Child Adolesc Psychiatry 1997;36(2):272–81.
30. Schanen NC. Epigenetics of autism spectrum disorders. Hum Mol Genet 2006; 15(2):R138–50.
31. Smalley SL, Loo SK, Yang MH, et al. Toward localizing genes underlying cerebral asymmetry and mental health. Am J Med Genet B Neuropsychiatr Genet 2005; 135(1):79–84.
32. Torrey EF, Hersh SP, McCabe KD. Early childhood psychosis and bleeding during pregnancy: a prospective study of gravid women and their offspring. J Autism Child Schizophr 1975;5(4):287–97.
33. Badawi N, Dixon G, Felix JF, et al. Autism following a history of newborn encephalopathy: more than a coincidence? Dev Med Child Neurol 2006;48(2):85–9.
34. Maimburg RD, Vaeth M. Perinatal risk factors and infantile autism. Acta Psychiatr Scand 2006;114(4):257–64.
35. Bilder D, Pinborough-Zimmerman J, Miller J, et al. Prenatal, perinatal, and neonatal factors associated with autism spectrum disorders. Pediatrics 2009; 123(5):1293–300.
36. Larsson HJ, Eaton WW, Madsen KM, et al. Risk factors for autism: perinatal factors, parental psychiatric history, and socioeconomic status. Am J Epidemiol 2005;161(10):916–25 [discussion: 26–8].
37. Schendel D, Bhasin TK. Birth weight and gestational age characteristics of children with autism, including a comparison with other developmental disabilities. Pediatrics 2008;121(6):1155–64.
38. Wier ML, Yoshida CK, Odouli R, et al. Congenital anomalies associated with autism spectrum disorders. Dev Med Child Neurol 2006;48(6):500–7.
39. Kolevzon A, Gross R, Reichenberg A. Prenatal and perinatal risk factors for autism: a review and integration of findings. Arch Pediatr Adolesc Med 2007; 161(4):326–33.

40. Brimacombe M, Ming X, Lamendola M. Prenatal and birth complications in autism. Matern Child Health J 2007;11(1):73–9.
41. Henderson H, Schwartz C, Mundy P, et al. Response monitoring, the error-related negativity, and differences in social behavior in autism. Brain Cogn 2006;61(1):96–109.
42. Glasson EJ, Bower C, Petterson B, et al. Perinatal factors and the development of autism: a population study. Arch Gen Psychiatry 2004;61(6):618–27.
43. Knoester M, Helmerhorst FM, van der Westerlaken LA, et al. Matched follow-up study of 5 8-year-old ICSI singletons: child behaviour, parenting stress and child (health-related) quality of life. Hum Reprod 2007;22(12):3098–107.
44. Hultman CM, Sparen P, Cnattingius S. Perinatal risk factors for infantile autism. Epidemiology 2002;13(4):417–23.
45. Niemitz EL, Feinberg AP. Epigenetics and assisted reproductive technology: a call for investigation. Am J Hum Genet 2004;74(4):599–609.
46. Weghofer A, Klein K, Stammler-Safar M, et al. Severity of prematurity risk in spontaneous and in vitro fertilization twins: does conception mode serve as a risk factor? Fertil Steril 2009 Jul 7.
47. Sunderam S, Chang J, Flowers L, et al. Assisted reproductive technology surveillance–United States, 2006. MMWR Surveill Summ 2009;58(5):1–25.
48. Sigurdsson E, Van Os J, Fombonne E. Are impaired childhood motor skills a risk factor for adolescent anxiety? Results from the 1958 U.K. birth cohort and the National Child Development Study. Am J Psychiatry 2002;159(6):1044–6.
49. Jones PB, Rantakallio P, Hartikainen AL, et al. Schizophrenia as a long-term outcome of pregnancy, delivery, and perinatal complications: a 28-year follow-up of the 1966 North Finland general population birth cohort. Am J Psychiatry 1998;155(3):355–64.
50. Botting N, Powls A, Cooke RW, et al. Attention deficit hyperactivity disorders and other psychiatric outcomes in very low birthweight children at 12 years. J Child Psychol Psychiatry 1997;38(8):931–41.
51. Whitaker AH, Van Rossem R, Feldman JF, et al. Psychiatric outcomes in low-birth-weight children at age 6 years: relation to neonatal cranial ultrasound abnormalities. Arch Gen Psychiatry 1997;54(9):847–56.
52. Hille ET, Dorrepaal C, Perenboom R, et al. Social lifestyle, risk-taking behavior, and psychopathology in young adults born very preterm or with a very low birthweight. J Pediatr 2008;152(6):793–800, e1–4.
53. Nadeau L, Boivin M, Tessier R, et al. Mediators of behavioral problems in 7-year-old children born after 24 to 28 weeks of gestation. J Dev Behav Pediatr 2001;22(1):1–10.
54. Hack M, Youngstrom EA, Cartar L, et al. Behavioral outcomes and evidence of psychopathology among very low birth weight infants at age 20 years. Pediatrics 2004;114(4):932–40.
55. Indredavik MS, Skranes JS, Vik T, et al. Low-birth-weight adolescents: psychiatric symptoms and cerebral MRI abnormalities. Pediatr Neurol 2005;33(4):259–66.
56. Hayes B, Sharif F. Behavioural and emotional outcome of very low birth weight infants: literature review. J Matern Fetal Neonatal Med 2009;1–8.
57. Cederlund M, Gillberg C. One hundred males with Asperger syndrome: a clinical study of background and associated factors. Dev Med Child Neurol 2004;46(10):652–60.
58. Msall ME. Supporting vulnerable preschool children: connecting the dots before kindergarten. Pediatrics 2004;114(4):1086.
59. Indredavik MS, Vik T, Skranes J, et al. Positive screening results for autism in ex-preterm infants. Pediatrics 2008;122(1):222 [author reply 3].

60. Robins DL, Dumont-Mathieu TM. Early screening for autism spectrum disorders: update on the modified checklist for autism in toddlers and other measures. J Dev Behav Pediatr 2006;27(2):S111–9.

61. Fombonne E. Autism and newborn encephalopathy [comment]. Dev Med Child Neurol 2006;48(2):84.

62. Limperopoulos C, Bassan H, Sullivan NR, et al. Positive screening for autism in ex-preterm infants: prevalence and risk factors. Pediatrics 2008;121(4): 758–65.

63. Kuban KC, O'Shea TM, Allred EN, et al. Positive screening on the Modified Checklist for Autism in Toddlers (M-CHAT) in extremely low gestational age newborns. J Pediatr 2009;154(4):535–40, e1.

64. Limperopoulos C, Bassan H, Gauvreau K, et al. Does cerebellar injury in premature infants contribute to the high prevalence of long-term cognitive, learning, and behavioral disability in survivors? Pediatrics 2007;120(3):584–93.

65. Limperopoulos C, Benson CB, Bassan H, et al. Cerebellar hemorrhage in the preterm infant: ultrasonographic findings and risk factors. Pediatrics 2005; 116(3):717–24.

66. Messerschmidt A, Brugger PC, Boltshauser E, et al. Disruption of cerebellar development: potential complication of extreme prematurity. AJNR Am J Neuroradiol 2005;26(7):1659–67.

67. Messerschmidt A, Fuiko R, Prayer D, et al. Disrupted cerebellar development in preterm infants is associated with impaired neurodevelopmental outcome. Eur J Pediatr 2008;167(10):1141–7.

68. Merrill JD, Piecuch RE, Fell SC, et al. A new pattern of cerebellar hemorrhages in preterm infants. Pediatrics 1998;102(6):E62.

69. Johnsen SD, Bodensteiner JB, Lotze TE. Frequency and nature of cerebellar injury in the extremely premature survivor with cerebral palsy. J Child Neurol 2005;20(1):60–4.

70. Courchesne E, Redcay E, Morgan JT, et al. Autism at the beginning: microstructural and growth abnormalities underlying the cognitive and behavioral phenotype of autism. Dev Psychopathol 2005;17(3):577–97.

71. Courchesne E, Pierce K, Schumann CM, et al. Mapping early brain development in autism. Neuron 2007;56(2):399–413.

72. Amaral DG, Schumann CM, Nordahl CW. Neuroanatomy of autism. Trends Neurosci 2008;31(3):137–45.

73. Skranes J, Vangberg TR, Kulseng S, et al. Clinical findings and white matter abnormalities seen on diffusion tensor imaging in adolescents with very low birth weight. Brain 2007;130(Pt 3):654–66.

74. Mori S, Wakana S, Nagae-Poetscher LM, et al. MRI atlas of human white matter. 1st edition. Amsterdam: Elsevier; 2005.

75. Barnea-Goraly N, Kwon H, Menon V, et al. White matter structure in autism: preliminary evidence from diffusion tensor imaging. Biol Psychiatry 2004;55(3): 323–6.

76. Casanova MF, Buxhoeveden DP, Brown C. Clinical and macroscopic correlates of minicolumnar pathology in autism. J Child Neurol 2002;17(9):692–5.

77. Casanova MF, van Kooten IA, Switala AE, et al. Minicolumnar abnormalities in autism. Acta Neuropathol 2006;112(3):287–303.

78. Limperopoulos C, Soul JS, Gauvreau K, et al. Late gestation cerebellar growth is rapid and impeded by premature birth. Pediatrics 2005;115(3):688–95.

79. Berry M, Bannister LH, Standring SM. Nervous system. In: Williams PL, editor. Gray's anatomy. 38th edition. Edinburgh: Churchill Livingstone; 1995. p. 901–1395.

80. Jacobson M. Developmental neurobiology. New York: Plenum Press; 1991.
81. Johnston MV. Selective vulnerability in the neonatal brain. Ann Neurol 1998;44(2): 155–6.
82. Limperopoulos C, du Plessis AJ. Disorders of cerebellar growth and development. Curr Opin Pediatr 2006;18(6):621–7.
83. Limperopoulos C, Soul JS, Haidar H, et al. Impaired trophic interactions between the cerebellum and the cerebrum among preterm infants. Pediatrics 2005;116(4): 844–50.
84. Srinivasan L, Allsop J, Counsell SJ, et al. Smaller cerebellar volumes in very preterm infants at term-equivalent age are associated with the presence of supratentorial lesions. AJNR Am J Neuroradiol 2006;27(3):573–9.
85. Palmen SJ, van Engeland H, Hof PR, et al. Neuropathological findings in autism. Brain 2004;127(Pt 12):2572–83.
86. Kemper TL, Bauman ML. The contribution of neuropathologic studies to the understanding of autism. Neurol Clin 1993;11(1):175–87.
87. Vargas DL, Nascimbene C, Krishnan C, et al. Neuroglial activation and neuroinflammation in the brain of patients with autism. Ann Neurol 2005;57(1):67–81.
88. Yip J, Soghomonian JJ, Blatt GJ. Decreased GAD67 mRNA levels in cerebellar Purkinje cells in autism: pathophysiological implications. Acta Neuropathol 2007;113(5):559–68.
89. Lee M, Martin-Ruiz C, Graham A, et al. Nicotinic receptor abnormalities in the cerebellar cortex in autism. Brain 2002;125(Pt 7):1483–95.
90. Riva D, Giorgi C. The cerebellum contributes to higher functions during development: evidence from a series of children surgically treated for posterior fossa tumours. Brain 2000;123(Pt 5):1051–61.
91. Schmahmann JD. Disorders of the cerebellum: ataxia, dysmetria of thought, and the cerebellar cognitive affective syndrome. J Neuropsychiatry Clin Neurosci 2004;16(3):367–78.
92. Levisohn PM. The autism-epilepsy connection. Epilepsia 2007;48(Suppl 9):33–5.
93. Grill J, Viguier D, Kieffer V, et al. Critical risk factors for intellectual impairment in children with posterior fossa tumors: the role of cerebellar damage. J Neurosurg 2004;101(2 Suppl):152–8.
94. Turkel SB, Shu Chen L, Nelson MD, et al. Case series: acute mood symptoms associated with posterior fossa lesions in children. J Neuropsychiatry Clin Neurosci 2004;16(4):443–5.
95. Schmahmann JD, Weilburg JB, Sherman JC. The neuropsychiatry of the cerebellum: insights from the clinic. Cerebellum 2007;6(3):254–67.

Advances in Near-Infrared Spectroscopy to Study the Brain of the Preterm and Term Neonate

Martin Wolf, PhD[a],*, Gorm Greisen, MD, DMSc[b]

KEYWORDS

- Near-infrared spectroscopy • Neonate • Brain
- Tissue oxygen saturation • Brain activity

Near-infrared spectroscopy (NIRS) and imaging (NIRI) are emerging diagnostic tools for the neonatal brain. Although the technology is approximately 30 years old, recent advances in quantification and instrumentation and the availability of commercial instruments have increased the interest in NIRS in clinical medicine, although so far its use in neonates is restricted to research.

From a clinical point of view, NIRS/NIRI is being tested as a tool to identify pathologies and thus predict or eventually prevent adverse outcomes, ie, cerebral palsy and other forms of neuro-psychological impairment. In general, two strategies of clinical use have been followed:

1. The measurement of cerebral autoregulation, blood volume, flow, and oxygenation. Here the future aim is to safeguard the brain by adjusting the blood and oxygen supply to the brain to adequate levels and to prevent brain lesions. This type of application is reviewed in the section "Cerebral autoregulation, blood volume, flow, and oxygenation."
2. The assessment of brain activity. Here the aim is to develop functional tests to understand neonatal brain activity. In the future, such tests may enable early detection and

---

For this review no specific funding was received.

[a] Biomedical Optics Research Laboratory, Clinic of Neonatology, University Hospital Zurich, Frauenklinikstr. 10, 8091 Zurich, Switzerland

[b] Department of Neonatology, Rigshospitalet, Copenhagen University, Blegdamsvej 9, 2100 Copenhagen Ø, Denmark

* Corresponding author.

E-mail address: martin.wolf@usz.ch (M. Wolf).

prognosis of disabilities and may help to guide therapy. This type of application is reviewed in the section "Assessment of neonatal brain activity by NIRS/NIRI."
3. The aim of this article is to review the progress and state of NIRS and NIRI instrumentation and their clinical applications from the perspective of the two mentioned strategies, which are addressed separately.

MATERIAL AND METHODS

The authors searched for papers on the database MEDLINE (PubMed) using the keywords: "near-infrared," "neonate" for cerebral autoregulation, blood volume, flow and oxygenation and "near-infrared spectroscopy," "neonate" and "brain" for brain activity up to May 2009. The references were screened and the full texts of relevant publications were retrieved. For non-English articles, the review was limited to the abstract. The review of instruments was restricted to NIRS oximetry and/or NIRI instrumentation. Web sites of commercial systems were searched and companies contacted if necessary. The retrieved data were attributed to studies of cerebral activity and oxygenation/circulation. All of the cited studies were investigational.

CEREBRAL AUTOREGULATION, BLOOD VOLUME, FLOW, AND OXYGENATION
Instrumentation

NIRS instruments are mostly portable, and with the rapid development of optics and electronics have become increasingly economical and robust.

In brief, measurement of deep tissues is made possible by the relative transparency of tissue in the range of wavelengths from 700 to 1000 nm, called the near-infrared (NIR) window. At shorter wavelengths, in the visible spectrum, the chromophore hemoglobin absorbs strongly and prevents a deeper look. At longer wavelengths, water absorbs increasingly. In the NIR spectrum, total optical density of tissue is about 1 to 2 per centimeter, meaning that for every centimeter of additional distance between the source and the sensor, light is attenuated by a factor of 10 to 100. For safe levels of light input, therefore, it is difficult to use source-detector distances of more than 5 cm. Furthermore, because of the random propagation of light in tissue, the depth of measurement is no more than 2 to 3 cm.[1] This depth is more than enough to measure signals within the newborn brain.

NIRS is useful to monitor tissue hemoglobin concentration (oxyhemoglobin [O_2Hb], deoxyhemoglobin [HHb], and total hemoglobin [$tHb = O_2Hb + HHb$]) and hemoglobin-oxygen saturation ($StO_2 = O_2Hb/tHb$), because O_2Hb and HHb are almost the only NIR-chromophores in tissue with a varying concentration.[2] Furthermore, they have different absorption spectra in the range 700 to 1000 nm, as they do in the visible spectrum.[2,3] Thus by NIRS it is relatively easy to measure the O_2Hb, HHb, and tHb concentration in tissue as well as its average StO_2. Cytochrome aa3 also absorbs in the NIR spectrum, and the absorption is oxidation-reduction state dependent.[4] This absorption of cytochrome aa3, however, does not in practice disturb the measurement of hemoglobin, partly because the absorption is less than 10%, partly because the cytochrome aa3 oxygenation dependent spectrum is relatively flat, and partly because cytochrome aa3 appears to reduce only at very low levels of oxygenation.[4]

The major problem in NIRS is the nonfocused nature of the measurement, being an average of the tissues from source to detector; on the head these represent skin, scalp, skull, subarachnoid space, and gray and white brain matter.[5,6] In the neonate, this type of measure is a relatively smaller problem because the skin, scalp, and skull are thin. Furthermore, NIRS is relatively less sensitive to blood in larger compared with smaller blood vessels.[7] As a result, the hemoglobin concentration measured by NIRS represents a somewhat different measure of tissue blood volume compared with other methods. Also, tissue StO_2 measured by NIRS represents a weighted average of arterial and venous saturation. This weighting factor is impossible to determine precisely, and may vary from tissue to tissue and over time.

Spectroscopy in the NIR spectrum can be performed in a variety of ways. Only two wavelengths are required to resolve the spectroscopic equations with two chromophores (O_2Hb and HHb), but some instruments use more wavelengths, allowing some quality control or the ability to account for other, minor chromophores such as cytochrome aa3[4] or bilirubin.[8]

Some instruments use laser diodes, each producing a very well defined wavelength (**Table 1**: O1, O4, O6, O7, O8, O9). In practice, this design means that the laser diodes sit in the instrument and light is carried to the skin through light fibers. They are switched on in sequence and thus a single detector can be used. Some instruments use light-emitting diodes (see **Table 1**: O2), each providing a small range of wavelengths with a bell-shaped curve. Still others use a white light source and broadband spectroscopy (see **Table 1**: O5). This design requires that the received light pass through a grid to produce a spectrum on a detector surface that is able to separate the spectral lines. Thus the sensitivity in these systems is less, and usually they can operate over short source-detector distances only, and therefore can be used only for superficial tissues.

Instruments performing spectroscopy with continuous light at one source-detector distance are called photometers. They usually measure changes only from an arbitrary set-point. They have not changed much over the past 20 years and will not be discussed further. In contrast, the oximeters are new and will therefore be described in some detail. They all provide a continuous measure of StO_2, ie, a measure of the oxygen saturation of the hemoglobin in the intravascular red blood cells. The important

Table 1
Overview of commercial NIRS oximetry instruments

No.	Instrument	Technique	No. of Channels	Neonatal Sensor	Company	Web site
O1	FORE-SIGHT	Spectral	1	Yes	Casmed, USA	www.casmed.com
O2	INVOS 5100 C	SRS	2 or 4	Yes	Somanetics, USA	www.somanetics.com
O3	NIMO	Spectral	4	Custom	NIROX, Italy	www.nirox.it
O4	NIRO 100, NIRO 200	SRS	2	Yes	Hamamatsu, Japan	www.hamamatsu.com
O5	O2 C	Spectral	2	Yes	LEA, Germany	www.lea.de
O6	OM-220	SRS	2		Shimadzu, Japan	www.med.shimadzu.co.jp
O7	OxiplexTS	SRS IM	2	Yes	ISS, USA	www.iss.com
O8	T.Ox	Spectral	2	Yes	ViOptix, USA	www.vioptix.com
O9	TRS-20	TRS	2	Yes	Hamamatsu, Japan	www.hamamatsu.com

Instruments O3 and O8 measure tissue oxygen saturation in muscle and not in brain. Instruments O6 and O9 are currently sold only in Japan.

Abbreviations: IM, intensity modulated frequency domain; SRS, spatially resolved spectroscopy; TRS, time resolved spectroscopy.

point is that the measurement is absolute on a scale from 0% to 100%. The instruments are in general designed for easy clinical use, and sales materials focus on the difference between saturation of arterial blood, important for delivery of oxygen to tissue, and tissue oxygenation as an expression of StO_2 sufficiency.

The principles of operation of oximeters differ among instruments. Briefly, some use spatially resolved spectroscopy (see **Table 1**: O2, O4, O6, O7), meaning that light is detected at two or more different distances from the source. If the StO_2 is calculated from the difference in intensity at the two positions, the influence of superficial layers of tissue on the value is reduced.[1,9] This approach may have advantages for some applications. Some instruments are based on the theory of light propagation in scattering media (diffusion approximation for semi-infinite boundary condition) and on some reasonable assumptions of the scattering properties at different wavelengths (eg, O4, O7, O9); others are based on empiric algorithms with calibration in vitro, in animals, or in humans (eg, O1, O2). Other instruments use wavelength-resolved spectroscopy and calibration factors (O1, O3, O5, and O8), meaning that more wavelengths are needed. Finally, some instruments use intensity modulation (O7) or time-of-flight (O9) to determine path length as well as optical density simultaneously. When this approach is taken at two or more distances, assumptions regarding the optical characteristics of tissue can be avoided altogether, and a real objective measurement is possible. Methodological and technical aspects are reviewed in more detail in the literature.[10]

Accuracy of Tissue Oximetry

Accuracy is important for putting a value into context. Accuracy cannot be assessed for tissue oximetry because there is no other way of measuring "tissue" StO_2. As a substitute, tissue oximetry has been compared with saturation in venous blood, in some instances to a weighted average of venous and arterial blood.

In principle, this comparison is problematic because the reference value, the venous blood saturation, is "flow weighted." That is, in case of heterogeneous microperfusion, (mean) venous saturation will be weighted toward those parts of the tissue that are most highly perfused. Think of a situation with 50% of the tissue perfused at 30 mL/100 g/min and 50% of the tissue at 10 mL/100 g/min, and assume that oxygen uptake per 100 g is equal and assume that arterial oxygen saturation is 95%. If the venous saturation of the blood from the highly perfused tissue now is 75% (corresponding to 20% oxygen extraction), the venous saturation of the lowly perfused tissue must be 35% (corresponding to an oxygen extraction of 60%). In this case, (mean) venous saturation would be (30 × 75% + 10 × 35%) / 40 = 65%, whereas tissue saturation, assuming the same blood volume in the two tissues and the same spatial representation in the oximetry sample volume, would simply be (75 + 35) / 2 = 55% (+ some unknown weighting of the arterial compartment). Furthermore, in the microcirculation there may be some arterio-venous diffusion of oxygen, in particular in tissue with parallel arrangement of small arteries and veins. Both of these considerations suggest that tissue oximetry may actually be more sensitive to hypoxia in the least well-perfused parts of the tissue.

In principle, tissue oximetry is "blood volume weighted." In other words, that tissue with a dense vascularization is more represented in the signal than is a tissue with fewer blood vessels. The human newborn brain is a very peculiar organ, particularly before term age. It is characterized by a large central volume of white matter with very little vasculature. Thus, it can be predicted that tissue oximetry will be rather insensitive to white matter hypoxia.

Accuracy of tissue oximetry has rarely been studied in newborn infants because of practical problems of blood sampling from brain veins.[11,12] In older children and in adults, however, this issue has been examined in many studies. Accuracy, as defined by the mean difference (bias) in Bland-Altman analysis,[13] is typically within 5%.[14–20] This finding is noteworthy for two reasons. First, there is no clear difference between oximeters that are based on theory of photon diffusion in tissue and those that are based on calibration in animals or humans. Second, because the bias is typically close to zero and not significantly positive, with the oximetry results biased by the contribution of 20% to 40% more highly saturated arterial blood, suggests that the perfusion of the tissue is indeed heterogeneous as described previously. Finally, the bias is typically the same, regardless of whether the venous blood was taken from the internal jugular vein (nearly strictly brain blood), the jugular bulb (intra + extracranial blood), the superior vena cava (head and upper part of the body), or lower vena cava or pulmonary artery. In the intensive care setting where these patients were studied, therefore, brain oxygenation, and hence brain perfusion, appear not to be significantly differentially regulated.

Precision of Tissue Oximetry

Precision, which tells us how likely it is to receive the same value when a measurement is repeated, is necessary to trust an individual value. In vitro precision of tissue oximetry is good. It is determined on optical phantoms and depends on optic and electronic limitations. This in vitro precision is 1% to 2%.

The problem is that in vivo precision is not so good. It is assessed by the limits of agreement of the Bland-Altman analysis (by the ability to come close to the comparison measurement at each measurement),[13] or by more conventional analysis of repeated measurements under stable conditions (repeatability, intraclass correlation coefficient). Neither approach is perfect; however, the following assumptions may be made: that a method with a low bias (good agreement of averages) also could be precise; that cerebral oxygenation is expected to be stable over time, as neither cerebral blood flow nor cerebral metabolic rate of oxygen is known to vary markedly spontaneously; and finally that cerebral oxygenation is expected to vary little from one brain region to another for the same reasons. In this light, it is remarkable that the limits of agreement in tissue oximetry are wide and the repeatability is poor, at least compared with pulse oximetry, another noninvasive method based on red/infrared light. Repeatability of pulse oximetry is 2% to 3%. For comparison, the standard deviation calculated from Bland-Altman analysis and the repeatability for NIRS oximetry is in the range of 5% to 8%.[12,21,22] The problem appears to be associated with the replacement of sensors. Possibly the sensors are sensitive to small local heterogeneities of the optical properties of tissue (hair, blood vessels, subarachnoidal space, gyral folding).[5] For clinical application, a precision less than 3% would be desirable.

Thresholds for Hypoxic-ischemic Brain Injury

A principal aim of life support and intensive care is to safeguard oxygen transport to tissue. Recently, two studies in newborn piglets have narrowed down the threshold for hypoxia-ischemia in the newborn piglet.[23,24] At an StO_2 of 35%, EEG is consistently affected and there is evidence of cellular energy failure. At exposure to 35% tissue saturation for 2 hours or more, there is neuronal loss at long term. This finding fits in very well with earlier cerebral blood flow work, showing that a reduction of blood flow to less than 50% of normal resting levels is necessary to affect electrical function and that at a moderate further decrease, several hours of exposure are necessary to induce cortical necrosis.[25] This finding also agrees with some evidence in the newborn infant with cyanotic heart disease where tissue saturation before operative correction below 35% predicted poor neurologic development.[26] In contrast, in a group of infants after Norwood repair of hypoplastic left heart, a mean postoperative cerebral StO_2 of less than 56% predicted later death in hospital, need for ECMO, or hospital stay exceeding 30 days.[27]

Thresholds for Hyperoxic Brain Injury

It is increasingly clear that hyperoxia is a threat to newborn infants, in particular to preterm infants. Arterial hyperoxia, however, has little effect on venous oxygen saturation, because of the S-shape of the hemoglobin-oxygen-dissociation curve. Tissue oximetry potentially can identify the combination of hyperperfusion with arterial hyperoxygenation, but it can be argued that a statistical relation between supranormal StO_2 and later brain injury is more likely to be attributable to a pathologically decreased oxygen metabolism or an uncoupling of flow from oxygen metabolism. Both would be indicators of a preceding brain injury, rather than the incident value of tissue saturation and indicator of ongoing risk.

Clinical Application in Neonatology

Photometers provide continuous signals of O_2Hb and HHb concentration, potentially at a very fast rate, up to 100 Hz. The limitation is that measurements are relative, ie, only available as changes from an arbitrary set-point. Whereas photometers may give qualitative information on changes in brain blood volume, or on relative brain oxygenation, their usefulness is severely limited by the inability always to distinguish between a change in blood volume or in saturation.[28] Therefore, while photometers have given and continue to provide important data for research, their use will not become a useful clinical method unless combined with other physiologic parameters in innovative ways.

Using a NIRS photometer along with challenges, either by increased oxygen concentration in inspired air or by obstructing venous outflow, it is possible to obtain good-quality data of cerebral blood volume, cerebral blood flow, and cerebro-venous saturation, as reviewed recently.[29] Again, this approach has been useful for research and still is used, but is too cumbersome for clinical practice. In principle, this approach could be automated, but that has not been attempted. A problem is that hyperoxygenation as well as impedance of venous outflow from the brain may not be absolutely without risks.

Co-registration of the oxygenation index, ie, O_2Hb-HHb, from a NIRS photometer and arterial blood pressure, makes it possible to determine continuously if blood pressure changes are reflected in cerebral oxygenation as estimated by NIRS.[30] An abnormally strong relation between the two signals can be taken as an indicator of lack of blood flow autoregulation. The association has usually been quantified by a measure of correlation in the frequency domain, called coherence. The measure used has been the coherence at very low frequencies, ie, the co-fluctuation within periods of 25 seconds to 3 minutes. High coherence (impaired autoregulation) has been found to vary from day to day under intensive care, and has been found associated with brain injury and death.[31,32] This method could also be automated, but first, artifacts have to be rejected, and second, it takes several hours to obtain a stable estimate of coherence, unless there are large spontaneous fluctuations in the blood pressure.

Thus, tissue oximetry is the most promising NIRS method for clinical use. The main problem with current technology is the low precision.[33] Nevertheless, much experience has been gathered in neonatology (**Table 2**) as well as in pediatric cardiology

(**Table 3**), and some technical improvements are possible. Furthermore, after Food and Drug Administration approval, commercial instruments are rapidly being put to clinical use, also in neonatology. Thus we will see a large volume of more or less well-planned clinical observations in the years to come. In the following discussion, a few of the questions addressed in the existing literature on tissue oximetry in neonatology are reviewed with a focus on limitations and potentials.

Severe hypoxic-ischemic encephalopathy is followed by cerebral hyperperfusion, as shown by Doppler ultrasound and xenon-clearance.[86,87] NIRS tissue oximetry has demonstrated that this event is in fact hyperperfusion, as StO_2 is abnormally high, and that this hyperoxygenation carries the same poor prognosis as does the hyperperfusion.[51] Prognosis, however, was determined only at the statistical level and was not feasible for individual infants. Large studies with long-term follow-up are necessary to compute sensitivity and specificity for poor outcome. NIRS is not going to replace EEG for early prediction and selection for cooling or other brain protective treatment because cerebral hyperoxygenation is a consequence of the secondary energy failure that comes late. In comparison, the EEG depression is a consequence of the primary insult.

A persistent arterial duct (PDA) is a frequent problem in very preterm infants. In spite of ever-improving sonographic diagnosis of the duct and quantification of the shunt, the best management of this problem is still debatable. Cerebral tissue oximetry is one way of quantifying the systemic hypoperfusion resulting from excessive left-to-right shunting. Indeed, PDA has been associated with decreased cerebral saturation[58] and its closure with normalization,[61] although the opposite has also been found.[52] This discrepancy is likely to represent different clinical severity at the time of surgical closure.

Extracorporeal membrane oxygenation is used relatively frequently in newborn infants, either to treat pulmonary failure following meconium aspiration, neonatal infection, or congenital diaphragmatic hernia, or to treat circulatory failure before or after surgery for congenital heart malformation. Cannulation usually takes place during maximal distress, and is performed using the right-sided neck vessels. StO_2 in the right frontal area fell in all of three patients following ligation of the right carotid artery during cannulation, whereas no change was seen over the left hemisphere.[47] StO_2 reflected episodes of desaturation,[11,12] and was recommended as clinical routine for extra safety in this high-risk treatment, as it has for bypass during cardiac surgery.[88]

Finally, newborn infants also suffer from congenital heart disease, an area where tissue oximetry is particularly appealing because of the large deviations in oxygenation and the frequency of neurologic deficits at follow-up. In general, the findings have been more substantial, compared with the results discussed above, and recently a clinical benefit in terms of simplification of preoperative treatment of infants with hypoplastic left heart syndrome monitored by tissue oximetry was shown by comparison with a historic group of controls.[82]

Discussion and Conclusion

The low precision of NIRS tissue oximetry is a problem for making clinical decisions by comparison of the reading in a single infant with a threshold for action. Furthermore, added value should be demonstrated, ie, that prediction is improved over and above that already possible by the use of conventional clinical data.

Future research should go in two directions. First, investigators must look for important new pathophysiology. It is no longer relevant to show that the brain, on average, is a little more or less oxygenated in this or that clinical situation. It is predictable that tissue oxygenation will vary with arterial saturation and pCO_2 over the normal range, and that tissue oxygenation will decrease in cases of severe circulatory compromise.

Table 2
Overview of clinical studies in newborn infants reporting data on cerebral tissue oxygen saturation (StO$_2$)

First Author	Year	Patients	No.	Main Finding of Cerebral StO$_2$
Isobe[34]	2000	Newborn	7	Rise from 18% at 1.5 min after birth to 55% at 5–6 min, then gradually to 65%
Wolf[35]	2000	Preterm	18	Average 71%, correlates with SaO$_2$ during variation of FiO$_2$
Isobe[36]	2002	Newborn	26	Normal rise, but secondary decrease in infants born by caesarian section
Schrod[37]	2002	<37 wk	36	2%–5% decrease during head-up tilt in infants < 1500 from day 2 to 8
Schulz[38]	2003	30 wk	20	Decrease during umbilical artery blood sampling
Huang[39]	2004	Term	41	Decreased in hypoxic-ischemic encephalopathy compared with controls
Naulaers[40]	2004	Preterm	8	Varying response during rewarming after admission to NICU
Shuhaiber[41]	2004	Newborn	1	Unilateral decrease during seizures due to tuberous sclerosis
Benni[11]	2005	ECMO	3	Average arterial-to-venous contribution to StO$_2$ is 30:70
Catelin[42]	2005	Newborn	15	Tended to be higher after environmental and behavioral intervention
Dotta[43]	2005	CDH	25	6% decrease during surgery
Elwell[44]	2005	Preterm	9	Metabolic rate of oxygen 0.95 and 0.88 mL/100 g/min on right and left hemispheres
Jjichi[45]	2005	Newborn	22	Average 70%, lower at higher gestational age
Zhao[46]	2005	Newborn	23	Average 59%
Ejike[47]	2006	ECMO	11	12%–25% drop over right hemisphere during cannulation
Lemmers[48]	2006	<32 wk	38	Not decreased but more variable in respiratory distress syndrome
Li[49]	2006	Term	103	Decreased in moderate/severe meconium aspiration syndrome
Petrova[50]	2006	<33 wk	10	Larger decrease over kidney than brain during desaturation
Rais-Bahrami[12]	2006	ECMO	17	Bias +0.6%, precision 5.1%
Sorensen[22]	2006	<33 wk	37	Average 75%, precision 5.2%, between-infant variation 6.9%
Toet[51]	2006	Term	18	Increased values 24 hours after birth asphyxia predicts poor outcome

Zaramella[52]	2006	PDA<35 wk	16	4% decrease after surgical closure
Baenziger[53]	2007	Preterm	39	4% higher after placental transfusion
Dani[54]	2007	<30 wk	14	Not affected by changing of nasal-CPAP pressure between 2 and 6 mbar
Huning[55]	2007	<32 wk	20	2% decrease during blood sampling from the umbilical vein catheter
Romeo[56]	2007	Newborn	25	Decrease by 12% during major surgery
Begum[57]	2008	<1600 g	16	Decreased variability during kangaroo care
Lemmers[58]	2008	<32 wk	40	10% lower in PDA, normalization 24 hours after medical closure
Sorensen[59]	2008	<33 wk	82	8.5% difference between average values obtained by two different probes
Sorensen[60]	2008	<33 wk	63	Not affected by foetal vasculitis
Vanderhaegen[61]	2008	PDA, preterm	10	Increase by 4% immediately after surgical closure, normalization at 1 hour
Wong[62]	2008	Very preterm	24	Covariation with arterial blood pressure predicts death
De Smet[63]	2009	Preterm	20	Covaries with arterial blood pressure as a measure of cerebral autoregulation
Lemmers[21]	2009	Preterm	36	Correlation 0.89 between simultaneous values from right and left hemisphere
Moran[64]	2009	<1500 g	27	Correlate with superior vena cave flow
Vanderhaegen[65]	2009	<1500 g	13	Correlate with pCO_2

Abbreviations: CDH, congenital diaphragmatic hernia; CPAP, continuous positive airway pressure; ECMO, extracorporeal membrane oxygenation; PDA, patent ductus arteriosus.

Table 3
Overview of clinical studies in newborns and small children with congenital heart disease reporting data on cerebral tissue oxygen saturation (StO_2)

First Author	Year	Patients	No.	Main Finding of Cerebral StO_2
Pigula[66]	2000	HLHS	6	Decrease with deep hypothermic circulatory arrest, normal during regional perfusion
Kurth[67]	2001	<7 years	110	68% in healthy children, in VSD and CAo, decreased in PDA, ToF, HLHS, and PA
Tabbutt[68]	2001	HLHS > 1 y	10	Unchanged by inhalation of 17% O_2, but increased by inhalation of 3% CO_2
Ramamoorthy[69]	2002	HLHS		Unchanged by inhalation of 17% O_2, but increased by inhalation of 3% CO_2
Andropoulos[70]	2003	CHD	20	Poor correlation between StO_2 and Doppler flow velocity during regional perfusion
Andropoulos[71]	2004	CHD	19	Right/left difference >10% during regional perfusion in 9 of 19 patients
Hoffman[72]	2004	HLHS	9	Normal during regional perfusion during surgery, decreased after rewarming
Kilpack[73]	2004	CHD	34	Normal values maintained by regional perfusion during aortic reconstruction
Hofer[74]	2005	HLHS	10	78% falling to 60% with reduction of regional perfusion from 30 to 10 mL/kg/min
Kussmann[75]	2005	CHD < 1 y	62	Similar values on right and left side, before, during and after surgery with bypass
Toet[26]	2005	CHD, TGA	20	Values below 35% before surgery predict poor neurologic outcome
Weiss[20]	2005	CHD < 1 y	155	Correlate with SvO_2 and "cardiac shunt" during postoperative days
Scholl[76]	2006	CHD	1	Rapid drop owing to displacement of arterial cannula during bypass
McQuillen[77]	2007	CHD < 1 y	70	Correlate with SvO_2 and pCO_2 in first postoperative days
Farouk[78]	2008	CAo	11	Decrease by aortic cross-clamping above the left carotid, normal otherwise
Li[79]	2008	HLHS	7	Increase by inhalation of CO_2
Li[80]	2008	HLHS	16	Correlate to systemic blood flow in the first postoperative days
Redlin[81]	2008	CHD < 10 kg	20	Poor correlation with superior vena cava saturation
Johnson[82]	2009	HLHS	92	Monitoring of StO_2 was associated with simplification of preoperative treatment
Maher[83]	2009	CHD	1	Rapid detection of postoperative cardiac tamponade
Mascio[84]	2009	CHD	16	Varying time taken to reach danger limit during deep hypothermic cardiac arrest
Phelps[27]	2009	HLHS	50	Mean value over 48 postoperative hours < 56% predict adverse outcome
Tobias[85]	2009	CHD < 1 y	8	Decrease to 53% ± 11% after 36 to 61 min of deep hypothermic circulatory arrest

Abbreviations: CAo, coarctation of the aorta; CHD, congenital heart disease; HLHS, hypoplastic left heart syndrome; PA, pulmonary atresia; PDA, patent ductus arteriosus; ToF, tetralogy of Fallot; TGA, transposition of the great arteries; VSD, ventricular septal defect.

Therefore, and secondly, large and if necessary collaborative trials should aim at defining the clinical role of cerebral tissue oximetry in neonatology. An important question here is how clinical staff understands and uses the data provided by tissue oximetry. Questions such as "what to do with a declining trend," "what is most significant: a deep, but brief desaturation, compared with a longer but less extreme," and, not least, "what to think about abnormally high levels of tissue oxygenation," need to be addressed. We do not want yet another expensive tool of uncertain value to complicate clinical care.

ASSESSMENT OF NEONATAL BRAIN ACTIVITY BY NIRS/NIRI

One important application of NIRS/NIRI is to study activity and function of the brain and its development. For this purpose, specific stimuli are applied and the response of the brain is recorded. Two types of optical signals associated with brain activity can be detected by NIRS/NIRI: the neuronal signal, which occurs within milliseconds and reflects optical changes in the neuron, and the hemodynamic signal, which occurs within seconds and is associated with an increase in blood flow to the activated brain region. Because brain activity is localized, both signals are localized. Therefore, although in many publications NIRS with one or two channels is used, it is more appropriate to make use of NIRI, which is able to give precise information about the localization. We will review NIRI instrumentation and its applications in neonates in the following sections.

Instrumentation

All instruments displayed in **Table 1** could be used for functional studies of the brain, if they measured changes in O_2Hb, HHb, and tHb. Most of these instruments, however, measure at only one location, and thus information on the localization of functional activity is absent. This absence may lead to false negative and false positive results, the former because a small area of activity can easily be missed, and the latter, because artifacts may lead to signals similar to activation. NIRI works similarly to NIRS except that NIRI uses a higher number of sources and detectors, which are arranged geometrically to interrogate a region of the brain. Thus, localized changes can be detected. NIRI generates an image of an area, and artifacts caused by systematic factors such as changes in arterial oxygenation, blood pressure, or pCO_2 can be identified more easily because they are not localized.

All instruments except I4 in **Table 4** are continuous wave instruments, ie, they usually rely on the modified Lambert-Beer law to quantify concentration changes in O_2Hb, HHb, and tHb. Instead of the modified Lambert-Beer law, instrument I1 applies a finite element reconstruction technique and thus is the only instrument that currently provides 3-dimensional (3D) images. All other NIRI devices provide images in 2D. I4 is a frequency domain instrument, which additionally measures the phase shift and thus in principle is able to measure the differential path length factor, which leads to more precise results also in imaging applications. This advantage is not as substantial as in oximetry, however.

All instruments except I3 in **Table 4** are based on fiber-optic sensors. The advantage of fiber optics is that they are electromagnetically inert and thus can be used for multimodal studies in combination with, for example, EEG. The disadvantage of fiber optics is that the fibers are often heavy and of limited flexibility, which may lead to discomfort. Instrument I3 has a sensor that includes electronics and electrical cables with enhanced comfort for the subject.

Table 4
Overview of commercially available near-infrared imaging instrumentation and their parameters

No.	Instrument	Technique	No. of Channels	Applicability in Neonates	Time Resolution Hz	Company	Web Site
I1	Dynot	CW	Up to 64	Yes	10 (90 single)	NIRx, USA	www.nirx.net
I2	ETG-4000	CW	48	Yes	10	Hitachi, Japan	www.hitachimed.com
I3	fNIR100	CW	16	Custom	2	Biopac, USA	www.biopac.com
I4	Imagent	IM	Up to 128	Custom	60 (variable)	ISS, USA	www.iss.com
I5	NIRS2 CE, CW6	CW	Up to 1024	Yes	100	TechEn, Inc, USA	www.nirsoptix.com
I6	OMM-3000	CW	64	Yes	40 (variable)	Shimadzu, Japan	www.med.shimadzu.co.jp
I7	OXYMON MkIII	CW	1-96	Custom	50	Artinis, The Netherlands	www.artinis.com

Abbreviations: CW, continuous wave; IM, intensity modulated frequency domain.

In general, the higher the number of channels of an instrument, the larger the area that can be interrogated by NIRI. How large the interrogated area needs to be depends on the application. The number of channels varies. Most of the instruments were conceived for applications in adults, ie, for a large head. Thus, in general the number of channels is sufficient for use in neonates and preterm infants. O4 has an imaging probe for adults, which is not applicable for neonates. However, this or earlier versions have often been used in studies in neonates (**Table 5**), by using just the two probes intended for oxygenation measurements, ie, by measuring at two locations only.

One important part of the instrument is its probe. Development of a suitable probe for the neonatal head is still quite a challenge, and many researchers consequently build their own probes. The probe has to fulfill several requirements. It has to be fixed tightly to the head, so that it does not slip during movement. At the same time, the probe needs to be flexible and soft to avoid pressure and associated pain or even lesions. Because dark hair interferes with the measurement, an intelligent probe design allows hair to be tucked away as in EEG. One major source of error may be light piping, ie, light reaching the detector that has not passed through the tissue. Light piping may occur when fibers are not in direct contact with the skin. The probe design thus needs to prevent light piping. In addition, the material of the probe needs to be robust, antiallergenic, and disinfectable. It is recommended that probes are tested before buying them. Whereas some manufactures (see **Table 4**) provide probes for neonates, others will build custom probes.

The time resolution varies among instruments. In I1, the time resolution depends on the number of optical fibers used. In general, a high time resolution has the advantage that the signals contain more information, such as the heart pulsation, which enables a more efficient signal analysis and thus yields a higher signal-to-noise ratio. The disadvantage is that the amount of data increases and the signal analysis is more time consuming. To directly detect neuronal signals, a time resolution of 50 Hz or more and an instrument with low noise is required.

In the future, more imagers providing 3D images will be developed. In addition, the spatial resolution of the images, which currently is approximately 1 cm, will be improved. Currently the data analysis between instruments varies considerably. It is expected that this process eventually will converge to an optimal solution.

Clinical Application

As mentioned, two major types of optical signals associated with brain activity can be detected by NIRI: the neuronal signal, which occurs within milliseconds, and the hemodynamic signal, which occurs within seconds.

The neuronal signal is related to optical changes directly associated with neuronal activity. This signal arises within milliseconds after the onset of the stimulation and has been studied at the cellular level, in animal studies, and in humans (see Wolf and colleagues[89] for a review). There is extensive literature on studies in single neurons and brain slices that demonstrate several optical changes associated with activity at the neuronal level. In addition, the neuronal signal is detectable in the exposed cortex of animals. Several research laboratories have therefore tried to detect the neuronal signal noninvasively in human subjects. Whether neuronal activity can be detected noninvasively in adult human subjects is still controversial.[89] To the best of our knowledge, in neonates and preterm infants nobody has attempted to detect neuronal activity so far.

The hemodynamic signal is related to increased blood perfusion in an area of activated neurons as a result of neurovascular coupling. Brain activity as a result of

Table 5
Overview of studies of functional brain activation in neonates

Author	Year	Stimulus	GA Weeks	PA (Days)	Excluded	N	Imaging	Instrument	TR Hz	IOD cm	N stim	O2Hb	HHb	tHb	StO2Hb diff	Criteria	State
Meek[96]	1998	Visual checkerboard 5 Hz		MD 52 (2–98)	38	20	No 1ch	O4		3.5	4–18	+90%	+90%			Sitting still >1 good cycle	Awake
Hoshi[97]	2000	Visual flashing 10 Hz	MD 38 (37–41)	MD 4 (4–5)	7		Yes 3ch	I6	2.5	1.5	2	+100%	+50%–21%	+100%		Increase O2Hb, t-test	Asleep
Taga[98]	2003	Visual flashing 14 Hz occipital cortex	term (36–41)		9	16	Yes	I2	10		10	nd56%	nd25%			Anova	Asleep
Taga[98]	2003	Visual flashing 14 Hz frontal cortex	Term (36–41)		9	16	Yes	I2	10		10	nd4%	nd50%			Anova	Asleep
Kusaka[99]	2004	Visual flashing 8 Hz	MD 29 (28–33)	MD 3 (1–5)		5	Yes	I6	7.5	2.0	8–11	–100%	+80%	–80%		Wilcoxon	Asleep
Bortfeld[100]	2007	Visual animation		MN 228 (186–275)	5	35	Yes	I5	20	2.0	5	+nd	–nd	+nd		None	Awake
Karen[101]	2008	Visual blinking 0.5/1 Hz	MD 39 (37–41)	MD 5 (2–9)	20	15	Yes	Custom	100	Variable	10	+67%	–33%			Wilcoxon	Asleep
Sakatani[102]	1999	Auditory piano music	MN 38.8 ±1.4	MN 3.1 ±0.3		28	No 1ch	O4		4.0	1	+93%–4%	+61%–32%	+93%–4%		None	
Zaramella[103]	2001	Auditory sweep 2 kHz to 4 kHz	MD 32 (28–41)	MD 15 (1–49)		19	No	O4	0.2	3.5	1	+63%–37%	+62%–38%	+68%–32%		Increase tHb	Variable
Chen[104]	2002	Auditory piano music healthy infants	Term			20	No	O4		4.0	1	+95%	+65%–30%	+95%		None	

Study	Year	Stimulus	GA	Age (days)	Sess	N	Probe								Stats	State
Chen[104]	2002	Auditory piano music HIE infants	Term			22 No	O4	10	4.0	1		+27%–64%	+68%–18%	+27%–64%	None	
Pena[105]	2003	Auditory forward/backward mother's voice	Term	MN 3 (2–5)	2	12 Yes	O4	10	3.0	10				+nd	None	Asleep
Nissila[106]	2004	Auditory 1.4kHz to 1 kHz	Term		2	8 Yes	Custom	0.3	2.5		+63%	–13%			t-test	
Kotilahti[107]	2005	Auditory sinus 1 kHz	MN 41 (38–42)	MN 2 (1–3)		20 Yes	Custom	1	2.5	≤30	+81%				t-test	Variable
Bortfeld[100]	2007	Auditory speech		MN 228 (186–275)		35 Yes	15	20	2.0	5	+nd	–nd		+nd	None	Awake
Saito[108]	2007	Auditory infant directed speech	Term	MN 4 (2–9)		20 No 2ch	O4	6		1	+nd				None	Asleep
Saito[108]	2007	Auditory adult directed speech	Term	MN 4 (2–9)		20 No 2ch	O4	6		1	–nd				None	Asleep
Saito[109]	2007	Auditory prosodic speech	Term	MN 5 (1–9)		22 No 2ch	O4	6		1	+nd				None	Asleep
Saito[109]	2007	Auditory monotonous speech	Term	MN 5 (1–9)		22 No 2ch	O4	6		1	–nd				None	Asleep
Nishida[110]	2008	Auditory word "Momotaro" 0.66 Hz	MD 31 (23–35)	MD 61 (36–163)		8 Yes	12		2.0	5–10	+100%	–100%		+100%	None	Asleep
Nishida[110]	2008	Auditory word "Momotaro" 0.66 Hz	MD 39 (37–41)	MD 5 (2–11)		10 Yes	12		2.0	5–10	+100%	+70% –30%		+100%	None	Asleep
Isobe[111]	2001	Somatosensory knee flexing 0.7 Hz	MD 30 (24–35)	MD 23 (3–57)		2 Yes	12	10	2.0	10	+100%	–86%		+100%	None	Sedated

(continued on next page)

Table 5 (continued)

Author	Year	Stimulus	GA Weeks	PA (Days)	Excluded	N	Imaging	Instrument	TR Hz	IOD cm	N stim	O₂Hb	HHb	tHb	StO₂Hb diff	Criteria	State
Hintz[112]	2001	Somatosensory arm flexing 1 Hz	MD 32 (24–33)	(14–75)		5	Yes	Custom	0.2–0.3	Variable	7	–nd	+nd			None	
Gibson[113]	2006	Somatosensory arm flexing 1 Hz	MD 29 (28–32)	30	2	4	3D	Custom	0.0015	Variable	1	+66%	+66%	+66%		Correct location	
Bartocci[114]	2006	Somatosensory tactile	MN 32 (28–36)	MN 1 (1–2)	6	40	No 2ch	O4	1	4.0	1	+nd				None	Awake
Bartocci[114]	2006	Somatosensory pain venipuncture	MN 32 (28–36)	MN 1 (1–2)	6	40	No 2ch	O4	1	4.0	1	+nd				None	Awake
Slater[115]	2006	Somatosensory contralateral pain heel lance	MN 28 (24–37)	MN 8 (5–134)		18	No 2ch	O4			1			+97%		None	
Slater[115]	2006	Somatosensory ipsilateral pain heel lance	MN 28 (24–37)	MN 8 (5–134)		18	No 2ch	O4			1			–84%		None	
Slater[116]	2008	Somatosensory pain heel lance	(24–35)	(5–134)		12	No 2ch	O4			1			+91%		None	

Study	Year	Stimulation	GA	PA	Excl	N		ch	O2		IOD	TR			Criteria	State
Begum[57]	2008	Somatosensory kangaroo care 1 h	MD 28 (24–33)	MD 56 (21–119)	3	16	No			1		1		−100%		Asleep
Bartocci[117]	2000	Olfactory vanilla	MN 39 (37–41)	MD 2 (0–8)	7	23	No	1ch	O4	2	4.0	1	+100%	+100%	None	Awake
Bartocci[117]	2000	Olfactory colostrum	MN 39 (37–41)	MD 2 (0–8)	7	23	No	1ch	O4	2	4.0	1	+9%	+100%	None	Awake
Bartocci[118]	2001	Olfactory unpleasant odor	MN 34 (30–37)	MN 13 (1–35)	10	20	No	2ch	O4	1	4.0	1	−85%	−85%	t-test	Awake
Zotter[119]	2007	Arousals	MN 32 ±2.3	MN 24 ±2.9		38	No	2ch	O4	2	4.0	3.2	ns	ns	None	Asleep

The response to stimulation is described as +, ie, an increase, or −, ie, a decrease in the respective parameter. The number indicates the percentage of infants who exhibited this kind of change. Often details about the results were only vaguely described and the mentioned parameters were not declared. Instrument codes can be found in **Table 1** or **4**; in some studies, earlier versions of the instruments were used.

Abbreviations: ch, channel/s; Criteria, criteria applied to determine whether an activation was present; GA, gestational age at birth; Hbdiff, $O_2Hb-HHb$; HIE, hypoxic-ischemic encephalopathy; IOD, interoptode distance; MD, median; MN, mean; N, number; nd, not declared; ns, not significant; PA, postnatal age; Excluded, number of infants excluded mostly because of movement artifacts; stim, stimulations; StO_2, tissue oxygen saturation; TR, time resolution.

a specific stimulation leads to an increase in the local oxygen consumption, immediately followed by an increase in blood flow that in turn changes the oxygenation and hemoglobin concentrations, ie, an increase in O_2Hb and tHb and a decrease in HHb. The relative local hyperoxygenation may be necessary to create a steeper gradient of oxygen concentration from capillary to mitochondrion, to drive the higher diffusion of oxygen needed by the increased metabolism. In adults, these changes occur within a few seconds after the onset of the stimulation, are reproducible[90,91] and highly localized,[92] and have been extensively studied by NIRI as well as by functional MR, using the BOLD (blood oxygen level dependent) effect (for reviews see Wolf and colleagues,[10] Hoshi,[93,94] and Obrig and Villringer).[95]

There are 26 reports in the literature on hemodynamic effects using NIRI in neonates (overview in **Table 5**). The stimuli can be divided into five categories: visual, auditory, somatosensory, and olfactory stimulations, and spontaneous arousals.

For visual stimulation in young infants, flashing or blinking light sources were used because infants were asleep and the stimulation had to occur through closed eyelids. Older and awake infants were exposed also to animations or reversing checkerboard patterns (for details see **Table. 5**). It is interesting to look at the changes observed. Most of the studies show an increase of O_2Hb as well as HHb (see **Table 5**). In adults, usually a decrease in HHb is observed.[10,95]

A wide variety of sounds were used for auditory stimulation: artificial sounds, music, and speech (see **Table 5**). According to **Table 5**, it seems that generally an increase in O_2Hb and tHb is observed during stimulation. Some studies show that the response depends on the type of stimulation; for example, adult-directed or monotonous speech leads to decreases in O_2Hb concentration.[108,109] The same can be observed in infants with hypoxic-ischemic encephalopathy. Again in these mostly term infants, an increase in HHb is observed.[104]

Somatosensory stimulation consists of flexing of limbs, pain, or tactile or kangaroo care (see **Table 5**). The response to tactile stimulation or flexing of a limb mostly consists of an increase in O_2Hb and tHb. The change in HHb is unclear and often not reported. The results of Hintz[112] are unusual, not only because O_2Hb decreases and HHb increases, but also because of the enormous size of the increase in HHb of 150 μM, twice the total hemoglobin concentration previously reported for preterm infants.[120] Pain leads to an increase in tHb and O_2Hb, whereas kangaroo care leads to a decrease in StO_2, which indicates a deactivation [57]

Pleasant olfactory stimulation leads to an increase in O_2Hb and tHb, whereas neutral stimuli like colostrum or water do not evoke detectable changes.[117] Unpleasant odors lead to the opposite, a decrease in O_2Hb and tHb. The latter is explained by the authors as a deactivation of the brain.[118]

Spontaneous arousals do not evoke any significant changes.[119] In many of the cited studies, effects were visible only in the group averages, which is fine for research applications. Thus, in the following we will discuss methodological issues that have to be solved.

Spontaneous changes in blood volume are common, eg, the so-called Mayer waves or slow vasomotion at 0.1 Hz. Such changes are approximately of the same size as functional activations and thus may be mistaken. It is vital that whenever possible, stimuli are repeated at least 10 times. In 8 of the 26 studies, stimuli were not repeated, although doing so would have been possible. By taking a time-triggered average, the influence of spontaneous changes, which are not synchronized with the stimulation, is reduced. In addition, the length of the recovery periods between stimulations should be randomly varied by a certain degree to avoid synchronization. Random variation of recovery period lengths leads to a more powerful time-triggered average.

Movement artifacts are a significant problem during functional NIRI studies, particularly because neonates will not always be quiet. Movement leads to changes in the hemoglobin concentration because the sensor locations shift, the light coupling between sensor and tissue changes, the sensor deforms geometrically, and/or blood volume in tissue alters. Often movement artifacts lead to abrupt concentration changes, which are easy to detect by eye. However, movement artifacts cannot be separated from real functional changes in all cases. In principle, movement can be detected by accelerometry, but none of the commercially available instruments includes this capability. Another, more sophisticated possibility is the recording of a video during the measurement.[107] Again, a sufficient number of repetitions of the stimulus will ensure that after the removal of sections with artifacts, a stable time-triggered average is obtained.

After data analysis, the question is how activation is identified. After a time-triggered average, there will always be some variation in the O_2Hb, HHb, and tHb traces. Thus, detection criteria are necessary. In 14 of the 26 studies, no such criteria were reported. Often statistical detection criteria were used, eg, a paired t test or Wilcoxon test that compares the last 10 seconds of the measurement before stimulation to the last 10 seconds of the period of stimulation.[101] Future studies should make use of such a criterion. From a clinical point of view, it would be worthwhile in the future also to generate criteria to identify areas without activation. If data analysis is performed online during the measurement, it would be ideal to use these criteria to adjust the lengths of a measurement until it is clear whether activation is identified or not.

A wealth of clinical and research applications of NIRI are envisioned. In the following we will characterize examples of interesting questions.

Kotilahti and colleagues[107] found that sleep stage affects functional activity. Begum and colleagues[57] found that kangaroo care reduced power spectral density in StO_2. This finding was most likely related to more quiet sleep, and more cardiorespiratory stability.

In contrast, pain[114,115,121] increases oxygenation and thus indicates higher activity. Pain is a very important area because iatrogenic pain is a major problem during neonatal intensive care and the study of pain in newborns is hampered by the lack of subjective report. We would like to point out, however, that it is very difficult to study pain with NIRI, because painful events invariably lead to many systemic changes and in particular to movement artifacts. We know of several groups (private communication) who attempted to study pain with NIRI and eventually gave up.

Chen and colleagues[104] found that the auditory functional response of healthy infants (both O_2Hb and total hemoglobin [tHb] increase) is highly significantly different from that of infants suffering from hypoxic-ischemic encephalopathy (in most of the infants, both O_2Hb and tHb decrease). This article clearly demonstrates that NIRI may supplement/replace evoked EEG potentials to assess and understand the effects of brain injury and possibly predict outcome.

Normal brain development is little studied (for a review, see Johnson[122]). Johnson[122] outlines three hypotheses (maturational development, interactive specialization, and skill learning) regarding how this development takes place, which are considerably different from one another. These differences emphasize how little is known. One of the key questions that remains is to what degree development is guided by extrinsic environmental and intrinsic factors. Functional NIRI is applied in several recent studies investigating the interaction between the infant and his or her environment, eg, learning to distinguish objects[123] or televised and real motion,[124] face recognition,[125] and language development.[100] Because of the relative simplicity of NIRI compared with functional MRI and its much greater ease in application for neonates and small infants, NIRI has tremendous potential to close this gap.

Maturational Effects on the Vascular Response to Functional Activation

From **Table 5** it is obvious that O_2Hb and tHb are more reliable markers of brain activity than HHb. Depending on the age of infants and possibly other unknown factors, the HHb sometimes increases or decreases during activation. The concentration changes are smaller than for O_2Hb or tHb. Consequently, fewer activations are detected in HHb than in O_2Hb or tHb. The physiologic reason for this fact is that during an activation, the blood flow usually increases. Because HHb is washed out, its concentration decreases. At the same time, the blood volume increases, which leads to an increase in HHb. Depending on the balance between blood flow and volume increase, HHb may increase, decrease, or remain the same. In conclusion, HHb is not a reliable marker for an activation. This conclusion also has important implications for MRI, which usually uses the BOLD signal to detect an activation. The BOLD signal corresponds to HHb and thus from the results we predict that the BOLD signal misses many activations in neonates.

In adults, the HHb usually decreases clearly, a situation that appears to be very different in the neonate and in particular in preterm infants. This difference may have several explanations. First, the cerebral blood flow in neonates is approximately three times lower than in adults[126]; cerebral blood volume is approximately half,[120,127] whereas resting venous oxygen saturation is similar.[128] This fact in itself is expected to result in a different ratio of the change of blood volume to blood flow.[129] Second, although the flow-metabolism coupling appears to operate even in the preterm,[130] many molecular mechanisms are involved, such as local pH, pCO_2, adenosine, NO, and collateral innervation of local blood vessels.[131,132] This redundancy makes sense for a vital function. But not all these mechanisms may mature at the same rate, and the results of the studies in **Table 5** indicate that maturation is still going on and affects the response to functional activity.

It has also been shown that age affects functional activity. For example, the latency of the hemodynamic response after the beginning of stimulation was found to decrease with age.[107,110] The interpretation was that this decrease may be related to myelinization of the afferent fibers and hence to the delay from sensory organ to the cortex. However, the delay latency decreased by a few seconds, which cannot be explained by the fraction of a second that is gained by myelinization. More likely there is a decreased latency in neurovascular coupling. Also, the HHb response in preterm infants seems to be similar to that in adults, whereas in older infants it is inversed, as pointed out previously. Thus, the development of the flow-metabolism coupling may be followed using NIRS.

Conclusion

NIRI is able to assess functioning and development of the brain noninvasively at the bedside, and the cited studies (see **Table 5**) demonstrate that NIRI is a potentially very powerful diagnostic tool. In many of the cited studies, effects were visible only in the group averages, which is fine for research applications. Before NIRI enters routine clinical procedure, however, it must necessarily provide reliable measurements in a single patient, which could be shown by repeatability studies similar to those performed for adults.[90,91]

Normal brain development is little studied. Because of the relative simplicity of NIRI compared with functional MRI and its much greater ease in application for neonates and small infants, NIRI has tremendous potential to close this gap.

SUMMARY

Near-infrared spectrometry (NIRS) and imaging (NIRI) to study preterm and newborn infants are reviewed. Two main applications of NIRS and NIRI are discussed:

1. The measurement of cerebral autoregulation, blood volume, flow, and oxygenation. Here the future aim is to safeguard the brain by adjusting the blood and oxygen supply to the brain to adequate levels and to prevent brain lesions. For this purpose, instrumentation, which provides absolute values of tissue oxygenation is available and discussed. So far, the low precision of NIRS tissue oximetry is a problem for making clinical decisions by comparison of the reading in a single infant to a threshold for action. Furthermore, added value should be demonstrated, ie, that prediction is improved over and above that already possible by the use of conventional clinical data.
2. The assessment of brain activity. This is the domain of NIRI instruments, which provide maps of functional brain activity and are discussed. Here the aim is to develop functional tests to understand neonatal brain activity. So far, interesting studies on cognitive function and brain development demonstrate the excellent value of NIRI as a research tool. This will grow in the future. Before applying NIRI in clinical routine, important aspects such as reproducibility, sensitivity, specificity, and prognostic value for individual patients have to be studied. In the future, such tests may enable an early detection and prognosis of disabilities and may help to guide therapy.

REFERENCES

1. Choi J, Wolf M, Toronov V, et al. Noninvasive determination of the optical properties of adult brain: near-infrared spectroscopy approach. J Biomed Opt 2004;9:221–9.
2. Wray S, Cope M, Delpy DT, et al. Characterization of the near infrared absorption spectra of cytochrome aa3 and haemoglobin for the non-invasive monitoring of cerebral oxygenation. Biochim Biophys Acta 1988;933:184–92.
3. Zijlstra WG, Buursma A, van Assendelft OW. Visible and near infrared absorption spectra of human and animal haemoglobin. Utrecht: VSP; 2000.
4. Cope M: The application of near infrared spectroscopy to non invasive monitoring of cerebral oxygenation in the newborn infant, in Department of Medical Physics and Bioengineering. London: University of London, 1991, Vol Ph D
5. Okada E, Delpy DT. The effect of overlying tissue on NIR light propagation in neonatal brain. In OSA TOPS on Advances in Optical Imaging and Photon Migration, Washington, 338–43.
6. Leung TS, Elwell CE, Delpy DT. Estimation of cerebral oxy- and deoxy-haemoglobin concentration changes in a layered adult head model using near-infrared spectroscopy and multivariate statistical analysis. Phys Med Biol 2005;50: 5783–98.
7. Liu H, Chance B, Hielscher AH, et al. Influence of blood vessels on the measurement of hemoglobin oxygenation as determined by time-resolved reflectance spectroscopy. Med Phys 1995;22:1209–17.

8. Madsen PL, Skak C, Rasmussen A, et al. Interference of cerebral near-infrared oximetry in patients with icterus. Anesth Analg 2000;90:489–93.

9. Franceschini MA, Fantini S, Paunescu LA, et al. Influence of a superficial layer in the quantitative spectroscopic study of strongly scattering media. Appl Opt 1998;37:7447–58.

10. Wolf M, Ferrari M, Quaresima V. Progress of near-infrared spectroscopy and topography for brain and muscle clinical applications. J Biomed Opt 2007;12:062104.

11. Benni PB, Chen B, Dykes FD, et al. Validation of the CAS neonatal NIRS system by monitoring vv-ECMO patients: preliminary results. Adv Exp Med Biol 2005;566:195–201.

12. Rais-Bahrami K, Rivera O, Short BL. Validation of a noninvasive neonatal optical cerebral oximeter in veno-venous ECMO patients with a cephalad catheter. J Perinatol 2006;26:628–35.

13. Bland JM, Altman DG. Statistical methods for assessing agreement between two methods of clinical measurement. Lancet 1986;1:307–10.

14. Bhutta AT, Ford JW, Parker JG, et al. Noninvasive cerebral oximeter as a surrogate for mixed venous saturation in children. Pediatr Cardiol 2007;28:34–41.

15. Daubeney PE, Pilkington SN, Janke E, et al. Cerebral oxygenation measured by near-infrared spectroscopy: comparison with jugular bulb oximetry. Ann Thorac Surg 1996;61:930–4.

16. Knirsch W, Stutz K, Kretschmar O, et al. Regional cerebral oxygenation by NIRS does not correlate with central or jugular venous oxygen saturation during interventional catheterisation in children. Acta Anaesthesiol Scand 2008;52:1370–4.

17. Nagdyman N, Fleck T, Barth S, et al. Relation of cerebral tissue oxygenation index to central venous oxygen saturation in children. Intensive Care Med 2004;30:468–71.

18. Ranucci M, Isgro G, De la Torre T, et al. Near-infrared spectroscopy correlates with continuous superior vena cava oxygen saturation in pediatric cardiac surgery patients. Paediatr Anaesth 2008;18:1163–9.

19. Shimizu N, Gilder F, Bissonnette B, et al. Brain tissue oxygenation index measured by near infrared spatially resolved spectroscopy agreed with jugular bulb oxygen saturation in normal pediatric brain: a pilot study. Childs Nerv Syst 2005;21:181–4.

20. Weiss M, Dullenkopf A, Kolarova A, et al. Near-infrared spectroscopic cerebral oxygenation reading in neonates and infants is associated with central venous oxygen saturation. Paediatr Anaesth 2005;15:102–9.

21. Lemmers PM, van Bel F. Left-to-right differences of regional cerebral oxygen saturation and oxygen extraction in preterm infants during the first days of life. Pediatr Res 2009;65:226–30.

22. Sorensen LC, Greisen G. Precision of measurement of cerebral tissue oxygenation index using near-infrared spectroscopy in preterm neonates. J Biomed Opt 2006;11:054005.

23. Hou X, Ding H, Teng Y, et al. Research on the relationship between brain anoxia at different regional oxygen saturations and brain damage using near-infrared spectroscopy. Physiol Meas 2007;28:1251–65.

24. Kurth CD, McCann JC, Wu J, et al. Cerebral oxygen saturation-time threshold for hypoxic-ischemic injury in piglets. Anesth Analg 2009;108:1268–77.

25. Jones TH, Morawetz RB, Crowell RM, et al. Thresholds of focal cerebral ischemia in awake monkeys. J Neurosurg 1981;54:773–82.

26. Toet MC, Flinterman A, Laar I, et al. Cerebral oxygen saturation and electrical brain activity before, during, and up to 36 hours after arterial switch procedure in neonates without pre-existing brain damage: its relationship to neurodevelopmental outcome. Exp Brain Res 2005;165:343–50.

27. Phelps HM, Mahle WT, Kim D, et al. Postoperative cerebral oxygenation in hypoplastic left heart syndrome after the Norwood procedure. Ann Thorac Surg 2009; 87:1490–4.

28. Skov L, Brun NC, Greisen G. Neonatal intensive care: an obvious yet difficult area for near infrared spectroscopy. J Biomed Opt 1997;2:7–14.

29. Wolfberg AJ, du Plessis AJ. Near-infrared spectroscopy in the fetus and neonate. Clin Perinatol 2006;33:707–28, viii.

30. Tsuji M, Saul JP, du Plessis A, et al. Cerebral intravascular oxygenation correlates with mean arterial pressure in critically ill premature infants. Pediatrics 2000;106:625–32.

31. Soul JS, Hammer PE, Tsuji M, et al. Fluctuating pressure-passivity is common in the cerebral circulation of sick premature infants. Pediatr Res 2007;61:467–73.

32. Wong FY, Barfield CP, Campbell L, et al. Validation of cerebral venous oxygenation measured using near-infrared spectroscopy and partial jugular venous occlusion in the newborn lamb. J Cereb Blood Flow Metab 2008;28:74–80.

33. Greisen G. Is near-infrared spectroscopy living up to its promises? Semin Fetal Neonatal Med 2006;11:498–502.

34. Isobe K, Kusaka T, Fujikawa Y, et al. Changes in cerebral hemoglobin concentration and oxygen saturation immediately after birth in the human neonate using full-spectrum near infrared spectroscopy. J Biomed Opt 2000;5:283–6.

35. Wolf M, von Siebenthal K, Keel M, et al. Tissue oxygen saturation measured by near infrared spectrophotometry correlates with arterial oxygen saturation during induced oxygenation changes in neonates. Physiol Meas 2000;21:481–91.

36. Isobe K, Kusaka T, Fujikawa Y, et al. Measurement of cerebral oxygenation in neonates after vaginal delivery and cesarean section using full-spectrum near infrared spectroscopy. Comp Biochem Physiol A Mol Integr Physiol 2002;132: 133–8.

37. Schrod L, Walter J. Effect of head-up body tilt position on autonomic function and cerebral oxygenation in preterm infants. Biol Neonate 2002;81:255–9.

38. Schulz G, Keller E, Haensse D, et al. Slow blood sampling from an umbilical artery catheter prevents a decrease in cerebral oxygenation in the preterm newborn. Pediatrics 2003;111:e73–6.

39. Huang L, Ding H, Hou X, et al. Assessment of the hypoxic-ischemic encephalopathy in neonates using non-invasive near-infrared spectroscopy. Physiol Meas 2004;25:749–61.

40. Naulaers G, Cossey V, Morren G, et al. Continuous measurement of cerebral blood volume and oxygenation during rewarming of neonates. Acta Paediatr 2004;93:1540–2.

41. Shuhaiber H, Bolton S, Alfonso I, et al. Cerebral regional oxygen fluctuations and decline during clinically silent focal electroencephalographic seizures in a neonate. J Child Neurol 2004;19:539–40.

42. Catelin C, Tordjman S, Morin V, et al. Clinical, physiologic, and biologic impact of environmental and behavioral interventions in neonates during a routine nursing procedure. J Pain 2005;6:791–7.

43. Dotta A, Rechichi J, Campi F, et al. Effects of surgical repair of congenital diaphragmatic hernia on cerebral hemodynamics evaluated by near-infrared spectroscopy. J Pediatr Surg 2005;40:1748–52.

44. Elwell CE, Henty JR, Leung TS, et al. Measurement of CMRO2 in neonates undergoing intensive care using near infrared spectroscopy. Adv Exp Med Biol 2005;566:263–8.
45. Ijichi S, Kusaka T, Isobe K, et al. Developmental changes of optical properties in neonates determined by near-infrared time-resolved spectroscopy. Pediatr Res 2005;58:568–73.
46. Zhao J, Ding HS, Hou XL, et al. In vivo determination of the optical properties of infant brain using frequency-domain near-infrared spectroscopy. J Biomed Opt 2005;10:024028.
47. Ejike JC, Schenkman KA, Seidel K, et al. Cerebral oxygenation in neonatal and pediatric patients during veno-arterial extracorporeal life support. Pediatr Crit Care Med 2006;7:154–8.
48. Lemmers PM, Toet M, van Schelven LJ, et al. Cerebral oxygenation and cerebral oxygen extraction in the preterm infant: the impact of respiratory distress syndrome. Exp Brain Res 2006;173:458–67.
49. Li ZG, Ye WF, Wen FQ, et al. [Regional cerebral oxygen saturation in neonates with meconium aspiration syndrome]. Zhongguo Dang Dai Er Ke Za Zhi 2006; 8:191–4 [in Chinese].
50. Petrova A, Mehta R. Near-infrared spectroscopy in the detection of regional tissue oxygenation during hypoxic events in preterm infants undergoing critical care. Pediatr Crit Care Med 2006;7:449–54.
51. Toet MC, Lemmers PM, van Schelven LJ, et al. Cerebral oxygenation and electrical activity after birth asphyxia: their relation to outcome. Pediatrics 2006;117:333–9.
52. Zaramella P, Freato F, Quaresima V, et al. Surgical closure of patent ductus arteriosus reduces the cerebral tissue oxygenation index in preterm infants: a near-infrared spectroscopy and Doppler study. Pediatr Int 2006;48:305–12.
53. Baenziger O, Stolkin F, Keel M, et al. The influence of the timing of cord clamping on postnatal cerebral oxygenation in preterm neonates: a randomized, controlled trial. Pediatrics 2007;119:455–9.
54. Dani C, Bertini G, Cecchi A, et al. Brain haemodynamic effects of nasal continuous airway pressure in preterm infants of less than 30 weeks' gestation. Acta Paediatr 2007;96:1421–5.
55. Huning BM, Horsch S, Roll C. Blood sampling via umbilical vein catheters decreases cerebral oxygenation and blood volume in preterm infants. Acta Paediatr 2007;96:1617–21.
56. Romeo DM, Betta P, Sanges G, et al. [Cerebral hemodynamics and major surgery]. Minerva Pediatr 2007;59:233–7 [in Italian].
57. Begum EA, Bonno M, Ohtani N, et al. Cerebral oxygenation responses during kangaroo care in low birth weight infants. BMC Pediatr 2008;8:51.
58. Lemmers PM, Toet MC, van Bel F. Impact of patent ductus arteriosus and subsequent therapy with indomethacin on cerebral oxygenation in preterm infants. Pediatrics 2008;121:142–7.
59. Sorensen LC, Leung TS, Greisen G. Comparison of cerebral oxygen saturation in premature infants by near-infrared spatially resolved spectroscopy: observations on probe-dependent bias. J Biomed Opt 2008;13:064013.
60. Sorensen LC, Maroun LL, Borch K, et al. Neonatal cerebral oxygenation is not linked to foetal vasculitis and predicts intraventricular haemorrhage in preterm infants. Acta Paediatr 2008;97:1529–34.
61. Vanderhaegen J, De Smet D, Meyns B, et al. Surgical closure of the patent ductus arteriosus and its effect on the cerebral tissue oxygenation. Acta Paediatr 2008;97:1640–4.

62. Wong FY, Leung TS, Austin T, et al. Impaired autoregulation in preterm infants identified by using spatially resolved spectroscopy. Pediatrics 2008;121: e604–11.

63. De Smet D, Vanderhaegen J, Naulaers G, et al. New measurements for assessment of impaired cerebral autoregulation using near-infrared spectroscopy. Adv Exp Med Biol 2009;645:273–8.

64. Moran M, Miletin J, Pichova K, et al. Cerebral tissue oxygenation index and superior vena cava blood flow in the very low birth weight infant. Acta Paediatr 2009;98:43–6.

65. Vanderhaegen J, Naulaers G, Vanhole C, et al. The effect of changes in tPCO2 on the fractional tissue oxygen extraction—as measured by near-infrared spectroscopy—in neonates during the first days of life. Eur J Paediatr Neurol 2009; 13:128–34.

66. Pigula FA, Nemoto EM, Griffith BP, et al. Regional low-flow perfusion provides cerebral circulatory support during neonatal aortic arch reconstruction. J Thorac Cardiovasc Surg 2000;119:331–9.

67. Kurth CD, Steven JL, Montenegro LM, et al. Cerebral oxygen saturation before congenital heart surgery. Ann Thorac Surg 2001;72:187–92.

68. Tabbutt S, Ramamoorthy C, Montenegro LM, et al. Impact of inspired gas mixtures on preoperative infants with hypoplastic left heart syndrome during controlled ventilation. Circulation 2001;104:I159–64.

69. Ramamoorthy C, Tabbutt S, Kurth CD, et al. Effects of inspired hypoxic and hypercapnic gas mixtures on cerebral oxygen saturation in neonates with univentricular heart defects. Anesthesiology 2002;96:283–8.

70. Andropoulos DB, Stayer SA, McKenzie ED, et al. Regional low-flow perfusion provides comparable blood flow and oxygenation to both cerebral hemispheres during neonatal aortic arch reconstruction. J Thorac Cardiovasc Surg 2003;126: 1712–7.

71. Andropoulos DB, Diaz LK, Fraser CD Jr, et al. Is bilateral monitoring of cerebral oxygen saturation necessary during neonatal aortic arch reconstruction? Anesth Analg 2004;98:1267–72, table of contents.

72. Hoffman GM, Stuth EA, Jaquiss RD, et al. Changes in cerebral and somatic oxygenation during stage 1 palliation of hypoplastic left heart syndrome using continuous regional cerebral perfusion. J Thorac Cardiovasc Surg 2004;127: 223–33.

73. Kilpack VD, Stayer SA, McKenzie ED, et al. Limiting circulatory arrest using regional low flow perfusion. J Extra Corpor Technol 2004;36:133–8.

74. Hofer A, Haizinger B, Geiselseder G, et al. Monitoring of selective antegrade cerebral perfusion using near infrared spectroscopy in neonatal aortic arch surgery. Eur J Anaesthesiol 2005;22:293–8.

75. Kussman BD, Wypij D, DiNardo JA, et al. An evaluation of bilateral monitoring of cerebral oxygen saturation during pediatric cardiac surgery. Anesth Analg 2005; 101:1294–300.

76. Scholl FG, Webb D, Christian K, et al. Rapid diagnosis of cannula migration by cerebral oximetry in neonatal arch repair. Ann Thorac Surg 2006;82:325–7.

77. McQuillen PS, Nishimoto MS, Bottrell CL, et al. Regional and central venous oxygen saturation monitoring following pediatric cardiac surgery: concordance and association with clinical variables. Pediatr Crit Care Med 2007;8:154–60.

78. Farouk A, Karimi M, Henderson M, et al. Cerebral regional oxygenation during aortic coarctation repair in pediatric population. Eur J Cardiothorac Surg 2008;34:26–31.

79. Li J, Zhang G, Holtby H, et al. Carbon dioxide—a complex gas in a complex circulation: its effects on systemic hemodynamics and oxygen transport, cerebral, and splanchnic circulation in neonates after the Norwood procedure. J Thorac Cardiovasc Surg 2008;136:1207–14.

80. Li J, Zhang G, Holtby H, et al. The influence of systemic hemodynamics and oxygen transport on cerebral oxygen saturation in neonates after the Norwood procedure. J Thorac Cardiovasc Surg 2008;135:83–90, 90 e81–2.

81. Redlin M, Koster A, Huebler M, et al. Regional differences in tissue oxygenation during cardiopulmonary bypass for correction of congenital heart disease in neonates and small infants: relevance of near-infrared spectroscopy. J Thorac Cardiovasc Surg 2008;136:962–7.

82. Johnson BA, Hoffman GM, Tweddell JS, et al. Near-infrared spectroscopy in neonates before palliation of hypoplastic left heart syndrome. Ann Thorac Surg 2009;87:571–9.

83. Maher KO, Phelps HM, Kirshbom PM. Near infrared spectroscopy changes with pericardial tamponade. Pediatr Crit Care Med 2009;10:e13–5.

84. Mascio CE, Myers JA, Edmonds HL, et al. Near-infrared spectroscopy as a guide for an intermittent cerebral perfusion strategy during neonatal circulatory arrest. ASAIO J 2009;55:287–90.

85. Tobias JD, Russo P, Russo J. Changes in near infrared spectroscopy during deep hypothermic circulatory arrest. Ann Card Anaesth 2009;12:17–21.

86. Levene MI, Sands C, Grindulis H, et al. Comparison of two methods of predicting outcome in perinatal asphyxia. Lancet 1986;1:67–9.

87. Pryds O, Greisen G, Lou H, et al. Vasoparalysis associated with brain damage in asphyxiated term infants. J Pediatr 1990;117:119–25.

88. Hoffman GM. Pro: near-infrared spectroscopy should be used for all cardiopulmonary bypass. J Cardiothorac Vasc Anesth 2006;20:606–12.

89. Wolf M, Morren G, Haensse D, et al. Near infrared spectroscopy to study the brain: an overview. Opto-Electron Rev 2008;16:413–9.

90. Plichta MM, Herrmann MJ, Baehne CG, et al. Event-related functional near-infrared spectroscopy (fNIRS): are the measurements reliable? Neuroimage 2006;31:116–24.

91. Kono T, Matsuo K, Tsunashima K, et al. Multiple-time replicability of near-infrared spectroscopy recording during prefrontal activation task in healthy men. Neurosci Res 2007;57:504–12.

92. Zeff BW, White BR, Dehghani H, et al. Retinotopic mapping of adult human visual cortex with high-density diffuse optical tomography. Proc Natl Acad Sci U S A 2007;104:12169–74.

93. Hoshi Y. Functional near-infrared optical imaging: utility and limitations in human brain mapping. Psychophysiology 2003;40:511–20.

94. Hoshi Y. Functional near-infrared spectroscopy: potential and limitations in neuroimaging studies. Int Rev Neurobiol 2005;66:237–66.

95. Obrig H, Villringer A. Beyond the visible—imaging the human brain with light. J Cereb Blood Flow Metab 2003;23:1–18.

96. Meek JH, Firbank M, Elwell CE, et al. Regional hemodynamic responses to visual stimulation in awake infants. Pediatr Res 1998;43:840–3.

97. Hoshi Y, Kohri S, Matsumoto Y, et al. Hemodynamic responses to photic stimulation in neonates. Pediatr Neurol 2000;23:323–7.

98. Taga G, Asakawa K, Hirasawa K, et al. Hemodynamic responses to visual stimulation in occipital and frontal cortex of newborn infants: a near-infrared optical topography study. Early Hum Dev 2003;75(Suppl):S203–10.

99. Kusaka T, Kawada K, Okubo K, et al. Noninvasive optical imaging in the visual cortex in young infants. Hum Brain Mapp 2004;22:122–32.

100. Bortfeld H, Wruck E, Boas DA. Assessing infants' cortical response to speech using near-infrared spectroscopy. Neuroimage 2007;34:407–15.

101. Karen T, Morren G, Haensse D, et al. Hemodynamic response to visual stimulation in newborn infants using functional near-infrared spectroscopy. Hum Brain Mapp 2008;29:453–60.

102. Sakatani K, Chen S, Lichty W, et al. Cerebral blood oxygenation changes induced by auditory stimulation in newborn infants measured by near infrared spectroscopy. Early Hum Dev 1999;55:229–36.

103. Zaramella P, Freato F, Amigoni A, et al. Brain auditory activation measured by near-infrared spectroscopy (NIRS) in neonates. Pediatr Res 2001;49:213–9.

104. Chen S, Sakatani K, Lichty W, et al. Auditory-evoked cerebral oxygenation changes in hypoxic-ischemic encephalopathy of newborn infants monitored by near infrared spectroscopy. Early Hum Dev 2002;67:113–21.

105. Pena M, Maki A, Kovacic D, et al. Sounds and silence: an optical topography study of language recognition at birth. Proc Natl Acad Sci U S A 2003;100:11702–5.

106. Nissila I, Kotilahti K, Huotilainen M, et al. Auditory hemodynamic studies of newborn infants using near-infrared spectroscopic imaging. Conf Proc IEEE Eng Med Biol Soc 2004;2:1244–7.

107. Kotilahti K, Nissila I, Huotilainen M, et al. Bilateral hemodynamic responses to auditory stimulation in newborn infants. Neuroreport 2005;16:1373–7.

108. Saito Y, Aoyama S, Kondo T, et al. Frontal cerebral blood flow change associated with infant-directed speech. Arch Dis Child Fetal Neonatal Ed 2007;92:F113–6.

109. Saito Y, Kondo T, Aoyama S, et al. The function of the frontal lobe in neonates for response to a prosodic voice. Early Hum Dev 2007;83:225–30.

110. Nishida T, Kusaka T, Isobe K, et al. Extrauterine environment affects the cortical responses to verbal stimulation in preterm infants. Neurosci Lett 2008;443:23–6.

111. Isobe K, Kusaka T, Nagano K, et al. Functional imaging of the brain in sedated newborn infants using near infrared topography during passive knee movement. Neurosci Lett 2001;299:221–4.

112. Hintz SR, Benaron DA, Siegel AM, et al. Bedside functional imaging of the premature infant brain during passive motor activation. J Perinat Med 2001;29:335–43.

113. Gibson AP, Austin T, Everdell NL, et al. Three-dimensional whole-head optical tomography of passive motor evoked responses in the neonate. Neuroimage 2006;30:521–8.

114. Bartocci M, Bergqvist LL, Lagercrantz H, et al. Pain activates cortical areas in the preterm newborn brain. Pain 2006;122:109–17.

115. Slater R, Cantarella A, Gallella S, et al. Cortical pain responses in human infants. J Neurosci 2006;26:3662–6.

116. Slater R, Cantarella A, Franck L, et al. How well do clinical pain assessment tools reflect pain in infants? PLoS Med 2008;5:e129.

117. Bartocci M, Winberg J, Ruggiero C, et al. Activation of olfactory cortex in newborn infants after odor stimulation: a functional near-infrared spectroscopy study. Pediatr Res 2000;48:18–23.

118. Bartocci M, Winberg J, Papendieck G, et al. Cerebral hemodynamic response to unpleasant odors in the preterm newborn measured by near-infrared spectroscopy. Pediatr Res 2001;50:324–30.

119. Zotter H, Urlesberger B, Kerbl R, et al. Cerebral hemodynamics during arousals in preterm infants. Early Hum Dev 2007;83:239–46.
120. Wolf M, Evans P, Bucher HU, et al. Measurement of absolute cerebral haemoglobin concentration in adults and neonates. Adv Exp Med Biol 1997;428:219–27.
121. Slater R, Fitzgerald M, Meek J. Can cortical responses following noxious stimulation inform us about pain processing in neonates? Semin Perinatol 2007;31: 298–302.
122. Johnson MH. Development of human brain functions. Biol Psychiatry 2003;54: 1312–6.
123. Wilcox T, Bortfeld H, Woods R, et al. Using near-infrared spectroscopy to assess neural activation during object processing in infants. J Biomed Opt 2005;10: 11010.
124. Shimada S, Hiraki K. Infant's brain responses to live and televised action. Neuroimage 2006;32:930–9.
125. Otsuka Y, Nakato E, Kanazawa S, et al. Neural activation to upright and inverted faces in infants measured by near infrared spectroscopy. Neuroimage 2007;34: 399–406.
126. Skov L, Pryds O, Greisen G. Estimating cerebral blood flow in newborn infants: comparison of near infrared spectroscopy and 133Xe clearance. Pediatr Res 1991;30:570–3.
127. Brun NC, Greisen G. Cerebrovascular responses to carbon dioxide as detected by near-infrared spectrophotometry: comparison of three different measures. Pediatr Res 1994;36:20–4.
128. Buchvald FF, Kesje K, Greisen G. Measurement of cerebral oxyhaemoglobin saturation and jugular blood flow in term healthy newborn infants by near-infrared spectroscopy and jugular venous occlusion. Biol Neonate 1999;75: 97–103.
129. Pryds O, Greisen G, Skov LL, et al. Carbon dioxide-related changes in cerebral blood volume and cerebral blood flow in mechanically ventilated preterm neonates: comparison of near infrared spectrophotometry and 133Xenon clearance. Pediatr Res 1990;27:445–9.
130. Greisen G, Hellstrom-Vestas L, Lou H, et al. Sleep-walking shifts and cerebral blood flow in stable preterm infants. Pediatr Res 1985;19:1156–9.
131. Koehler RC, Gebremedhin D, Harder DR. Role of astrocytes in cerebrovascular regulation. J Appl Physiol 2006;100:307–17.
132. Phillis JW. Adenosine and adenine nucleotides as regulators of cerebral blood flow: roles of acidosis, cell swelling, and KATP channels. Crit Rev Neurobiol 2004;16:237–70.

Hypoxic-Ischemic Encephalopathy in the Term Infant

Ali Fatemi, MD, Mary Ann Wilson, PhD, Michael V. Johnston, MD*

KEYWORDS

- Hypoxia-ischemia • Neonatal encephalopathy • Apoptosis
- Oxidative stress • Hypothermia

Hypoxia-ischemia in the perinatal period is an important cause of cerebral palsy and associated disabilities in children. Cerebral palsy is one of the most costly neurologic disabilities because of its frequency (2/1000 births) and persistence over the life span.[1] In the term infant, the most common mechanism of hypoxic injury is intrauterine asphyxia brought on by circulatory problems, such as clotting of placental arteries, placental abruption, or inflammatory processes.[2] These factors result in perinatal depression, leading to diminished exchange of oxygen and carbon dioxide and severe lactic acidosis.[2] A recent study by Graham and colleagues[3] showed that the incidence of neonatal neurologic morbidity and mortality for term infants born with cord pH less than 7.0 is approximately 25%. Reduced cardiac output in the setting of hypoxia is referred to as hypoxia-ischemia (HI).[4] If an episode of HI is severe enough to damage the brain, it leads within 12 to 36 hours to a neonatal encephalopathy known as hypoxic-ischemic encephalopathy (HIE).[5] This clinical syndrome includes seizures, epileptic activity on electroencephalogram (EEG), hypotonia, poor feeding, and a depressed level of consciousness that typically lasts from 7 to 14 days.[6] Pathology studies of term neonates who sustained a profound hypoxic-ischemic event show relative cortical sparing and deep gray matter injury, particularly involving hippocampi, lateral geniculate nuclei, putamen, ventrolateral thalami, and dorsal mesencephalon.[7] There is no effective pharmacologic therapy, although hypothermia has shown promise in several clinical trials.[8,9] Magnetic resonance imaging (MRI) has markedly improved the understanding of the patterns of brain injury from perinatal asphyxia. The pattern produced by so-called near-total asphyxia is easily recognized on MRI scans and includes selective injury to the putamen, thalamus, and perirolandic cerebral cortex, and often involves the brainstem as well.[10] This pattern is similar to

Support received from NIH R01-NS028208-17A2.

Kennedy Krieger Institute, Department of Neurology, Johns Hopkins Medical Institutions, 707 N Broadway, Baltimore, MD 21205, USA

* Corresponding author.

E-mail address: Johnston@kennedykrieger.org (M. V. Johnston).

the pathologic pattern of diencephalic and brainstem injury described by Myers in a model of acute total asphyxia in nonhuman primates, developed in the early 1970s.[11] This injury can be distinguished from that produced by a partial prolonged insult that results in more extensive cortical injury. In most infants, white matter is relatively spared, although a transient increase in the T2-weighted MRI signal is often seen in the posterior internal capsule soon after injury.[12] Infants who demonstrate this pattern of insult may require vigorous resuscitation to survive, and have severe metabolic acidosis in the umbilical cord blood.[13] Metabolic derangements leading to oxidative stress, inflammatory factors, excitotoxicity, and perhaps genetic factors are thought to contribute to brain injury after HIE.

DELAYED CELL DEATH IN HIE

Clinical and experimental observations demonstrate that HIE is not a single "event" but is rather an evolving process. The clinical signs of HIE reflect the evolution of a delayed cascade of molecular events triggered by the initial insult. MRI studies show progression of lesion size over the first few days after injury (**Fig. 1**).[14] Initial findings within the first few hours after near-total asphyxia are subtle and often seen only on diffusion-weighted imaging, which shows restricted diffusion typically starting as small lesions in the putamen and thalami, and usually progressing over the next 3 to 4 days to involve more extensive areas of the brain.[14] MR spectroscopy shows a similar pattern of progression, with an increase in lactic acid and reduction of N-acetyl-aspartate over the first few days after initial insult (**Fig. 2**).[15] Studies of animal models of HIE show that during the period after the insult, many neurons and other cells "commit" to die or survive over a period of days to weeks.[16] Many of them might be rescued during this "window of opportunity." Along with this notion, hypothermia has shown beneficial effect in HIE,[9] suggesting that intervention after birth is still helpful, possibly by preventing delayed cell death. Therefore, it is crucial to investigate molecular pathways involved in this event to identify potential therapeutic interventions.

Animal studies have led to new insights into HIE. Rodent models combine unilateral carotid artery ligation with exposure to a period of hypoxia to replicate the combination of hypoxemia and ischemia seen in human infants after asphyxia.[17] Comparison of histology from the animal model with MRI of human term infants after near-total asphyxia reveals remarkably similar patterns of injury to the basal ganglia and cerebral cortex.[10,13,16] Unilateral carotid ligation plus hypoxia results in predominant injury on one side with modest or no injury on the other.[18] These studies show that during the initial phase of HI there is rapid depletion of adenosine triphosphate (ATP),[19,20] leading to failure of Na/K-pump and depolarization of the cell, with severe cell swelling and cytoplasmic calcium accumulation, further leading to necrosis and activation of multiple cascades that eventually result in more cell death.

The form of cell death depends on the severity of ischemic injury.[21] Necrosis predominates in more severe cases, whereas apoptosis occurs in areas with milder ischemic injury, often days after the initial insult.[22] The authors have shown that activation of the proapoptotic protein, caspase-3, in a neonatal rodent model of cerebral hypoxia-ischemia is prolonged and that moderate to high levels of activated caspase-3 persist for at least 7 days after hypoxic-ischemic injury.[16] The regional and temporal patterns of caspase-3 activation correspond well with those for apoptosis,[16] lending further support for a prolonged role of apoptosis in hypoxic-ischemic injury in the neonatal brain. The newborn brain is primed to respond to various insults with activation of apoptotic cascades, due to the importance of programmed cell death in the

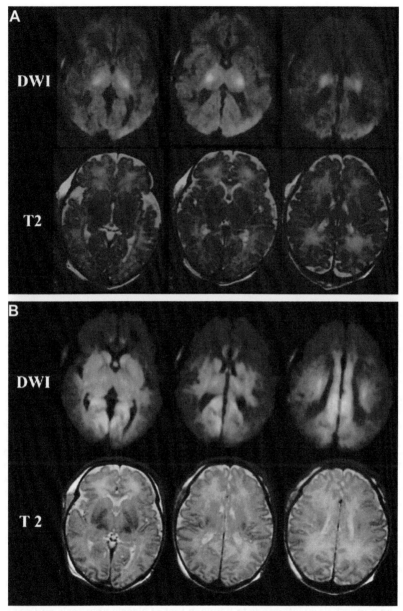

Fig. 1. Diffusion-weighted imaging (DWI) and T2-weighted imaging in a neonate with HIE 24 hours (*A*) and 3 days (*B*) after birth. DWI at 24 hours shows hyperintensities in the bilateral thalami and posterior limbs of the internal capsule (left > right), which are not recognized on T2-weighted images at the same levels. Repeat DWI at 3 days of life demonstrates diffuse hyperintensities in the bilateral basal ganglia and thalami as well as the internal capsule. Gyral enhancement consistent with cortical injury is observed in multiple areas, and is most prominent in the bilateral medial temporal and occipital lobes, and less evident in the parasagittal frontal and parietal lobes. These changes are present but much less prominent on T2-weighted images at the same levels. (*Modified from* Takeoka M, Soman TB, Yoshii A, et al. Diffusion-weighted images in neonatal cerebral hypoxic-ischemic injury. Pediatr Neurol 2002;26(4):277; with permission.)

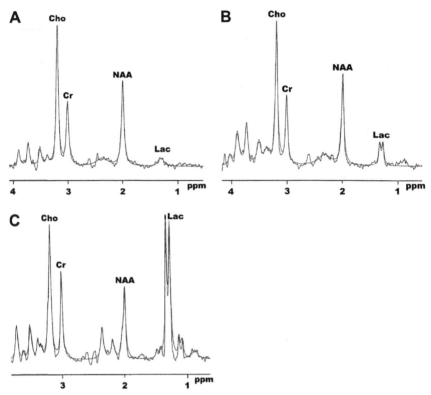

Fig. 2. Proton magnetic resonance spectroscopy in newborn infants after HI, showing choline (Cho), creatine (Cr), N-acetyl-aspartate (NAA), and lactate (Lac). (*A*) Spectra of a healthy newborn showing normal NAA to Creatine ratio, and minimum lactate double peak. (*B*) Newborn with moderate HIE, showing normal NAA, but elevated lactate double peak. (*C*) Newborn with severe HIE showing low NAA and markedly increased lactate. (*Modified from* Cheong JLY, Cady EB, Penrice J, et al. Proton MR spectroscopy in neonates with perinatal cerebral hypoxic-ischemic injury: metabolite peak-area ratios, relaxation times, and absolute concentrations. AJNR Am J Neuroradiol 2006;27:1549; with permission. Copyright © by American Society of Neuroradiology.)

normal development of the central nervous system (CNS).[23] Proapoptotic proteins are highly expressed in the developing brain,[24] and caspase-3 and -9 deficient mice present with severe brain overgrowth malformations.[25,26]

In addition to necrosis and apoptosis, neurons in rodents subjected to neonatal HI display morphologic features along an apoptosis-necrosis continuum.[16,27] Cells showing a morphology intermediate between that of classic apoptosis and necrosis, referred to as "hybrid" cells, are observed.[27] The nuclei of such cells have large, irregularly shaped chromatin clumps, similar to apoptotic neurons, but the cytoplasm shows changes similar to necrotic neurons (**Fig. 3**A, A1). A study by Northington and colleagues[28] showed that the evolution of this morphology coincides with mitochondrial bioenergetic and structural failure superimposed on activation of apoptotic pathways after neonatal HI. Bioenergetic failure likely prevents execution of a full apoptotic phenotype. Evidence that apoptotic pathways are activated following neonatal HI coexists with evidence for incomplete execution of these pathways, energy failure, and biochemical evidence of necrosis.[28] It is presumed that mitochondrial failure

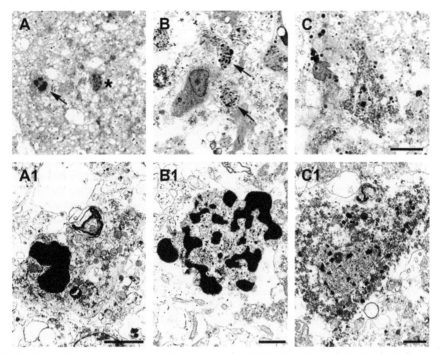

Fig. 3. Necrosis-apoptosis spectrum in neurons after HI in the neonatal rat. Nuclear changes in degenerating cells in cortex 48 hours after HI. Light microscopic photographs of 1 mm, Nissl-stained sections (*A–C*) and electron micrographs (*A1–C1*) are shown. An intermediate type of degenerating neurons was found, hybrid cells (*arrow* in A, A1) with large, chromatin clumps in the nucleus that were similar in size to those found in cells undergoing apoptosis but that were more irregular in shape. Typical necrotic neurons had smaller clumps of irregularly shaped, condensed chromatin (*asterisk* in A; *arrows* in B, B1). Necrotic neurons, which had a relatively homogeneous nucleus with a few irregular chromatin clumps and condensed granular cytoplasm (*C, C1*), and were typically found in adult ischemic models, were rarely identified in this model. *Scale bars*: A–C, 10 mm; A1, C1, 2 mm; B1, 1 mm. (*Reprinted from* Nakajima W, Ishida A, Lange MS, et al. Apoptosis has a prolonged role in the neurodegeneration after hypoxic ischemia in the newborn rat. J Neurosci 2000;20(21):8001; with permission.)

may interrupt apoptotic cascades initiated by injury to the immature rodent brain and result in the hybrid phenotype of neuronal cell death.

ROLE OF NEUROTRANSMITTER RECEPTORS AND EXCITOTOXICITY IN HYPOXIA-ISCHEMIA

Excitotoxicity has emerged as an important mechanism of injury in the brain, and the concept is important for understanding perinatal brain pathology. Glutamate is the predominant excitatory amino acid neurotransmitter in the brain, and most neurons and many glia possess receptors for glutamate.[29] Neuronal pathways that use glutamate as their neurotransmitter are ubiquitous in the brain, mediating vision, hearing, somatosensory function, learning and memory, and other functions.[30] The development of excitatory neuronal circuits, as well as expression of specific glutamate receptor subtypes in excitatory synapses, are dynamic in the perinatal brain, and these changes can be related to changing patterns of pathology at different gestational ages.[31,32] There are 3 major groups of glutamate receptors within the post-synaptic membrane that operate ion channels, so-called ionotropic receptors, and a group of G-protein linked metabotropic glutamate receptors. The 3 major types of ionotropic receptors are the N-methyl-D-aspartate (NMDA), α-amino-3-hydroxy-5-methylisoazole-4-propionic acid (AMPA), and kainic acid receptors. Glutamate normally is contained within the presynaptic nerve terminal until release is stimulated by neuronal depolarization[33]; when release into the synaptic cleft does occur, the neurotransmitter is quickly taken up by high-capacity glutamate transporters in astroglia that surround synapses and nerve terminals.[33] Glutamate taken up into the astroglia is converted to glutamine before being transported back into the nerve terminal to recycle glutamate neurotransmitter.[34] The glutamate transporter is dependent on a sodium gradient created by Na^+/K^+ ATPase that is powered by anaerobic glucose metabolism, and impaired delivery of glucose to the brain by ischemia or hypoglycemia impairs glutamate removal from the synapse.[35,36] Severe hypoxia associated with HI or ischemia also leads to reversal of glutamate transporters, presumably via a nuclear factor (NF)-κB mediated mechanism, leading to additional accumulation of synaptic glutamate.[37] Elevations in extracellular glutamate have been measured in animal models of perinatal HI using intracerebral microdialysis.[38,39] Whereas the accumulation of glutamate within synapses and in the brain's extracellular space is a generic phenomenon that occurs in most regions of the brain where glutamate-containing pathways are present, the toxic effect of this accumulation is determined by the local repertoire of postsynaptic glutamate receptors. The distribution and molecular characteristics of NMDA-type glutamate receptors seem to be an especially important determinant of the pattern of neuronal injury in the perinatal brain.[31] The NMDA receptor requires coactivation by both glutamate and glycine.[40,41] The NMDA receptor channel is blocked by magnesium at rest, and requires depolarization of the postsynaptic membrane for the channel to release this block and allow calcium to flux inward.[42] These special features allow the NMDA receptor to play a role in activity-dependent synaptic plasticity, including long-term potentiation (LTP) and refinement of synaptic connections.[31,43] However, failure of ATP-dependent Na^+ transport during HI disrupts membrane potentials, which can overcome the magnesium block and allow Ca^{2+} influx through the NMDA channels.[44,45] Drugs that block NMDA receptors or channels, such as dizocilpine (MK-801),[46] dextromethorphan,[47] ketamine,[48] or magnesium,[42] are strongly protective against hypoxic-ischemic injury if given before or shortly after HI or other insults in neonatal rodent models. At around 7 days of age the rodent brain is much more sensitive to direct intracerebral injections of NMDA, ibotenic acid, HI, or trauma than the adult brain.[17] Hypersensitivity to NMDA receptor activation during the neonatal period can be correlated with molecular features of the immature NMDA receptor channels that allow them to open more easily and flux more calcium than their adult counterparts.[40,49] NMDA receptors probably mediate much of the injury to neurons in structures such as cerebral cortex, basal ganglia, hippocampus, and thalamus, associated with hypoxic-ischemic injury in animal models.[29,50]

Activation of AMPA receptors, which primarily flux sodium and mediate most of the fast excitatory activity in the brain, also contribute to injury.[51] From a developmental standpoint, NMDA receptors are the first glutamate receptors to appear at new synapses, followed by AMPA receptors associated with increasing neuronal activity.[52,53] Immature AMPA receptor channels flux calcium similar to NMDA receptors, but increasing expression of GluR2 receptor subunits and RNA editing over the first 2 postnatal weeks in rodents shift the balance toward calcium-impermeable AMPA receptors in the mature brain.[51,54] Direct injection of AMPA agonists at various postnatal ages produces greater injury during the postnatal period than during adult-hood,[55] with a peak several days after that for NMDA. Calcium flooding through open NMDA and calcium-permeable AMPA receptor channels triggers a cascade of intra-cellular events that mediate cell death, including generation of reactive oxygen species (ROS) and activation of apoptotic pathways (**Fig. 4**).

AMPA antagonist drugs are not as protective against hypoxic-ischemic neuronal injury as NMDA antagonists in the perinatal period,[56] although the AMPA antagonist topiramate has been shown to be protective in combination with hypothermia in a model of hypoxic-ischemic injury in infant rats.[57] The molecular features of both NMDA and AMPA receptors during the perinatal period that enhance Ca^{2+} entry allow them to support activity-dependent neuronal plasticity and development. One indica-tion of their importance for normal development is the observation that prolonged blockade of NMDA receptors causes apoptosis in cell culture and animal models.[58] However, their vital role and enhanced function in the perinatal period also make

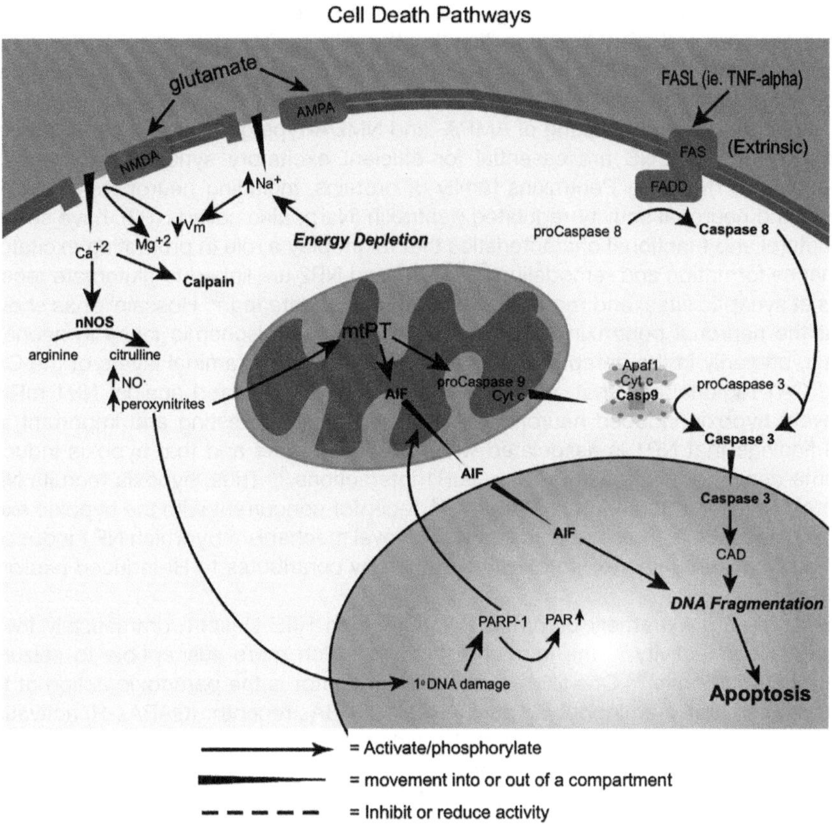

Cell Death Pathways

= Activate/phosphorylate

= movement into or out of a compartment

= Inhibit or reduce activity

Fig. 4. Cell death pathways involved in hypoxic-ischemic brain injury. AIF, apoptosis-inducing factor; AMPA, α-amino-3-hydroxy-5-methylisoazole-4-propionic acid; Apaf1, apoptotic protease activating factor 1; CAD, caspase-activated deoxyribonuclease; Casp9, caspase-9; Cyt c, cytochrome c; FADD, Fas-associated protein with death domain; FAS, Fas; FASL, Fas ligand; mtPT, mitochondrial permeability transition; NMDA, N-methyl-D-aspartate; NO, nitric oxide; nNOS, neuronal nitric oxide synthase; PAR, poly(ADP-ribose); PARP-1, poly(ADP-ribose) polymerase 1; TNF, tumor necrosis factor.

neurons more vulnerable to excitotoxicity, thus creating a paradox: the immature brain can withstand longer periods of energy deprivation than the adult brain because of its low energy requirement, yet when a critical threshold of energy deprivation is reached, excitotoxic injury is enhanced because of developmentally enhanced excitatory pathways.

In contrast to the probable role that NMDA receptors play in perinatal damage to the cerebral cortex, thalamus, and basal ganglia, AMPA and kainate receptors are implicated most strongly in perinatal damage to the brainstem.[29] Autoradiographic studies in human postmortem tissue indicate that AMPA or kainate receptor binding is elevated in these vulnerable regions in the midgestation fetus and neonate[59,60] and then declines at later ages, whereas NMDA receptor binding is undetectable at midgestation and then matures in the postnatal period. Elevated levels of AMPA/kainate receptors in the griseum pontis at midgestation and early infancy may be relevant to pontosubicular necrosis from HI during the last trimester and early infancy.[60] AMPA receptors probably mediate the stimulus of breathing movements via the nucleus of the solitary tract during the fetal period, whereas NMDA receptors likely mediate stimulation of this nucleus in response to hypoxia and sustained ventilation in the newborn and infant,[60] suggesting that the vulnerability of these brainstem structures to injury is related to the adaptive roles that the different types of glutamate receptors play in normal neuronal development and plasticity.

The targeting and clustering of AMPA- and NMDA-type glutamate receptors to the synapses in the CNS are essential for efficient excitatory synaptic transmission. Members of the Long Pentraxins family of proteins, including neuronal pentraxin 1 (NP1) and neuronal activity-regulated pentraxin (Narp, also called NP2), have several structural and functional characteristics that might play a role in promoting excitatory synapse formation and remodeling.[61,62] NP1 and NP2 are linked to glutamate receptors at synaptic sites, and regulate AMPA receptor clustering.[62] Hossain[61] has shown that the neuronal pentraxin NP1 is induced in hypoxic-ischemic injury in neonatal brain, primarily in the cerebral cortex and hippocampal pyramidal layers of the CA3 and CA1 regions, and that antisense oligonucleotides directed against NP1 mRNA prevent hypoxia-induced neuronal death. Particularly interesting and important are the findings that NP1 is associated with AMPA receptors and that hypoxia induces a time-dependent increase in NP1-GluR1 interactions.[62] Thus, hypoxia recruits NP1 protein to the GluR1 subunit of the AMPA receptor concurrent with the hypoxic excitotoxic cascade.[61] These results suggest a novel mechanism by which NP1 induction during HI accentuates excitotoxicity and thereby contributes to HI-induced neuronal death.

Seizures are extremely common in infants with HIE. Despite dramatically lower synaptic connectivity,[63] the immature brain is much more susceptible to seizures than the adult brain.[64] One likely proconvulsant factor is the paradoxic action of the neurotransmitter γ-aminobutyric acid (GABA). $GABA_A$ receptor ($GABA_A$-R) activation is inhibitory in the adult brain, both by virtue of the membrane hyperpolarization induced by chloride (Cl) influx through the $GABA_A$ ionophore and by virtue of shunting of dendritic excitatory inputs.[65] In the fetal and neonatal periods, however, the transmembrane chloride gradient is reversed.[65] As a result, $GABA_A$-R activation depolarizes the neuronal membrane. $GABA_A$ receptor-mediated synaptic currents with depolarizing reversal potentials are common in the embryonic and neonatal brain,[66] and are most likely explained by a high intracellular chloride concentration.[67] GABAergic synapses are established first and exert an excitatory action, as measured by the capacity for $GABA_A$ receptor activation to trigger action potentials in the postsynaptic cells.[68] In addition to triggering action potentials, the depolarizing action of GABA in the neonatal brain may induce Ca^{2+} entry through voltage-dependent Ca^{2+} channels,[69] contribute to removal of the Mg^{2+} block from NMDA channels, and further enhance glutamate excitotoxicity.

INFLAMMATORY MECHANISMS INVOLVED IN HYPOXIA-ISCHEMIA

Inflammatory cytokines have been associated with neonatal hypoxic-ischemic encephalopathy, and are significantly elevated in term infants who later develop cerebral palsy.[70] Elevated levels of interleukin (IL)-6 and IL-8 in the cerebrospinal fluid of term newborns have been correlated with an increased degree of encephalopathy and poor neurodevelopmental outcome.[71] A study employing MR spectroscopy demonstrated a correlation between elevated lactic acid level in the basal ganglia and serum IL-1, IL-6, IL-8, and tumor necrosis factor (TNF)-α levels in infants with HIE.[72] Studies in newborn mice subjected to unilateral carotid artery ligation demonstrate upregulation of many inflammatory genes associated with cellular activation in the injured hemisphere.[73] Inflammatory gene expression is evident at 8 hours and increases further at 24 to 72 hours post HI, and the set of genes that is expressed suggests activation of microglia and other inflammatory cells.[73] There is also increased chemokine expression and infiltration of inflammatory cells around the lesion.[74] Microglial aggregation in the dentate gyrus has been observed in human infants after HI insults.[75] Microglia may contribute to secondary brain injury through the production of proinflammatory cytokines, proteases, reactive oxygen species (ROS), nitric oxide (NO), complement factors, and excitotoxic neurotransmitters such as quinolinic acid.

There is now substantial experimental evidence that preexisting intrauterine inflammation can exacerbate HIE.[76,77] Lipopolysaccharide (LPS), also referred to as endotoxin, has been used extensively to induce an inflammatory response in animal models for HIE.[78–81] LPS binds to Toll-like receptor 4[76] and myeloid differentiation factor 88[82] to activate downstream signaling, including activation and nuclear translocation of the nuclear transcription factor NF-κB,[83] which promotes transcription of proinflammatory cytokines such as IL-1β, IL-6, TNF-α, prostaglandins, and a variety of adhesion molecules and acute-phase proteins.[84] NF-κB has been found in various cell populations in the brain including microglia, astrocytes, and neurons.[85] Wang and colleagues[80] demonstrated an upregulation of NF-κB in the fetal brain at an early stage after LPS administration. The timing of NF-κB elevation in this study corresponded with the cytokine changes that occur after intrauterine LPS administration. NF-κB has also been found to be involved in preconditioning-induced neuroprotection.[86] LPS treatment leads to activation of microglia with increased production of ROS and NO.[87] Astrocytes also play a significant role in inflammation following HI.[88,89] Astrocytes are the major source of IL-6 in CNS injury and inflammation.[89] Reactive astrocytes also release TNF-α and IL-6 through a carrier-dependent mechanism, which can result in sustained modulatory action on neighboring neurons.[88,90]

Low-dose treatment with intrauterine LPS, applied between the chorionic and amniotic membranes, dramatically increased the severity of injury after HI in neonatal mice but conferred protection against HI in adult rodents.[80] It seems, therefore, that inflammatory processes may either potentiate HI-induced injury or exert a neuroprotective effect in a time-dependent manner.

ROLE OF OXIDATIVE STRESS IN HYPOXIA-ISCHEMIA

Fetal life elapses in a low oxygen environment, with a mean intrauterine arterial oxygen saturation (SpO_2) under physiologic conditions of 40% to 45%.[91] In the first minutes of life, an abrupt increase of SpO_2 to 80% to 90% occurs, which creates a prooxidant condition.[92] This condition facilitates activation of specific metabolic pathways.[93] Under pathologic conditions, such as birth asphyxia, a series of pathophysiologic events, such as excess calcium influx via glutamate receptors, leads to severe oxidative stress.[94] There is accumulation of hydrogen peroxide (H_2O_2) after HI in neonatal mice but not in adult mice.[95] H_2O_2 may be the critical mediator in determining whether downstream signaling will favor cell death or repair. Repeated episodes of hypoxia cause purine derivatives, such as adenosine or hypoxanthine, to accumulate and promote specific changes that predispose cells to enhanced damage on reoxygenation.[96] Activation of oxidases and nitric oxide synthase (NOS), and upregulation of hypoxia-inducible factor-1α (HIF-1α), as well as downregulation of antioxidant enzymes, such as superoxide dismutases, catalases, and glutathione peroxidases, generate a burst of ROS on reoxygenation.[97] There is a marked increase in neuronal NOS (nNOS) immunoreactivity in nerve fibers for more than a week after HI in regions such as the thalamus.[98]

Nitric oxide synthase comprises a family of enzymes that produces NO. In addition, $\bullet$OH can react with NO to form a powerful oxidant and nitrosylating agent in the CNS, peroxynitrite.[99,100] Mitochondria seem to be a major target of ROS attack, and the immature brain is particularly susceptible to free radical injury because of its poorly developed scavenging systems and high availability of iron for the catalytic formation of hydroxyl radicals.[101] Formation of ROS in the brain after various insults is respiration dependent, mitochondria in vitro are sensitive to ROS and peroxynitrite, and most data suggest that oxidative stress contributes to the postischemic impairment of mitochondrial respiration.[102,103] When the ROS levels exceed the capacity of the cell in general and the mitochondria in particular to scavenge and render them harmless, the resulting oxidative stress may initiate mitochondrial permeability transition (mtPT),[104] which in turn potentiates the oxidative stress.[101] The mitochondrial permeability transition dissipates the proton motive force, uncoupling oxidative phosphorylation, and causes mitochondrial swelling.[105] Rupture of the outer membrane allows the release of mitochondrial intermembrane proteins with the potential to activate the initial steps of apoptosis (see **Fig. 4**).[101,105]

Consistent with the notion that excessive NO in the neonate may be detrimental, Ferriero and colleagues have shown that nNOS knockout mice are protected from neonatal HI-induced histopathological brain damage.[106] Continuing production of nitric oxide during the period after injury is probably important in the evolution of injury, and it was shown that doses of the nNOS inhibitor 7-nitroindazole (7-NI) that inhibited nNOS by more than 50% over 9 to 12 hours were more effective in reducing brain injury than transient inhibition.[107] After maternal administration in a rabbit model of intrauterine HI, selective nNOS inhibitors were found to distribute to fetal brain and inhibit nNOS activity in vivo.[108] There was a reduction of NO concentration in fetal brain, and dramatic reduction of deaths and the number of newborn kittens exhibiting signs of cerebral palsy.[108] One has to note, however, that NO generated by endothelial NOS (eNOS) plays an important role in maintaining blood flow and blood pressure.[109] Animals that lack the eNOS gene have enlarged cerebral infarcts after HI.[110] Therefore, NO may play a dual role in HIE.

The free radical scavenging agent N-acetylcysteine (NAC) is able to cross the placenta[111]; it is considered safe during pregnancy and, therefore, of potential therapeutic value in humans, and has been shown to reduce oxidative stress and inflammation.[112] NAC has been shown to provide marked neuroprotection in a clinically relevant model of combined LPS/HI in neonatal rats.[113] The protective effect of NAC was much more pronounced than that produced by another free radical scavenger, melatonin, when administered before and after LPS/HI.[113] NAC was also effective when administered directly after HI[113] (3 days after LPS). In addition to reducing total tissue loss, NAC reduced white matter injury. The mechanism of NAC neuroprotection seems to be related to reduced oxidative stress, as indicated by lower levels of iso-prostane and nitrotyrosine, preservation of the scavengers glutathione and Trx2, attenuated activation of apoptotic proteases (caspase-3, calpain), and reduced inflammation as indicated by attenuated activation of microglia and caspase-1.[113]

APOPTOTIC MECHANISMS INVOLVED IN HYPOXIA-ISCHEMIA

Multiple apoptotic pathways have been shown to be involved in neonatal hypoxic-ischemic cell death. Excitotoxicity, oxidative stress, and other factors lead to injury of the mitochondrial membrane. Mitochondrial permeability transition plays an impor-tant role as an event that marks the point of no return in multiple pathways to cell death.[101] The opening of the permeability transition pore (PTP) in the inner mitochon-drial membrane, a process enhanced by cyclophilin D (CypD), is believed to be responsible for mtPT in the adult brain.[114] However, Wang and colleagues[114] recently demonstrated that in the developing brain, the proapoptotic Bcl-2 associated X protein (Bax) plays a more prominent role in mtPT. It is thought that Bax plays a central role in regulating apoptosis in early development.[115] mtPT leads to release of several proapoptotic factors into the cytoplasm including cytochrome c, apoptosis-inducing factor (AIF), caspase-9, and endonuclease G.[116] Release of cytochrome c and procas-pase-9 into the cytoplasm leads to activation of caspase-9 between 3 and 24 hours after the insult, and is followed by conversion of procaspase-3 to active caspase-3 between 6 and 48 hours after injury.[16,117] Caspase-3 activation results in proteolysis of essential cellular proteins, including cytoskeletal proteins and kinases, and can commit the cell to the morphologic changes characteristic of apoptosis, including nuclear fragmentation.[118] This cytochrome c mediated pathway is also referred to as the intrinsic pathway. Activated caspase-3 has been shown in human postmortem brain tissue of full-term neonates with severe perinatal asphyxia.[119]

Several cell surface receptors respond to cytokine (inflammatory) stimulation, re-sulting in activation of cell death signaling programs.[23] The Tumor Necrosis Factor Receptor Superfamily (TNFRSF) belongs to this group of cytokine-responsive recep-tors.[120] Fas death receptor is one of the most extensively studied TNFRSF members.[121] The apoptotic pathway that is regulated by Fas receptor involves cas-pase-8 and is referred to as the extrinsic pathway.[121] Caspase-8 leads then to cas-pase-3 activation.[122] Lack of a functional Fas death receptor is neuroprotective in adult models of HI.[123] Hypoxia-ischemia also activates Fas death receptor signaling in the neonatal brain.[124] Depending on the type of stimulus applied, a cell may undergo apoptosis, necrosis, or survival and proliferation in response to activation of the Fas death receptor.[121] In addition to activation of the extrinsic caspase-directed apoptosis cascade in the presence of increased Fas ligand,[124] there is abundant evidence that the intrinsic apoptosis cascade is also activated following Fas death receptor signaling, and functions to amplify Fas-mediated cell death.[121] Inhibitors of both cas-pase-9 and caspase-8, given immediately after the hypoxic period in the neonatal rat HI model, result in long-term neuroprotection.[125,126]

A caspase-independent apoptotic pathway has also been extensively studied. Poly(ADP-ribose) polymerase (PARP-1) is a nuclear enzyme that transfers adenosine diphosphate (ADP) ribose groups from nicotinamide adenine dinucleotide (NAD$^+$) to nuclear proteins and facilitates DNA repair.[127] Mandir and colleagues[128] reported that PARP mediates neuronal cell death caused by NMDA but not non-NMDA excito-toxicity. Ducrocq and colleagues[129] found that the PARP inhibitor 3-aminobenzamide reduced infarct size in a neonatal model of focal ischemia. DNA damage caused by hydrogen peroxide in PC12 cells also stimulated PARP-1, and 3-aminobenzamide decreased both apoptosis and necrosis in this model.[130] PARP activation consumes NAD^+ needed for mitochondrial energy production, which in turn triggers release of cytochrome c and activation of caspases.[127] However, PARP's primary effect is to activate movement of AIF from mitochondria into the nucleus, a caspase-independent mechanism of cell death.[127] The translocation of AIF to the nucleus is preceded by increasing translocation of the proapoptotic bcl-2 family member Bid (BH3-interacting domain death agonist) to mitochondria, perinuclear accumulation of Bid-loaded mitochondria, and loss of mitochondrial membrane integrity.[131] AIF translocation leads to release from the nucleus of molecular signals that impair mitochondrial function and ATP production.[132,133] Movement of AIF into the nucleus is greater in the immature brain than in the adult.[134] Recent reports also indicate that PARP-1 has important molecular roles beyond DNA repair, including regulation of chromatin structure and transcription.[135] PARP-1 represses transcription by DNA polymerase II at specific loci, but is released from chromatin when activated by NAD^+, allowing derepression.[135] These new data supplement older results indicating that PARP-1 can alter gene transcription by modifying histones, and provide an explanation for its recently reported role in learning and memory.[135,136]

The authors made the unexpected observation that knocking out the Parp1 gene in mice reduced brain damage from HI in 7-day-old male but not female mice.[137] It was also found that NAD levels were significantly lower in males but not in female wild-type neonatal mice after HI.[137] The authors planned this experiment because PARP-1 is downstream in the NMDA activated excitotoxicity pathway, and is activated by DNA strand breaks caused by nitric oxide radical ($NO^•$) production.[128] Knocking out this gene in adult mice had been shown to protect the brain from damage from middle cerebral artery stroke,[127] and the authors wanted to determine if the protective effect was also present in neonates subjected to HI. Turtzo and McCullough[138] confirmed these results on sexual dimorphism in adult mice. The effect of sex had been missed in the initial report on Parp1 knockout on stroke in mice because only males had been used in those experiments.[138] McCullough and colleagues[139] found a more striking difference between males and females in adults than was found by the authors in neonates: males were protected, but injury in females was even greater in the Parp1 knockout animals. McCullough and colleagues also showed that the effect of pharmacologic inhibition of nNOS was sexually dimorphic. These gender differences are consistent with data from Li and colleagues,[140] who reported that inhibition of nNOS with 7-nitroindazole reduced injury from oxygen-glucose deprivation in male but not female neurons in culture. Male neurons also produced more nitrite and nitrate than female neurons in this study.

Du and colleagues[141] reported that the cell death in response to cytotoxic challenge proceeds by different cell death pathways in male and female rat neurons cultured separately. These investigators reported that XY neurons are more sensitive to nitrosative stress and glutamate excitotoxicity, whereas XX neurons are more sensitive to etoposide and staurosporine, agents that activate caspase-dependent apoptosis. These results showed that male neurons die predominantly through activation of an AIF-dependent pathway, whereas female neurons preferentially release cytochrome c from mitochondria and die as a result of subsequent activation of caspase-3. Male neurons also had lower levels of glutathione following nitrosative stress than neurons from females. The finding by the authors that Parp1 knockout protects males, but not females, is consistent with the preferential activation of the NMDA→NO→ PARP-1→AIF release in males.[137] Two recent articles confirmed that these sex-related differences in cell death pathways are present in neonatal mice and rats in vivo.[142,143] The first article by Zhu and colleagues studied 9-day-old mice subjected to HI.[142] This article reported that there was no difference in injury between males and females at 9 days, but there was greater translocation of AIF from mitochondria to nuclei in males and greater activation of caspase-3 in females. The second article by Nijboer and colleagues[143] reported that HI in 7-day-old rat pups caused transloca-tion of AIF only in males, and 2-iminobiotin treatment was neuroprotective and reduced cytochrome c release and caspase activation only in females. These studies support the hypothesis that gender-specific cell death pathways are conserved across species in the perinatal brain. The authors have also shown that the glutamate antagonist dextromethorphan is protective against stroke in male but not female mice at 12 days of age.[144] This finding also supports the greater influence of the excitotoxic pathway in immature males.

This new information about gender differences in neuronal death pathways in exper-imental models is probably directly relevant to gender differences reported in the response of infants and children to brain injuries. The 2005 surveillance of cerebral palsy in Europe study reported that male babies are at higher risk for cerebral palsy than females.[145] This finding agrees with the observation that arterial stroke and cere-bral sinovenous thrombosis are more commonly diagnosed in boys than in girls in the neonatal period.[146,147] This observation is consistent with earlier data showing that the cognitive and motor outcome of brain injury is worse in male than in female low birth weight infants.[146] Quantitative imaging showed that male premature infants are more vulnerable than girls to white matter injury from intraventricular hemorrhage, but girls are more vulnerable to gray matter injury.[148] It follows directly from this information that an infant's sex could influence the efficacy of neuroprotective agents and the cell types most at risk. A striking example of this effect was reported from the prospec-tive indomethacin intraventricular hemorrhage prevention trial.[149] In this study, indo-methacin eliminated parenchymal hemorrhage and improved verbal scores in boys at age 3 to 8 years, but had no effect on girls. As stated in the editorial that accompa-nied publication of this article, "it is becoming increasingly clear that gender differ-ences are not simply a result of hormonal influence but are profound properties of individual cells."

MECHANISMS OF HYPOTHERMIC PROTECTION IN HYPOXIA-ISCHEMIA

Although several different agents have shown a neuroprotective effect in animal models of HI, hypothermia is the only therapeutic intervention that has been exten-sively investigated in the newborn patient population.[8,150–153] This clinical investiga-tion was preceded by a large number of preclinical studies in multiple animal models that demonstrated a neuroprotective effect.[90,154–159] Clinical studies have shown an overall reduction in mortality accompanied by a reduction in disability among newborns with HIE who were enrolled in hypothermia protocols within the first day of life.[9] Further supportive information comes from MRI studies that suggested both head cooling and total body cooling were associated with a reduced incidence of basal ganglia/thalamic brain lesions. To date, 2 large randomized controlled trials and 1 large pilot study that evaluated hypothermia in infants with HIE have been completed. The multicenter Cool Cap Study involved 243 infants with moderate or severe encephalopathy and an abnormal amplitude-integrated EEG (aEEG), who were either cooled to a temperature of 34° to 35°C for 72 hours or treated with temper-ature maintenance in normothermia range with conventional care.[160] The effect of head cooling for infants with the most severe aEEG changes was not protective; on the other hand, the effect of head cooling for infants with less severe aEEG changes was protective. The National Institute of Child Health and Human Development Neonatal Research Network trial evaluated 102 infants randomized to hypothermia with whole body cooling to 33.5°C for 72 hours compared with 106 control infants randomized to conventional care.[161] Death or moderate/severe disability at 18 months of age was noted in 44% of infants in the hypothermia group compared with 62% of infants in the control group. The mode of cooling used in each trial was different, and it is unknown if one cooling regimen (head cooling vs whole body hypothermia) is superior to the other. Current meta-analyses suggest that the only consistent adverse effects of hypothermia are clinically benign physiologic sinus bradycardia and increased thrombocytopenia, and there seems to be a borderline increase in inotropic support but no increase in the incidence or degree of hypotension, or other major adverse events.[9] Eicher and colleagues[162] demonstrated an increase in intraventricular hemorrhage, but this finding was not confirmed in 2 other larger randomized trials. It is reassuring that in piglet studies in which the cortex was cooled significantly (to <30°C), no cerebral hemorrhages were seen, and a recent retrospective case series suggests that hypothermia may be safe even down to rectal temperatures as low as 30°C.[163,164]

The remarkable neuroprotective effect of mild hypothermia against ischemic brain injury is likely attributed to its broad inhibitory actions on a variety of harmful cellular processes induced by HI. Among the proposed key mechanisms underlying hypothermic neuroprotection is the inhibition of intracellular signaling events that initiate the cell death cascade. Under injury conditions, hypothermia decreases loss of high-energy organic phosphates, slows the rates of metabolite consumption and lactic acid accumulation, and reduces oxygen consumption.[163,165]

Hypothermia was originally thought to protect the brain by reducing cerebral metabolism during conditions of reduced substrate availability and increased anaerobic glycolysis. However, hypothermia slows but does not completely prevent the eventual depletion of ATP, and several other studies suggest that metabolism is not significantly altered despite remarkable neuroprotection.[166–168] For example, rodents subjected to 20 minutes of forebrain ischemia showed marked protection, but brain levels of various metabolites were no different from normothermic ischemic controls. Thus, the influence of hypothermia on cerebral metabolism probably does not fully explain its protective effect. Mild hypothermia during ischemia diminishes oxidative DNA damage in the brain after severe focal ischemia and reperfusion in adult rats.[50] Furthermore, hypothermia inhibits the activation of apoptotic signaling pathways in the ischemic brain.[159] Hypothermia has also been shown to reduce inflammation triggered by ischemia.[169] Postischemic hypothermia reduces IL-18 expression and suppresses microglial activation accompanied by decreased loss of MAP-2 (a marker of neuronal integrity) immunoreactivity.[169] In adult rats treated with hypothermia after HI, a reduction in volume of infarct and neuronal loss was also associated with a marked reduction of astrocytosis, and of TNF-α, and IL-6 mRNA, and protein levels in the ipsilateral hippocampus.[90] In summary, it is likely that hypothermia influences multiple pathways, ultimately leading to neuroprotection.

FUTURE DIRECTIONS

There has been significant research progress in HIE over the last 2 decades, and many new molecular mechanisms have been identified. Despite all these advances, therapeutic interventions are still limited. As mentioned in this review, hypothermia is slowly becoming a promising approach to reduce the degree of injury and perhaps allow a longer window of opportunity to intervene. One of the difficulties with evaluation of therapeutics is the limited availability of surrogate markers for outcome as well as ethical dilemmas associated with clinical trials in newborns. However, the authors are hopeful that there will be significant progress in this field soon. First, the addition of advanced MRI methods has not only contributed to a better understanding of the pathologic events but also allows quantitative monitoring of disease progression that may guide decisions regarding interventions. In addition, recent advances in stem cell engineering may soon lead to cell-based interventions in HIE. The authors' group and others have demonstrated a protective effect of neural stem cell transplantation in rodents with neonatal HI, and recently reports have been published on a similar protective effect by systemic injection of cord blood cells. There is currently an ongoing trial to assess the role of cord blood transplantation in infants with HI. Finally, given the number of different pathways involved in HIE, it is likely that the best outcome will be achieved by a multimodal therapeutic approach such as a combination of glutamate receptor antagonists with antioxidants and hypothermia.

REFERENCES

1. Johnston MV, Hoon AH Jr. Cerebral palsy. Neuromolecular Med 2006;8(4): 435–50.
2. Locatelli A, Incerti M, Ghidini A, et al. Factors associated with umbilical artery acidemia in term infants with low Apgar scores at 5 min. Eur J Obstet Gynecol Reprod Biol 2008;139(2):146–50.
3. Graham EM, Ruis KA, Hartman AL, et al. A systematic review of the role of intrapartum hypoxia-ischemia in the causation of neonatal encephalopathy. Am J Obstet Gynecol 2008;199(6):587–95.
4. Liu J, Li J, Gu M. The correlation between myocardial function and cerebral hemodynamics in term infants with hypoxic-ischemic encephalopathy. J Trop Pediatr 2007;53(1):44–8.
5. Volpe JJ. Perinatal brain injury: from pathogenesis to neuroprotection. Ment Retard Dev Disabil Res Rev 2001;7(1):56–64.
6. Shah PS, Perlman M. Time courses of intrapartum asphyxia: neonatal characteristics and outcomes. Am J Perinatol 2009;26(1):39–44.
7. Folkerth RD. Neuropathologic substrate of cerebral palsy. J Child Neurol 2005; 20(12):940–9.
8. Shankaran S, Pappas A, Laptook AR, et al. Outcomes of safety and effectiveness in a multicenter randomized, controlled trial of whole-body hypothermia for neonatal hypoxic-ischemic encephalopathy. Pediatrics 2008;122(4):e791–8.
9. Shankaran S. Neonatal encephalopathy: treatment with hypothermia. J Neurotrauma 2009;26(3):437–43.
10. Barkovich AJ, Westmark K, Partridge C, et al. Perinatal asphyxia: MR findings in the first 10 days. AJNR Am J Neuroradiol 1995;16(3):427–38.
11. Myers RE. Two patterns of perinatal brain damage and their conditions of occurrence. Am J Obstet Gynecol 1972;112(2):246–76.
12. Rutherford M, Srinivasan L, Dyet L, et al. Magnetic resonance imaging in perinatal brain injury: clinical presentation, lesions and outcome. Pediatr Radiol 2006;36(7):582–92.
13. Okereafor A, Allsop J, Counsell SJ, et al. Patterns of brain injury in neonates exposed to perinatal sentinel events. Pediatrics 2008;121(5):906–14.
14. Takeoka M, Soman TB, Yoshii A, et al. Diffusion-weighted images in neonatal cerebral hypoxic-ischemic injury. Pediatr Neurol 2002;26(4):274–81.

15. Zhu W, Zhong W, Qi J, et al. Proton magnetic resonance spectroscopy in neonates with hypoxic-ischemic injury and its prognostic value. Transl Res 2008;152(5):225–32.
16. Nakajima W, Ishida A, Lange MS, et al. Apoptosis has a prolonged role in the neurodegeneration after hypoxic ischemia in the newborn rat. J Neurosci 2000;20(21):7994–8004.
17. Johnston MV, Ferriero DM, Vannucci SJ, et al. Models of cerebral palsy: which ones are best? J Child Neurol 2005;20(12):984–7.
18. Rice JE 3rd, Vannucci RC, Brierley JB. The influence of immaturity on hypoxic-ischemic brain damage in the rat. Ann Neurol 1981;9(2):131–41.
19. Brillault J, Lam TI, Rutkowsky JM, et al. Hypoxia effects on cell volume and ion uptake of cerebral microvascular endothelial cells. Am J Physiol Cell Physiol 2008;294(1):C88–96.
20. Hausmann R, Seidl S, Betz P. Hypoxic changes in Purkinje cells of the human cerebellum. Int J Legal Med 2007;121(3):175–83.
21. Bonfoco E, Krainc D, Ankarcrona M, et al. Apoptosis and necrosis: two distinct events induced, respectively, by mild and intense insults with N-methyl-D-aspartate or nitric oxide/superoxide in cortical cell cultures. Proc Natl Acad Sci U S A 1995;92(16):7162–6.
22. Stroemer RP, Rothwell NJ. Exacerbation of ischemic brain damage by localized striatal injection of interleukin-1beta in the rat. J Cereb Blood Flow Metab 1998; 18(8):833–9.
23. Blomgren K, Leist M, Groc L. Pathological apoptosis in the developing brain. Apoptosis 2007;12(5):993–1010.
24. Zhu C, Wang X, Xu F, et al. The influence of age on apoptotic and other mechanisms of cell death after cerebral hypoxia-ischemia. Cell Death Differ 2005; 12(2):162–76.
25. Kuida K, Zheng TS, Na S, et al. Decreased apoptosis in the brain and premature lethality in CPP32-deficient mice. Nature 1996;384(6607):368–72.
26. Kuida K, Haydar TF, Kuan CY, et al. Reduced apoptosis and cytochrome c-mediated caspase activation in mice lacking caspase 9. Cell 1998;94(3): 325–37.
27. Portera-Cailliau C, Price DL, Martin LJ. Excitotoxic neuronal death in the immature brain is an apoptosis-necrosis morphological continuum. J Comp Neurol 1997;378(1):70–87.
28. Northington FJ, Zelaya ME, O'Riordan DP, et al. Failure to complete apoptosis following neonatal hypoxia-ischemia manifests as "continuum" phenotype of cell death and occurs with multiple manifestations of mitochondrial dysfunction in rodent forebrain. Neuroscience 2007;149(4):822–33.
29. Johnston MV. Excitotoxicity in perinatal brain injury. Brain Pathol 2005;15(3): 234–40.
30. Johnston MV, Coyle JT. Development of central neurotransmitter systems. Ciba Found Symp 1981;86:251–70.
31. Johnston MV. Neurotransmitters and vulnerability of the developing brain. Brain Dev 1995;17(5):301–6.
32. Johnston MV. Developmental aspects of NMDA receptor agonists and antagonists in the central nervous system. Psychopharmacol Bull 1994;30(4):567–75.
33. Santos MS, Li H, Voglmaier SM. Synaptic vesicle protein trafficking at the glutamate synapse. Neuroscience 2009;158(1):189–203.
34. Yang CZ, Zhao R, Dong Y, et al. Astrocyte and neuron intone through glutamate. Neurochem Res 2008;33(12):2480–6.

35. Brongholi K, Souza DG, Bainy AC, et al. Oxygen-glucose deprivation decreases glutathione levels and glutamate uptake in rat hippocampal slices. Brain Res 2006;1083(1):211–8.

36. Thomazi AP, Boff B, Pires TD, et al. Profile of glutamate uptake and cellular viability in hippocampal slices exposed to oxygen and glucose deprivation: developmental aspects and protection by guanosine. Brain Res 2008;1188: 233–40.

37. Boycott HE, Wilkinson JA, Boyle JP, et al. Differential involvement of TNF alpha in hypoxic suppression of astrocyte glutamate transporters. Glia 2008;56(9): 998–1004.

38. Fraser M, Bennet L, Van Zijl PL, et al. Extracellular amino acids and lipid peroxidation products in periventricular white matter during and after cerebral ischemia in preterm fetal sheep. J Neurochem 2008;105:2219–23.

39. Silverstein FS, Naik B, Simpson J. Hypoxia-ischemia stimulates hippocampal glutamate efflux in perinatal rat brain: an in vivo microdialysis study. Pediatr Res 1991;30(6):587–90.

40. Wilson MA, Kinsman SL, Johnston MV. Expression of NMDA receptor subunit mRNA after MK-801 treatment in neonatal rats. Brain Res Dev Brain Res 1998;109(2):211–20.

41. McDonald JW, Johnston MV. Nonketotic hyperglycinemia: pathophysiological role of NMDA-type excitatory amino acid receptors. Ann Neurol 1990;27(4): 449–50.

42. McDonald JW, Silverstein FS, Johnston MV. Magnesium reduces N-methyl-D-aspartate (NMDA)-mediated brain injury in perinatal rats. Neurosci Lett 1990; 109(1–2):234–8.

43. Ai J, Baker A. Long-term potentiation of evoked presynaptic response at CA3-CA1 synapses by transient oxygen-glucose deprivation in rat brain slices. Exp Brain Res 2006;169(1):126–9.

44. Quintana P, Alberi S, Hakkoum D, et al. Glutamate receptor changes associated with transient anoxia/hypoglycaemia in hippocampal slice cultures. Eur J Neurosci 2006;23(4):975–83.

45. Windelborn JA, Lipton P. Lysosomal release of cathepsins causes ischemic damage in the rat hippocampal slice and depends on NMDA-mediated calcium influx, arachidonic acid metabolism, and free radical production. J Neurochem 2008;106(1):56–69.

46. McDonald JW, Silverstein FS, Johnston MV. Neuroprotective effects of MK-801, TCP, PCP and CPP against N-methyl-D-aspartate induced neurotoxicity in an in vivo perinatal rat model. Brain Res 1989;490(1):33–40.

47. McDonald JW, Johnston MV. Pharmacology of N-methyl-D-aspartate-induced brain injury in an in vivo perinatal rat model. Synapse 1990;6(2):179–88.

48. McDonald JW, Roeser NF, Silverstein FS, et al. Quantitative assessment of neuroprotection against NMDA-induced brain injury. Exp Neurol 1989;106(3): 289–96.

49. Nakanishi N, Tu S, Shin Y, et al. Neuroprotection by the NR3A subunit of the NMDA receptor. J Neurosci 2009;29(16):5260–5.

50. Mueller-Burke D, Koehler RC, Martin LJ. Rapid NMDA receptor phosphorylation and oxidative stress precede striatal neurodegeneration after hypoxic ischemia in newborn piglets and are attenuated with hypothermia. Int J Dev Neurosci 2008;26(1):67–76.

51. Talos DM, Fishman RE, Park H, et al. Developmental regulation of alpha-amino-3-hydroxy-5-methyl-4-isoxazole-propionic acid receptor subunit expression in

forebrain and relationship to regional susceptibility to hypoxic/ischemic injury. I. Rodent cerebral white matter and cortex. J Comp Neurol 2006;497(1):42–60.

52. Blue ME, Johnston MV. The ontogeny of glutamate receptors in rat barrel field cortex. Brain Res Dev Brain Res 1995;84(1):11–25.

53. McCarran WJ, Goldberg MP. White matter axon vulnerability to AMPA/kainate receptor-mediated ischemic injury is developmentally regulated. J Neurosci 2007;27(15):4220–9.

54. Deng W, Rosenberg PA, Volpe JJ, et al. Calcium-permeable AMPA/kainate receptors mediate toxicity and preconditioning by oxygen-glucose deprivation in oligodendrocyte precursors. Proc Natl Acad Sci U S A 2003;100(11):6801–6.

55. McDonald JW, Trescher WH, Johnston MV. Susceptibility of brain to AMPA induced excitotoxicity transiently peaks during early postnatal development. Brain Res 1992;583(1–2):54–70.

56. McDonald JW, Johnston MV. Excitatory amino acid neurotoxicity in the developing brain. NIDA Res Monogr 1993;133:185–205.

57. Noh MR, Kim SK, Sun W, et al. Neuroprotective effect of topiramate on hypoxic ischemic brain injury in neonatal rats. Exp Neurol 2006;201(2):470–8.

58. Ikonomidou C, Bosch F, Miksa M, et al. Blockade of NMDA receptors and apoptotic neurodegeneration in the developing brain. Science 1999; 283(5398):70–4.

59. Panigrahy A, Sleeper LA, Assmann S, et al. Developmental changes in heterogeneous patterns of neurotransmitter receptor binding in the human interpeduncular nucleus. J Comp Neurol 1998;390(3):322–32.

60. Panigrahy A, Rosenberg PA, Assmann S, et al. Differential expression of glutamate receptor subtypes in human brainstem sites involved in perinatal hypoxia-ischemia. J Comp Neurol 2000;427(2):196–208.

61. Hossain MA. Hypoxic-ischemic injury in neonatal brain: involvement of a novel neuronal molecule in neuronal cell death and potential target for neuroprotection. Int J Dev Neurosci 2008;26(1):93–101.

62. Bjartmar L, Huberman AD, Ullian EM, et al. Neuronal pentraxins mediate synaptic refinement in the developing visual system. J Neurosci 2006;26(23): 6269–81.

63. Bayer SA. Development of the hippocampal region in the rat. I. Neurogenesis examined with 3H-thymidine autoradiography. J Comp Neurol 1980;190(1): 87–114.

64. Holmes GL. Epilepsy in the developing brain: lessons from the laboratory and clinic. Epilepsia 1997;38(1):12–30.

65. Staley KJ, Soldo BL, Proctor WR. Ionic mechanisms of neuronal excitation by inhibitory GABAA receptors. Science 1995;269(5226):977–81.

66. Smith RL, Clayton GH, Wilcox CL, et al. Differential expression of an inwardly rectifying chloride conductance in rat brain neurons: a potential mechanism for cell-specific modulation of postsynaptic inhibition. J Neurosci 1995;15(5 Pt 2): 4057–67.

67. Dzhala VI, Talos DM, Sdrulla DA, et al. NKCC1 transporter facilitates seizures in the developing brain. Nat Med 2005;11(11):1205–13.

68. Staley KJ, Mody I. Shunting of excitatory input to dentate gyrus granule cells by a depolarizing GABAA receptor-mediated postsynaptic conductance. J Neurophysiol 1992;68(1):197–212.

69. Leinekugel X, Tseeb V, Ben-Ari Y, et al. Synaptic GABAA activation induces Ca^{2+} rise in pyramidal cells and interneurons from rat neonatal hippocampal slices. J Physiol 1995;487(Pt 2):319–29.

70. Dammann O, O'Shea TM. Cytokines and perinatal brain damage. Clin Perinatol 2008;35(4):643–63, v.
71. Savman K, Blennow M, Gustafson K, et al. Cytokine response in cerebrospinal fluid after birth asphyxia. Pediatr Res 1998;43(6):746–51.
72. Bartha AI, Foster-Barber A, Miller SP, et al. Neonatal encephalopathy: association of cytokines with MR spectroscopy and outcome. Pediatr Res 2004;56(6):960–6.
73. Bona E, Andersson AL, Blomgren K, et al. Chemokine and inflammatory cell response to hypoxia-ischemia in immature rats. Pediatr Res 1999;45(4 Pt 1): 500–9.
74. Hedtjarn M, Mallard C, Hagberg H. Inflammatory gene profiling in the developing mouse brain after hypoxia-ischemia. J Cereb Blood Flow Metab 2004; 24(12):1333–51.
75. Del Bigio MR, Becker LE. Microglial aggregation in the dentate gyrus: a marker of mild hypoxic-ischaemic brain insult in human infants. Neuropathol Appl Neurobiol 1994;20(2):144–51.
76. Lehnardt S, Massillon L, Follett P, et al. Activation of innate immunity in the CNS triggers neurodegeneration through a Toll-like receptor 4-dependent pathway. Proc Natl Acad Sci U S A 2003;100(14):8514–9.
77. Eklind S, Mallard C, Arvidsson P, et al. Lipopolysaccharide induces both a primary and a secondary phase of sensitization in the developing rat brain. Pediatr Res 2005;58(1):112–6.
78. Girard S, Kadhim H, Beaudet N, et al. Developmental motor deficits induced by combined fetal exposure to lipopolysaccharide and early neonatal hypoxia/ ischemia: a novel animal model for cerebral palsy in very premature infants. Neuroscience 2009;158(2):673–82.
79. Girard S, Kadhim H, Larouche A, et al. Pro-inflammatory disequilibrium of the IL-1 beta/IL-1ra ratio in an experimental model of perinatal brain damages induced by lipopolysaccharide and hypoxia-ischemia. Cytokine 2008;43(1):54–62.
80. Wang X, Hagberg H, Nie C, et al. Dual role of intrauterine immune challenge on neonatal and adult brain vulnerability to hypoxia-ischemia. J Neuropathol Exp Neurol 2007;66(6):552–61.
81. Mallard C, Hagberg H. Inflammation-induced preconditioning in the immature brain. Semin Fetal Neonatal Med 2007;12(4):280–6.
82. Bhattacharyya S, Dudeja PK, Tobacman JK. Lipopolysaccharide activates NF-kappaB by TLR4-Bcl10-dependent and independent pathways in colonic epithelial cells. Am J Physiol Gastrointest Liver Physiol 2008;295(4):G784–90.
83. Lehnardt S, Lachance C, Patrizi S, et al. The toll-like receptor TLR4 is necessary for lipopolysaccharide-induced oligodendrocyte injury in the CNS. J Neurosci 2002;22(7):2478–86.
84. Ridder DA, Schwaninger M. NF-kappaB signaling in cerebral ischemia. Neuroscience 2009;158(3):995–1006.
85. Nijboer CH, Heijnen CJ, Groenendaal F, et al. A dual role of the NF-kappaB pathway in neonatal hypoxic-ischemic brain damage. Stroke 2008;39(9): 2578–86.
86. Marini AM, Jiang X, Wu X, et al. Preconditioning and neurotrophins: a model for brain adaptation to seizures, ischemia and other stressful stimuli. Amino Acids 2007;32(3):299–304.
87. Wang X, Rousset CI, Hagberg H, et al. Lipopolysaccharide-induced inflammation and perinatal brain injury. Semin Fetal Neonatal Med 2006;11(5):343–53.
88. Sen E, Levison SW. Astrocytes and developmental white matter disorders. Ment Retard Dev Disabil Res Rev 2006;12(2):97–104.

89. Svedin P, Guan J, Mathai S, et al. Delayed peripheral administration of a GPE analogue induces astrogliosis and angiogenesis and reduces inflammation and brain injury following hypoxia-ischemia in the neonatal rat. Dev Neurosci 2007;29(4–5):393–402.

90. Xiong M, Yang Y, Chen GQ, et al. Post-ischemic hypothermia for 24h in P7 rats rescues hippocampal neuron: association with decreased astrocyte activation and inflammatory cytokine expression. Brain Res Bull 2009;79:351–7.

91. East CE, Dunster KR, Colditz PB. Fetal oxygen saturation and uterine contractions during labor. Am J Perinatol 1998;15(6):345–9.

92. Stiller R, von Mering R, Konig V, et al. How well does reflectance pulse oximetry reflect intrapartum fetal acidosis? Am J Obstet Gynecol 2002;186(6):1351–7.

93. Widmer R, Engels M, Voss P, et al. Postanoxic damage of microglial cells is mediated by xanthine oxidase and cyclooxygenase. Free Radic Res 2007; 41(2):145–52.

94. Forder JP, Tymianski M. Postsynaptic mechanisms of excitotoxicity: Involvement of postsynaptic density proteins, radicals, and oxidant molecules. Neuroscience 2009;158(1):293–300.

95. Lafemina MJ, Sheldon RA, Ferriero DM. Acute hypoxia-ischemia results in hydrogen peroxide accumulation in neonatal but not adult mouse brain. Pediatr Res 2006;59(5):680–3.

96. Hagberg H, Andersson P, Lacarewicz J, et al. Extracellular adenosine, inosine, hypoxanthine, and xanthine in relation to tissue nucleotides and purines in rat striatum during transient ischemia. J Neurochem 1987;49(1):227–31.

97. Guglielmotto M, Aragno M, Autelli R, et al. The up-regulation of BACE1 mediated by hypoxia and ischemic injury: role of oxidative stress and HIF1alpha. J Neurochem 2009;108(4):1045–56.

98. Ishida A, Ishiwa S, Trescher WH, et al. Delayed increase in neuronal nitric oxide synthase immunoreactivity in thalamus and other brain regions after hypoxic-ischemic injury in neonatal rats. Exp Neurol 2001;168(2):323–33.

99. Vinas JL, Sola A, Hotter G. Mitochondrial NOS upregulation during renal I/R causes apoptosis in a peroxynitrite-dependent manner. Kidney Int 2006;69(8): 1403–9.

100. Zhu C, Wang X, Qiu L, et al. Nitrosylation precedes caspase-3 activation and translocation of apoptosis-inducing factor in neonatal rat cerebral hypoxia-ischaemia. J Neurochem 2004;90(2):462–71.

101. Blomgren K, Hagberg H. Free radicals, mitochondria, and hypoxia-ischemia in the developing brain. Free Radic Biol Med 2006;40(3):388–97.

102. Teshima Y, Akao M, Li RA, et al. Mitochondrial ATP-sensitive potassium channel activation protects cerebellar granule neurons from apoptosis induced by oxidative stress. Stroke 2003;34(7):1796–802.

103. Blomgren K, Zhu C, Hallin U, et al. Mitochondria and ischemic reperfusion damage in the adult and in the developing brain. Biochem Biophys Res Commun 2003;304(3):551–9.

104. Boya P, Gonzalez-Polo RA, Poncet D, et al. Mitochondrial membrane permeabilization is a critical step of lysosome-initiated apoptosis induced by hydroxychloroquine. Oncogene 2003;22(25):3927–36.

105. Nakai A. Role of mitochondrial permeability transition in the immature brain following intrauterine ischemia. J Nippon Med Sch 2007;74(3):190–201.

106. Ferriero DM, Holtzman DM, Black SM, et al. Neonatal mice lacking neuronal nitric oxide synthase are less vulnerable to hypoxic-ischemic injury. Neurobiol Dis 1996;3(1):64–71.

107. Muramatsu K, Sheldon RA, Black SM, et al. Nitric oxide synthase activity and inhibition after neonatal hypoxia ischemia in the mouse brain. Brain Res Dev Brain Res 2000;123(2):119–27.
108. Silverman RB. Design of selective neuronal nitric oxide synthase inhibitors for the prevention and treatment of neurodegenerative diseases. Acc Chem Res 2009; 42:439–51.
109. Kaminski A, Kasch C, Zhang L, et al. Endothelial nitric oxide synthase mediates protective effects of hypoxic preconditioning in lungs. Respir Physiol Neurobiol 2007;155(3):280–5.
110. Huang Z, Huang PL, Ma J, et al. Enlarged infarcts in endothelial nitric oxide synthase knockout mice are attenuated by nitro-L-arginine. J Cereb Blood Flow Metab 1996;16(5):981–7.
111. Aremu DA, Madejczyk MS, Ballatori N. N-acetylcysteine as a potential antidote and biomonitoring agent of methylmercury exposure. Environ Health Perspect 2008;116(1):26–31.
112. Lee TF, Tymafichuk CN, Bigam DL, et al. Effects of postresuscitation N-acetylcysteine on cerebral free radical production and perfusion during reoxygenation of hypoxic newborn piglets. Pediatr Res 2008;64(3):256–61.
113. Wang X, Svedin P, Nie C, et al. N-acetylcysteine reduces lipopolysaccharide-sensitized hypoxic-ischemic brain injury. Ann Neurol 2007;61(3):263–71.
114. Wang X, Carlsson Y, Basso E, et al. Developmental shift of cyclophilin D contribution to hypoxic-ischemic brain injury. J Neurosci 2009;29(8):2588–96.
115. Brenner C, Cadiou H, Vieira HL, et al. Bcl-2 and Bax regulate the channel activity of the mitochondrial adenine nucleotide translocator. Oncogene 2000; 19(3):329–36.
116. Cao G, Xing J, Xiao X, et al. Critical role of calpain I in mitochondrial release of apoptosis-inducing factor in ischemic neuronal injury. J Neurosci 2007;27(35): 9278–93.
117. Gill R, Soriano M, Blomgren K, et al. Role of caspase-3 activation in cerebral ischemia-induced neurodegeneration in adult and neonatal brain. J Cereb Blood Flow Metab 2002;22(4):420–30.
118. Wang X, Karlsson JO, Zhu C, et al. Caspase-3 activation after neonatal rat cerebral hypoxia-ischemia. Biol Neonate 2001;79(3–4):172–9.
119. Rossiter JP, Anderson LL, Yang F, et al. Caspase-3 activation and caspase-like proteolytic activity in human perinatal hypoxic-ischemic brain injury. Acta Neuropathol 2002;103(1):66–73.
120. Collette Y, Gilles A, Pontarotti P, et al. A co-evolution perspective of the TNFSF and TNFRSF families in the immune system. Trends Immunol 2003;24(7):387–94.
121. Strasser A, Jost PJ, Nagata S. The many roles of FAS receptor signaling in the immune system. Immunity 2009;30(2):180–92.
122. Le DA, Wu Y, Huang Z, et al. Caspase activation and neuroprotection in caspase-3-deficient mice after in vivo cerebral ischemia and in vitro oxygen glucose deprivation. Proc Natl Acad Sci U S A 2002;99(23):15188–93.
123. Rosenbaum DM, Gupta G, D'Amore J, et al. Fas (CD95/APO-1) plays a role in the pathophysiology of focal cerebral ischemia. J Neurosci Res 2000;61(6):686–92.
124. Northington FJ, Ferriero DM, Flock DL, et al. Delayed neurodegeneration in neonatal rat thalamus after hypoxia-ischemia is apoptosis. J Neurosci 2001; 21(6):1931–8.
125. Feng Y, Fratkin JD, LeBlanc MH. Inhibiting caspase-8 after injury reduces hypoxic-ischemic brain injury in the newborn rat. Eur J Pharmacol 2003; 481(2–3):169–73.

126. Feng Y, Fratkin JD, LeBlanc MH. Inhibiting caspase-9 after injury reduces hypoxic ischemic neuronal injury in the cortex in the newborn rat. Neurosci Lett 2003;344(3):201–4.

127. Andrabi SA, Dawson TM, Dawson VL. Mitochondrial and nuclear cross talk in cell death: parthanatos. Ann N Y Acad Sci 2008;1147:233–41.

128. Mandir AS, Poitras MF, Berliner AR, et al. NMDA but not non-NMDA excitotoxicity is mediated by Poly(ADP-ribose) polymerase. J Neurosci 2000;20(21):8005–11.

129. Ducrocq S, Benjelloun N, Plotkine M, et al. Poly(ADP-ribose) synthase inhibition reduces ischemic injury and inflammation in neonatal rat brain. J Neurochem 2000;74(6):2504–11.

130. Cole KK, Perez-Polo JR. Poly(ADP-ribose) polymerase inhibition prevents both apoptotic-like delayed neuronal death and necrosis after H(2)O(2) injury. J Neurochem 2002;82(1):19–29.

131. Landshamer S, Hoehn M, Barth N, et al. Bid-induced release of AIF from mitochondria causes immediate neuronal cell death. Cell Death Differ 2008;15(10): 1553–63.

132. Zhu C, Wang X, Huang Z, et al. Apoptosis-inducing factor is a major contributor to neuronal loss induced by neonatal cerebral hypoxia-ischemia. Cell Death Differ 2007;14(4):775–84.

133. Baud O, Li J, Zhang Y, et al. Nitric oxide-induced cell death in developing oligodendrocytes is associated with mitochondrial dysfunction and apoptosis-inducing factor translocation. Eur J Neurosci 2004;20(7):1713–26.

134. Zhu C, Qiu L, Wang X, et al. Involvement of apoptosis-inducing factor in neuronal death after hypoxia-ischemia in the neonatal rat brain. J Neurochem 2003;86(2):306–17.

135. Caiafa P, Guastafierro T, Zampieri M. Epigenetics: poly(ADP-ribosyl)ation of PARP-1 regulates genomic methylation patterns. FASEB J 2009;23(3):672–8.

136. Clark RS, Vagni VA, Nathaniel PD, et al. Local administration of the poly(ADP-ribose) polymerase inhibitor INO-1001 prevents NAD+ depletion and improves water maze performance after traumatic brain injury in mice. J Neurotrauma 2007;24(8):1399–405.

137. Hagberg H, Wilson MA, Matsushita H, et al. PARP-1 gene disruption in mice preferentially protects males from perinatal brain injury. J Neurochem 2004; 90(5):1068–75.

138. Turtzo LC, McCullough LD. Sex differences in stroke. Cerebrovasc Dis 2008; 26(5):462–74.

139. McCullough LD, Zeng Z, Blizzard KK, et al. Ischemic nitric oxide and poly (ADP-ribose) polymerase-1 in cerebral ischemia: male toxicity, female protection. J Cereb Blood Flow Metab 2005;25(4):502–12.

140. Li H, Pin S, Zeng Z, et al. Sex differences in cell death. Ann Neurol 2005;58(2): 317–21.

141. Du L, Hickey RW, Bayir H, et al. Starving neurons show sex difference in autophagy. J Biol Chem 2009;284(4):2383–96.

142. Zhu C, Xu F, Wang X, et al. Different apoptotic mechanisms are activated in male and female brains after neonatal hypoxia-ischaemia. J Neurochem 2006;96(4): 1016–27.

143. Nijboer CH, Groenendaal F, Kavelaars A, et al. Gender-specific neuroprotection by 2-iminobiotin after hypoxia-ischemia in the neonatal rat via a nitric oxide independent pathway. J Cereb Blood Flow Metab 2007;27(2):282–92.

144. Comi AM, Highet BH, Mehta P, et al. Dextromethorphan protects male but not female mice with brain ischemia. Neuroreport 2006;17(12):1319–22.

145. Jarvis S, Glinianaia SV, Arnaud C, et al. Case gender and severity in cerebral palsy varies with intrauterine growth. Arch Dis Child 2005;90(5):474–9.
146. Johnston MV, Hagberg H. Sex and the pathogenesis of cerebral palsy. Dev Med Child Neurol 2007;49(1):74–8.
147. Wood NS, Costeloe K, Gibson AT, et al. The EPICure study: associations and antecedents of neurological and developmental disability at 30 months of age following extremely preterm birth. Arch Dis Child Fetal Neonatal Ed 2005; 90(2):F134–40.
148. Thompson DK, Warfield SK, Carlin JB, et al. Perinatal risk factors altering regional brain structure in the preterm infant. Brain 2007;130(Pt 3):667–77.
149. Ment LR, Vohr BR, Makuch RW, et al. Prevention of intraventricular hemorrhage by indomethacin in male preterm infants. J Pediatr 2004;145(6):832–4.
150. Ziino A. Moderate hypothermia in neonatal encephalopathy [comment]. Pediatr Neurol 2006;34(2):169.
151. Wilkinson DJ, Casalaz D, Watkins A, et al. Hypothermia: a neuroprotective therapy for neonatal hypoxic-ischemic encephalopathy. Pediatrics 2007; 119(2):422–3.
152. Wyatt JS, Gluckman PD, Liu PY, et al. Determinants of outcomes after head cooling for neonatal encephalopathy. Pediatrics 2007;119(5):912–21.
153. Shankaran S, Laptook AR. Hypothermia as a treatment for birth asphyxia. Clin Obstet Gynecol 2007;50(3):624–35.
154. Xie YC, Li CY, Li T, et al. Effect of mild hypothermia on angiogenesis in rats with focal cerebral ischemia. Neurosci Lett 2007;422(2):87–90.
155. Thoresen M, Satas S, Puka-Sundvall M, et al. Post-hypoxic hypothermia reduces cerebrocortical release of NO and excitotoxins. Neuroreport 1997;8(15): 3359–62.
156. Trescher WH, Ishiwa S, Johnston MV. Brief post-hypoxic-ischemic hypothermia markedly delays neonatal brain injury. Brain Dev 1997;19(5):326–38.
157. Redmond JM, Zehr KJ, Blue ME, et al. AMPA glutamate receptor antagonism reduces neurologic injury after hypothermic circulatory arrest. Ann Thorac Surg 1995;59(3):579–84.
158. Nishi H, Nakatsuka T, Takeda D, et al. Hypothermia suppresses excitatory synaptic transmission and neuronal death induced by experimental ischemia in spinal ventral horn neurons. Spine 2007;32(25):E741–7.
159. Gressens P, Dingley J, Plaisant F, et al. Analysis of neuronal, glial, endothelial, axonal and apoptotic markers following moderate therapeutic hypothermia and anesthesia in the developing piglet brain. Brain Pathol 2008;18(1):10–20.
160. Gluckman PD, Wyatt JS, Azzopardi D, et al. Selective head cooling with mild systemic hypothermia after neonatal encephalopathy: multicentre randomised trial. Lancet 2005;365(9460):663–70.
161. Higgins RD, Raju TN, Perlman J, et al. Hypothermia and perinatal asphyxia: executive summary of the National Institute of Child Health and Human Development workshop. J Pediatr 2006;148(2):170–5.
162. Eicher DJ, Wagner CL, Katikaneni LP, et al. Moderate hypothermia in neonatal encephalopathy: safety outcomes. Pediatr Neurol 2005;32(1):18–24.
163. O'Brien FE, Iwata O, Thornton JS, et al. Delayed whole-body cooling to 33 or 35 degrees C and the development of impaired energy generation consequential to transient cerebral hypoxia-ischemia in the newborn piglet. Pediatrics 2006; 117(5):1549–59.
164. Compagnoni G, Bottura C, Cavallaro G, et al. Safety of deep hypothermia in treating neonatal asphyxia. Neonatology 2008;93(4):230–5.

165. Andrews P. Effect of hypothermia on brain tissue oxygenation in patients with severe head injury. Br J Anaesth 2003;90(2):251 [author reply 251–2].
166. Krafft P, Frietsch T, Lenz C, et al. Mild and moderate hypothermia (alpha-stat) do not impair the coupling between local cerebral blood flow and metabolism in rats. Stroke 2000;31(6):1393–400 [discussion: 1401].
167. Frietsch T, Krafft P, Piepgras A, et al. Relationship between local cerebral blood flow and metabolism during mild and moderate hypothermia in rats. Anesthesiology 2000;92(3):754–63.
168. Zhang H, Zhou M, Zhang J, et al. Initiation time of post-ischemic hypothermia on the therapeutic effect in cerebral ischemic injury. Neurol Res 2009;31(4):336–9.
169. Fukui O, Kinugasa Y, Fukuda A, et al. Post-ischemic hypothermia reduced IL-18 expression and suppressed microglial activation in the immature brain. Brain Res 2006;1121(1):35–45.

Neuroprotection in the Newborn Infant

Fernando F. Gonzalez, MD[a,c], Donna M. Ferriero, MD[a,b,c,*]

KEYWORDS

- Neonatal stroke • Hypoxia • Ischemia • Neuroprotection
- Neurogenesis

Causes of early brain injury include stroke, birth trauma, metabolic or genetic disorders, status epilepticus, and asphyxial events. Perinatal asphyxia presents as encephalopathy, or hypoxic ischemic encephalopathy, occurring in 3 to 5 in 1000 live births,[1] whereas stroke studies conservatively estimate an incidence of 1 in 4000 live births.[2] It is classically thought that hypoxic-ischemic (HI) injury leads to periventricular white matter damage in premature infants, whereas term infants develop cortical/subcortical lesions,[3] but more recent evidence suggests that this distinction in injury type may not be so clear.[4] Although many suffering from perinatal brain injury die during early life, most survivors exhibit neurologic deficits that persist, such as cerebral palsy, mental retardation, or epilepsy.[5] Aside from hypothermia, no established therapies exist, and treatment and care for the sequelae of early brain injury requires significant resources. Even after maximal care, there is often little improvement in an individual's overall abilities, with long-term effects on the family, health care system, and society.[6]

A search for therapies that can prevent injury progression or enhance repair of the immature brain continues, with the goal of improving long-term motor and cognitive outcomes. Because the neonatal and adult brain do not respond to insults in the same manner, secondary to differences in gene regulation during hypoxia and altered susceptibility to oxidative stress and excitotoxicity, alternate therapies must be sought.[7] Damage occurs via multiple pathways, and repair occurs over a period of days to weeks, if not months.[8] Although some therapies that manipulate injury pathways show promise, not all neonates will benefit from treatment. Damage may be so severe or prolonged that repair may not be possible, or survivors may be particularly devastated.[9]

[a] Department of Pediatrics, University of California, 521 Parnassus Avenue, C215, Box 0663, San Francisco, CA 94143, USA
[b] Department of Neurology, University of California, 521 Parnassus Avenue, C215, Box 0663, San Francisco, CA 94143, USA
[c] Neonatal Brain Disorders Laboratory, University of California, 521 Parnassus Avenue, C215, Box 0663, San Francisco, CA 94143, USA
* Corresponding author. Neonatal Brain Disorders Laboratory, University of California, San Francisco, 521 Parnassus Avenue C215, Box 0663, San Francisco, CA 94143.
E-mail address: ferrierod@neuropeds.ucsf.edu (D.M. Ferriero).

Clin Perinatol 36 (2009) 859–880
doi:10.1016/j.clp.2009.07.013 **perinatology.theclinics.com**
0095-5108/09/$ – see front matter © 2009 Elsevier Inc. All rights reserved.

The term "neuroprotection" is frequently used to describe the treatment response to brain injury, but should we think only about protecting neurons? Optimizing therapy for early brain injury requires capitalizing on multiple pathways that not only prevent cell death, but also enhance cell growth, differentiation, and long-term integration into neural networks. In addition to neuronal damage, injury to non-neuronal cell types, such as oligodendrocytes and astrocytes, adversely affects development and results in long-term morbidity. By targeting the response to injury, the goal is to use selected pharmacotherapies to salvage cells that would otherwise die, protect cells from becoming injured or at risk for death by increasing tolerance, and also repair injured cells and enhance neurogenesis. Recent evidence suggests that therapies may be combined to enhance the protective and reparative processes, and thought must be given to the best time to administer these interventions. Clearly, because injury evolves over long periods of time with different mechanistic phases, therapies will also need to be administered over long periods of time, with different drugs aimed at these temporally evolving targets.

To maximize the efficacy of post-injury treatment, we need to identify quickly those neonates who will benefit from these therapies. A variety of clinical predictors have been used to identify those at risk for hypoxic brain injury. These include low Apgar scores, cord blood or early arterial acidosis, and seizures or the presence of encephalopathy on examination.[10] Cerebral function monitoring using bedside amplitude integrated EEG (aEEG) has provided an efficient means for identifying encephalopathy or prolonged seizure,[11] but it does not replace full EEG.[12] Brain imaging with magnetic resonance imaging (MRI), including newer techniques such as spectroscopy (MRS), diffusion-weighted (DWI) and diffusion tensor imaging (DTI), and volumetric analyses, provides the most accurate assessment of injury.[13] These techniques allow determination of the severity and evolution of brain injury, with specific injury patterns being associated with poor outcomes such as loss of gray/white differentiation, watershed injury, and thalamic or basal ganglia injury.[14] However, early and sequential imaging in neonates is often not possible because of scanner availability or difficulty in transporting these critically ill patients. Biomarkers for oxidative stress and inflammation, or indicators of injury to other organ systems, are currently being studied but are of equivocal value in identifying early neonatal brain injury. Given all of the available evidence, a combination of encephalopathic physical examination and seizures provides the best estimate of infants who may be at risk for brain injury.[10] This review will focus on recent developments in treating neonatal brain injury, as well as on combination therapy that will potentially enhance repair and optimize long-term outcomes.

HYPOTHERMIA

Therapeutic hypothermia has now become standard of care for neonatal HI brain injury. Multiple animal models of perinatal brain injury demonstrate histologic and functional benefit of early initiation of hypothermia (**Table 1**).[15–19] Brief hypothermia provides partial neuroprotection,[20,21] but prolonged moderate hypothermia to 32 to 34°C for 24 to 72 hours results in sustained improvement in behavioral performance in both newborn and adult animals.[18,19] The only complications noted are transient effects on heart rate and blood pressure.[22]

Studies of therapeutic hypothermia in human neonates show a reduction in mortality and long-term neurodevelopmental disability at 12 to 24 months of age, with the most benefit seen in moderately encephalopathic infants.[9,23–25] Sustained protection depends on the dose of hypothermia, with maximum benefit obtained with cooling

Table 1
Hypothermia studies (discussed in text)

Study	Species	Type of Cooling	Primary Outcome
Laptook et al, 1994	Pig	Whole body	Decreased histologic/behavioral impairment
Towfigh et al, 1994	Rat	Head	Improved histology
Thoresen et al, 1995	Pig	Whole body	Improved MRI measures
Gunn et al, 1997	Ovine	Head	Improved EEG/histology
Laptook et al, 1997	Pig	Whole body	Less encephalopathy/histologic damage
Bona et al, 1998	Rat	Whole body	Improved histology/no change in sensorimotor function
Gunn et al, 1998	Human	Head	Safe for mild systemic/moderate head cooling
Azzopardi et al, 2000	Human	Whole body	Only mild abnormalities in VS seen with cooling
Thoresen & Whitelaw, 2000	Human	Head	Non-hazardous changes in HR/BP with cooling
Eicher et al, 2005	Human	Whole body	Mild-mod abnormalities with cooling, improved outcomes
Gluckman et al, 2005	Human	Head	Beneficial in infants with less severe EEG changes
Shankaran et al, 2005	Human	Head	Reduced death/disability, trend toward improvement at 18–22 months
Wyatt et al, 2007	Human	Head	Less death/disability at 18 months
Battin et al, 2009	Human	Whole body	No effect on mean arterial blood pressure
Sarkar et al, 2009	Human	Both	Pulmonary dysfunction common but not severe
Robertson et al, 2009	Human	Whole body	Demonstrates ability to cool in low-resource setting

Abbreviations: BP, blood pressure; EEG, electroencephalogram; HR, heart rate; mod, moderate; MRI, magnetic resonance imaging; VS, vital signs.

to 33 to 34°C, as well as on limited delay to treatment initiation.[18,26] Mild hypothermia to this level appears to be well tolerated without serious adverse effects if initiated within the first 6 hours of life.[23,27–29] Recent evidence shows that there are no changes in arterial blood pressure,[30] but there may be some mild changes in blood gas parameters.[31] There also appears to be an increased risk of pulmonary hypertension in cooled infants, although generally not severe.[32] In selective head cooling, treatment benefits infants with moderate, but not severe, aEEG changes, improving survival without severe neurodevelopmental deficits or an increase in complications.[9] In addition to severity of encephalopathy, larger infants appear to be more responsive to hypothermia and at more risk for injury if hyperthermic at any point.[33,34] In a second multicenter trial, whole-body cooling to 33.5°C initiated within 6 hours and continued for 72 hours resulted in fewer deaths and less severe disability at 18 to 22 months.[35] Whole-body cooling may be more effective in reducing temperature in the deep brain structures,[36] and may be more feasible in certain clinical settings.[37]

GROWTH FACTORS

The response of the immature brain to milder forms of injury can help us learn about mechanisms the brain uses to protect itself from insults. Animals treated with sublethal stress are protected from subsequent insults that would otherwise be deadly.[38,39] For example, immature rats that are exposed to hypoxia have reduced brain injury following HI that occurs 24 hours after this preconditioning stimulus, with protection that persists 1 to 3 weeks later.[40,41] It is possible that injury may only be delayed, and protection may not be permanent; however, hypoxic preconditioning does provide long-lasting histologic and functional protection for up to 8 weeks after neonatal rodent HI.[42]

Hypoxia-inducible factor 1α (HIF-1α) activation is a key modulator of the protection against subsequent HI injury that is induced by hypoxic preconditioning.[38,43] HIF-1α is a neuronal transcription factor that stabilizes during hypoxia by binding to HIF-1β. Following stabilization, it produces a variety of downstream targets that are neuroprotective, including insulin-like growth factor-1 (IGF-1), vascular endothelial growth factor (VEGF), and erythropoietin (EPO).

EPO is a 34-kDa glycoprotein that was originally identified for its role in erythropoiesis, but has since been found to have a variety of other roles. Functions include modulation of the inflammatory and immune responses,[44] vasogenic and proangiogenic effects through its interaction with VEGF,[45,46] as well as effects on central nervous system (CNS) development and repair. EPO and EPO receptor are expressed by a variety of different cell types in the CNS, with changing patterns during development.[47] EPO plays a vital role in neural differentiation and neurogenesis early in development, promoting neurogenesis in vitro and in vivo.[48]

Increasing evidence suggests that exogenously administered EPO has a protective effect in a variety of different models of brain injury. Postinjury treatment protocols in newborn rodents have demonstrated both short- and long-term histologic and behavioral improvement.[49] A single dose of EPO given immediately after neonatal HI injury in rats significantly reduces infarct volume and improves long-term spatial memory.[50] Single- and multiple-dose treatment regimens of EPO following neonatal focal ischemic stroke in rats reduce infarct volume[51] and improve both short-term sensorimotor[52] and long-term cognitive[53] outcomes, but there may be more long-lasting behavioral benefit in female rats.[54] EPO treatment initiated 24 hours after neonatal HI also decreases brain injury.[55] In addition, EPO enhances neurogenesis and directs multipotential neural stem cells toward a neuronal cell fate.[45,48,56] Following transient ischemic stroke, there is a temporary precursor-cell proliferation in the rodent subventricular zone (SVZ), a source of endogenous precursor cells throughout the life of the rodent, with this precursor-cell proliferation and differentiation favoring gliogenesis.[57] EPO has been shown to enhance neurogenesis in vivo in the SVZ following stroke in the adult rat.[45] Neurogenesis has also been demonstrated following EPO treatment, with an increase in newly generated cells from precursors[45,48,58] and possibly also an effect on cell fate commitment in vitro.[45,48]

In humans, EPO is safely used for treatment of anemia in premature infants.[59] EPO for neuroprotection is given in much higher doses (1000–5000 U/kg/dose) than for anemia, to enable crossing of the blood-brain barrier,[52,60,61] with unknown pharmacokinetics in humans. Recently, extremely low birth weight infants tolerated doses between 500 and 2500 U/kg/dose (**Table 2**),[62] and studies are ongoing.

VEGF is a regulator of angiogenesis that is also involved in neuronal cell proliferation and migration.[63] The endothelial microenvironment establishes a vascular niche that promotes survival and proliferation of progenitor cells, events that are tightly

Table 2
Human studies of neuroprotectants (discussed in text)

Treatment	Mechanism	Study	Primary Outcome
Hypothermia	multiple	(see Table 1)	
EPO	Growth factor	Juul et al, 2008	High-dose EPO safe in ELBW infants
Inhaled nitric oxide	Antioxidant	Schreiber et al, 2003	Lower incidence of severe IVH and PVL
		Ballard et al, 2006	Decreased neurodevelopmental disability
Melatonin	Antioxidant	Gitto et al, 2004	Decreased proinflammatory markers, nitrates/nitrites
		Gitto et al, 2005	Reduced proinflammatory cytokines, improved clinical outcome
Allopurinol	Antioxidant	Clancy et al, 2001	Neurocardiac protection in HLHS infants
		Benders et al, 2006	Postnatal treatment had no effect
Magnesium sulfate	↓ excitotoxicity	Levene et al, 2002	Increased Mg dose associated with hypotension
		Groenendaal et al, 2002	No positive effect on aEEG patterns
		Crowther et al, 2003	May improve pediatric outcomes when given to mothers during pregnancy
		Khashaba et al, 2006	No effect on postnatal level of EAA

Abbreviations: aEEG, amplitude integrated EEG; EAA, excitatory amino acids; ELBW, extremely low birth weight; HLHS, hypoplastic left heart syndrome; IVH, intraventricular hemorrhage; Mg, magnesium; PVL, periventricular leukomalacia.

coordinated with angiogenesis.[64] VEGF-A is the most important member of a family of growth factors that also includes placental growth factor (PLGF) and VEGFs B, C, and D. VEGF-A is expressed in cortical neurons during early development, switching to mature glial cells near vessels during maturation. Following exposure to hypoxia, there is increased neuronal and glial expression of VEGF-A,[65] directing vascularization and stimulating proliferation of neuronal and non-neuronal cell types.[66–68] VEGF also has chemotactic effects on neurogenic zones in the brain,[69] increasing migration of stem cells during anoxia.[70,71] VEGF knockout mice have severe impairments in vascularization, neuronal migration, and survival.[72]

In adult ischemia models, intravenous VEGF administered 1 hour after insult increases blood-brain barrier leakage and lesion size, but late administration 48 hours after ischemia enhances angiogenesis and functional performance.[73] Both topical and intracerebroventricular injection reduced infarct volume,[74,75] and benefit has been shown in neurodegenerative and traumatic models of injury as well. VEGF-overexpressing mice also show benefit from direct neuroprotection resulting from inhibition of apoptotic pathways.[63]

Other trophic factors have also shown promise, but given their role in normal neurodevelopment the effects of treatment are not known. IGF-1 is important for growth and maturation of the fetal brain as well as differentiation of oligodendrocyte precursors.[76] IGF-1 has prosurvival properties that can prevent perinatal hypoxic and excitotoxic injury,[77,78] and is also effective after intranasal administration.[79] Brain-derived neurotrophic factor (BDNF) is a neurotrophin that also provides neuroprotection in neonatal HI.[80–83] BDNF prevents spatial learning and memory impairments after injury, but its effectiveness is limited by the stage of development.[82,83] Although protective in mice when given on postnatal day 5 (P5), BDNF has no effect at later time points and actually exacerbates excitotoxicity if given on the day of birth.[82]

STEM CELL THERAPY

Neural stem cells (NSCs) are multipotent precursors that self-renew and retain the ability to differentiate into a variety of neuronal and non-neuronal cell types in the CNS. They reside in neurogenic zones throughout life, such as the SVZ and the dentate gyrus of the hippocampus in rodents, and are responsible for maintaining baseline turnover of cells as well as replacing injured cells through migration to penumbral tissue after injury. NSC transplantation has shown potential as a therapeutic strategy in adult animal models of brain injury. Implanted cells integrate into injured tissue,[84] decreasing volume loss[85–87] and improving behavioral outcomes.[88,89] In neonatal models, intraventricular implantation of NSCs after HI results in their migration to injured areas[86,87] and differentiation into neurons, astrocytes, oligodendrocytes, and undifferentiated progenitors. These cells promote regeneration, angiogenesis, and neuronal cell survival in both rodent and primate models, and non-neuronal progeny inhibit inflammation and scar formation.[90,91] Although complications of implantation have not been noted in these models, efficacy does depend on time of implantation, and the therapeutic window is not known. More recent technology enables labeling of stem cells, which can then be tracked from the site of implantation through their migratory path into the ischemic tissue,[92–95] making their identification and eventual outcome in humans possible.

ANTIOXIDANTS

Oxidative stress is an important component of early injury to the neonatal brain,[96] resulting from the excess formation of free radicals (FR) (reactive oxygen species [ROS] and reactive nitrogen species [RNS]) under pathologic conditions. These include superoxide anion (O_2^-), hydroxyl radical (OH), singlet oxygen ($^1O_2$), and hydrogen peroxide (H_2O_2).[97,98] Antioxidant defenses such as superoxide dismutase (SOD), glutathione peroxidase (GPx), catalase, and compounds such as vitamins A, C, and E; beta carotene; glutathione; and ubiquinones scavenge FRs under normal conditions. Damage occurs when there is an imbalance between their generation and uptake.[97] Following HI, there is an increase in superoxide and hydroxyl radical production and rapid depletion of antioxidant stores, which leads to cell membrane damage, excitotoxic energy depletion, cytosolic calcium accumulation, and activation of pro-apoptotic genes that cause damage to cellular components and result in cell death.[99]

The neonatal brain has a high rate of oxygen consumption and low concentration of antioxidants, making it susceptible to damage.[100,101] In the rat, total GPx activity increases between embryonic day 18 (E18) and postnatal day 1 (P1), but is still at lower levels than that seen in the mature brain.[102] In humans, mature oligodendrocytes carry increased antioxidant enzymes compared with the oligodendrocyte precursors present in the immature brain, which may partially explain the susceptibility of premature infants to white matter damage.[103–105]

In an effort to reduce oxidative damage to the neonate, a number of strategies have been used, including ROS scavengers, lipid peroxidation inhibitors, FR reducers, and nitric oxide synthase inhibitors. Nitric oxide synthase (NOS) catalyzes the synthesis of nitric oxide (NO) from the conversion of arginine to citrulline.[106] NO plays an important role in pulmonary, systemic, and cerebral vasodilation, and is constitutively produced in response to increased intracellular calcium by endothelial nitric oxide synthase (eNOS) in endothelial cells and by neuronal nitric oxide synthase (nNOS) in astrocytes and neurons. An inducible isoform of nitric oxide synthase (iNOS) also produces NO in response to cellular stress, which initiates neuronal damage when converted to secondary reactive nitrogen species that facilitate nitration and nitrosylation reactions.[107] Early endothelial NO is protective by maintaining blood flow, but early neuronal NO and late inducible NO promote cell death.[108] Brain iNOS is induced in multiple cell types during up-regulation of the proinflammatory pathway after brain injury,[109] modifying binding to N-methyl-D-aspartate (NMDA) receptors and enhancing excitotoxicity.[110]

Selective inhibition of nNOS or iNOS has shown potential as a neuroprotective strategy.[111] Regions expressing nNOS correspond to those that are susceptible to excitoxicity, expressing NMDA receptors in vivo and in vitro.[112–114] Destruction of neurons containing nNOS or targeted disruption of the nNOS gene protects animals from HI injury,[113,115] but nonspecific blockade of nNOS and eNOS is not protective.[116] There have been few studies in human newborns examining cerebral NO production. Cerebrospinal fluid (CSF) NO levels increase with severity of HI encephalopathy at 24 to 72 hours after asphyxia,[117] with increased NO and nitrotyrosine levels in the spinal cord as well.[118] Initial results in premature infants treated with inhaled NO for prevention of bronchopulmonary dysplasia show reductions in ultrasound-diagnosed brain injury and improvements in neurodevelopmental outcomes at 2 years of age, but long-term results are still pending.[119,120]

Several other antioxidant strategies that either block FR production or increase antioxidant defenses are being studied. Melatonin is an indoleamine that is formed in higher quantities in adults and functions as a direct scavenger of ROS and NO. It has been found to provide long-lasting neuroprotection in experimental HI and focal cerebral ischemic injury,[121,122] and human neonates treated with melatonin were also found to have decreased proinflammatory cytokines.[123,124] Allopurinol has mixed effects that have shown promise in animal and human studies. Xanthine oxidase–derived superoxide and H_2O_2 react with NO to form damaging RNS. Allopurinol reduces FR production by inhibiting xanthine oxidase while also scavenging hydroxyl radicals. High-dose allopurinol given 15 minutes after HI in P7 rats decreases acute edema and long-term infarct volume.[125] Short-term benefits have also been seen in neonates undergoing cardiac surgery for hypoplastic left heart syndrome.[126] Early allopurinol in asphyxiated infants improved short-term neurodevelopmental outcomes and decreased serum NO levels after administration; however, there may be only a brief window for benefit, as no improvement in long-term outcomes was seen with later treatment after birth asphyxia.[127] Deferoxamine (DFO) is an iron chelator that decreases FR production by binding with iron and decreasing the production of OH that occurs via the Fenton reaction,[128,129] while also stabilizing HIF-1α to produce its downstream products VEGF and EPO.[128] DFO is protective during exposure to H_2O_2 or excitotoxicity in vitro,[130] and in animal models of HI and transient ischemic stroke in vivo.[128,131,132] N-acetylcysteine (NAC) is a glutathione precursor and FR scavenger that attenuates lipopolysaccharide-induced white matter injury in newborn rats,[133,134] but results for other antioxidant compounds, such as vitamin E, have been inconclusive.[135]

EXCITOTOXICITY

Glutamate plays an important role in progenitor cell proliferation, differentiation, migration, and survival in the developing brain. Excitotoxicity refers to excessive glutamatergic activation that leads to cell injury and death.[136] Glutamate accumulates in the brain after HI[137] from a variety of causes, including vesicular release[138] and reversal of glutamate transporters.[139,140] Glutamatergic receptors include NMDA, alpha-3-amino-hydroxy-5-methyl-4-isoxazole propionic acid (AMPA), and kainate. NMDA receptor activation, although important for synaptic plasticity,[141] can increase intracellulular calcium and pro-apoptotic pathways via caspase-3 activation if overactivated.[142,143] Excitotoxicity has long been known to play a part in the progression of HI brain injury, and differences in receptor expression contribute to the vulnerability of the developing brain.[144] NMDA, as well as AMPA and kainate, receptors on oligodendrocyte precursors play a large part in their susceptibility to damage in premature HI-induced white matter injury.[145–147]

There has long been a search for agents that decrease brain injury by decreasing excitotoxicity. Dizocilpine (MK801) is a noncompetitive NMDA receptor antagonist that has been studied in humans, but is poorly tolerated and has also been shown to increase apoptosis and decrease neuronal migration in animal models.[148] Memantine is a low-affinity noncompetitive NMDA receptor antagonist that is well tolerated in adults for Alzheimer's-type dementia.[149] Post-HI treatment with memantine attenuates acute white matter injury in P6 rats, resulting in long-term histologic improvement in vivo and restoring neuronal migration in vitro.[150–152] Another method to decrease excitotoxicity is the use of topiramate, an AMPA-kainate receptor antagonist that is an FDA-approved anti-epileptic for patients older than 2 years. It has been shown to protect newborn rodents from excitotoxic brain lesions,[153] reducing brain damage and cognitive impairment when administered within 2 hours of the insult.[154] An intravenous (IV) preparation of topiramate does not yet exist for human use, but this treatment shows potential as a therapy for early newborn seizure and injury. Cannabinoids have also shown promise as a treatment for neurodegenerative disorders[155] and in adult models of ischemia[156] or trauma.[157] They are involved in control of synaptic transmission, and their receptors (CB1 and CB2) are expressed on neurons and glia.[158,159] In the immature brain, cannabinoids have effects on excitotoxic lesions,[160] and the agonist WIN 55,212-2 reduces short-term brain injury when administered after neonatal HI.[161]

Magnesium sulfate has shown some benefit in preventing white matter damage in animal models,[162–164] and one possible mechanism of its neuroprotection is the blockade of NMDA receptors.[165] In a multicenter clinical trial of mothers treated with magnesium who were at risk for preterm delivery, no perinatal side effects were seen and there was some benefit in the neurodevelopment of survivors.[166] However, magnesium administered to asphyxiated term neonates did not result in improvements in aEEG patterns, and when given in larger doses was associated with profound hypotension.[167,168]

ANTI-INFLAMMATORY THERAPY

Maternal infection is a known risk factor for white matter damage and poor outcomes, such as cerebral palsy.[169–171] The inflammatory response and cytokine production that accompany infection may play a large role in cell damage and loss.[172] Local microglia are activated early and produce proinflammatory cytokines such as tumor necrosis factor (TNF)-α, interleukin (IL)-1β and IL-6, as well as glutamate, FRs, and NO. Systemic administration of these cytokines increases excitotoxic lesions,[173] whereas therapies that block microglial activation and cytokine release protect the brain from excitotoxic damage.[174]

Minocycline is a tetracycline derivative that crosses the blood-brain barrier and has anti-inflammatory effects, including decreasing microglial activation and caspase-3 expression,[175,176] lipid peroxidation,[177] and other pro-inflammatory activity[178] while increasing anti-apoptotic gene expression.[179,180] Minocycline has shown promise in a number of animal models of neurodegenerative or ischemic disease.[175,181–185] In the neonatal brain, minocycline appears to decrease tissue damage and caspase-3 activation in rodents when given immediately before or after injury, but results are inconsistent.[186–188] Low- and high-dose regimens were effective in reducing short-term HI-induced inflammation, protecting developing oligodendrocytes[188] and myelin content in neonatal rats,[189] but this effect was only transient in another study of neonatal rodent stroke.[187] Delayed therapy was found to decrease TNF-α and matrix metalloproteinase MMP-12, but efficacy was lost when treatment was extended for a week after stroke.[190] These effects also appear to be species dependent, with an increase in injury in developing C57B1/6 mice.[191]

CELL DEATH INHIBITORS

Apoptosis is a critical component of normal brain development. Although necrosis plays a major role in early neuronal death in both the immature and mature brain following injury,[192] a spectrum of cell death that includes apoptosis occurs within the first 24 hours following neonatal HI,[193] and may result in heterogeneous responses to anti-apoptotic therapies.[194] It is also probable that apoptosis and cleavage and activation of caspase-3 are responsible for more of the cell death that occurs in delayed phases of injury and neurodegeneration.[195]

Specific and nonspecific inhibition of caspases or cysteine proteases, which are highly activated after HI, has been attempted with some success.[196–199] For example, calpain or caspase-3 inhibitors such as MDL 28710 and M826 protect neonatal rats after HI.[197,200] Pretreatment with the hormone 17β-estradiol is neuroprotective in immature rats, and appears to work through both anti-apoptotic and FR scavenging pathways.[201] In addition, the nuclear enzyme poly (ADP-ribose) polymerase (PARP) is activated during stress and enables DNA repair; however, the PARP-1 isoform also contributes to ischemic neuronal injury by depleting energy stores and activating microglia, leading to cell death. PARP-1 is more abundant in the immature brain, and its blockade protects against excitotoxicity and ischemic injury.[202] The PARP-1 inhibitor 3-aminobenzamide reduces injury after focal ischemia in P7 rats,[203] but PARP-1 blockade appears to protect males preferentially.[202]

COMBINATION THERAPY

Single therapy that attacks any of the aforementioned injury pathways often results in only mild improvement. For example, therapeutics targeting apoptosis may prevent delayed cell death, but would not effect earlier necrotic and excitotoxic injury. Hypothermia has become the standard of care in many institutions since showing benefit in moderately encephalopathic newborns; however, it does not completely protect or repair an injured brain, and benefits may not necessarily be long lasting,[204,205] so the search for adjuvant therapies continues. Combinatorial therapy may provide more long-lasting neuroprotection, salvaging the brain from severe injury and deficits while also enhancing repair and regeneration, hopefully providing additive, if not synergistic, protection.

Xenon is approved for use as a general anesthetic in Europe and has shown promise as a protective agent. It is an NMDA antagonist, preventing progression of excitotoxic damage. It appears to be superior to other NMDA antagonists, possibly through inhibition of AMPA and kainate receptors, reduction of neurotransmitter release, or effects on other ion channels.[206–208] Combination xenon and hypothermia initiated 4 hours after neonatal HI provided synergistic histologic and functional protection when evaluated at 30 days after injury.[209] Hypothermia does reduce glutamate and glycine release,[210] and NMDA receptor antagonism may explain these effects. More recently, an additive effect was shown after HI in P7 rats that were cooled to 32°C and received 50% xenon, with improvement in long-term histology and functional performance that exceeded the individual benefit of either.[211] More extensive studies on xenon use in human neonates are necessary.

N-acetylcysteine (NAC) is a medication approved for neonates that is a scavenger of oxygen radicals and restores intracellular glutathione levels, attenuating reperfusion injury and decreasing inflammation and NO production in adult models of stroke.[212,213] Adding NAC therapy to systemic hypothermia reduced brain volume loss at both 2 and 4 weeks after neonatal rodent HI, with increased myelin expression and improved reflexes.[214] Inhibition of inflammation with MK-801 has also been effective when combined with hypothermia in neonatal rats post HI injury.[215] In P7 rats that underwent HI followed by early topiramate and delayed hypothermia, improved short-term histology and function were seen.[216] The inhibition of inflammation may provide a window for protection if hypothermia is delayed, which is possible given difficulty in initiation of cooling if infants are born at an outside hospital or transport is delayed.

SUMMARY

Most studies have focused on singular mechanisms of injury, such as oxidative stress, inflammation, and excitotoxicity. More recent evidence suggests that injury occurs over long periods of time and that therapies may need to be administered over much longer periods than have been previously entertained. Although hypothermia and single pharmacotherapies show promise, combined therapy may be necessary to increase the therapeutic time window for protection and repair, making recovery possible.

REFERENCES

1. Wu YW, Backstrand KH, Zhao S, et al. Declining diagnosis of birth asphyxia in California: 1991–2000. Pediatrics 2004;114(6):1584–90.
2. Nelson KB, Lynch JK. Stroke in newborn infants. Lancet Neurol 2004;3(3):150–8.
3. Gressens P, Luton D. Fetal MRI: obstetrical and neurological perspectives. Pediatr Radiol 2004;34(9):682–4.
4. Miller SP, McQuillen PS, Hamrick S, et al. Abnormal brain development in newborns with congenital heart disease. N Engl J Med 2007;357(19):1928–38.
5. Dilenge ME, Majnemer A, Shevell MI, et al. Long-term developmental outcome of asphyxiated term neonates. J Child Neurol 2001;16(11):781–92.
6. Ferriero DM. Neonatal brain injury. N Engl J Med 2004;351(19):1985–95.
7. McQuillen PS, Ferriero DM. Selective vulnerability in the developing central nervous system. Pediatr Neurol 2004;30(4):227–35.
8. Geddes R, Vannucci RC, Vannucci SJ, et al. Delayed cerebral atrophy following moderate hypoxia-ischemia in the immature rat. Dev Neurosci 2001;23(3):180–5.
9. Gluckman PD, Wyatt JS, Azzopardi D, et al. Selective head cooling with mild systemic hypothermia after neonatal encephalopathy: multicentre randomised trial. Lancet 2005;365(9460):663–70.
10. Miller SP, Latal B, Clark H, et al. Clinical signs predict 30-month neurodevelopmental outcome after neonatal encephalopathy. Am J Obstet Gynecol 2004;190(1):93–9.

11. Hellstrom-Westas L, Rosen I. Continuous brain-function monitoring: state of the art in clinical practice. Semin Fetal Neonatal Med 2006;11(6):503–11.
12. Shellhaas RA, Soaita AI, Clancy RR, et al. Sensitivity of amplitude-integrated electroencephalography for neonatal seizure detection. Pediatrics 2007; 120(4):770–7.
13. Chau V, Clement JF, Robitaille Y, et al. Congenital axonal neuropathy and encephalopathy. Pediatr Neurol 2008;38(4):261–6.
14. Miller SP, Ramaswamy V, Michelson D, et al. Patterns of brain injury in term neonatal encephalopathy. J Pediatr 2005;146(4):453–60.
15. Laptook AR, Corbett RJ, Sterett R, et al. Modest hypothermia provides partial neuroprotection for ischemic neonatal brain. Pediatr Res 1994;35(4 Pt 1): 436–42.
16. Laptook AR, Corbett RJ, Sterett R, et al. Modest hypothermia provides partial neuroprotection when used for immediate resuscitation after brain ischemia. Pediatr Res 1997;42(1):17–23.
17. Thoresen M, Penrice J, Lorek A, et al. Mild hypothermia after severe transient hypoxia-ischemia ameliorates delayed cerebral energy failure in the newborn piglet. Pediatr Res 1995;37(5):667–70.
18. Gunn AJ, Gunn TR, de Haan HH, et al. Dramatic neuronal rescue with prolonged selective head cooling after ischemia in fetal lambs. J Clin Invest 1997;99(2): 248–56.
19. Gunn AJ, Gunn TR, Gunning MI, et al. Neuroprotection with prolonged head cooling started before postischemic seizures in fetal sheep. Pediatrics 1998; 102(5):1098–106.
20. Towfighi J, Housman C, Heitjan DF, et al. The effect of focal cerebral cooling on perinatal hypoxic-ischemic brain damage. Acta Neuropathol 1994;87(6): 598–604.
21. Laptook AR, Corbett RJ. The effects of temperature on hypoxic-ischemic brain injury. Clin Perinatol 2002;29(4):623–49, vi.
22. Thoresen M, Whitelaw A. Cardiovascular changes during mild therapeutic hypothermia and rewarming in infants with hypoxic-ischemic encephalopathy. Pediatrics 2000;106(1 Pt 1):92–9.
23. Gunn AJ, Gluckman PD, Gunn TR, et al. Selective head cooling in newborn infants after perinatal asphyxia: a safety study. Pediatrics 1998;102(4 Pt 1): 885–92.
24. Eicher DJ, Wagner CL, Katikaneni LP, et al. Moderate hypothermia in neonatal encephalopathy: efficacy outcomes. Pediatr Neurol 2005;32(1):11–7.
25. Shankaran S, Laptook AR, Ehrenkranz RA, et al. Whole-body hypothermia for neonates with hypoxic-ischemic encephalopathy. N Engl J Med 2005;353(15): 1574–84.
26. Bona E, Hagberg H, Loberg EM, et al. Protective effects of moderate hypothermia after neonatal hypoxia-ischemia: short- and long-term outcome. Pediatr Res 1998;43(6):738–45.
27. Azzopardi D, Robertson NJ, Cowan FM, et al. Pilot study of treatment with whole body hypothermia for neonatal encephalopathy. Pediatrics 2000; 106(4):684–94.
28. Thoresen M. Cooling the newborn after asphyxia—physiological and experimental background and its clinical use. Semin Neonatol 2000;5(1):61–73.
29. Shankaran S, Laptook A, Wright LL, et al. Whole-body hypothermia for neonatal encephalopathy: animal observations as a basis for a randomized, controlled pilot study in term infants. Pediatrics 2002;110(2 Pt 1):377–85.

30. Battin MR, Thoresen M, Robinson E, et al. Does head cooling with mild systemic hypothermia affect requirement for blood pressure support? Pediatrics 2009; 123(3):1031–6.
31. Groenendaal F, De Vooght KM, van Bel F. Blood gas values during hypothermia in asphyxiated term neonates. Pediatrics 2009;123(1):170–2.
32. Sarkar S, Barks JD, Bhagat I, et al. Pulmonary dysfunction and therapeutic hypothermia in asphyxiated newborns: whole body versus selective head cooling. Am J Perinatol 2009;26(4):265–70.
33. Wyatt JS, Gluckman PD, Liu PY, et al. Determinants of outcomes after head cooling for neonatal encephalopathy. Pediatrics 2007;119(5):912–21.
34. Laptook A, Tyson J, Shankaran S, et al. Elevated temperature after hypoxic-ischemic encephalopathy: risk factor for adverse outcomes. Pediatrics 2008; 122(3):491–9.
35. Shankaran S, Pappas A, Laptook AR, et al. Outcomes of safety and effectiveness in a multicenter randomized, controlled trial of whole-body hypothermia for neonatal hypoxic-ischemic encephalopathy. Pediatrics 2008;122(4): e791–8.
36. Van Leeuwen GM, Hand JW, Lagendijk JJ, et al. Numerical modeling of temperature distributions within the neonatal head. Pediatr Res 2000;48(3):351–6.
37. Robertson NJ, Nakakeeto M, Hagmann C, et al. Therapeutic hypothermia for birth asphyxia in low-resource settings: a pilot randomised controlled trial. Lancet 2008;372(9641):801–3.
38. Bergeron M, Gidday JM, Yu AY, et al. Role of hypoxia-inducible factor-1 in hypoxia-induced ischemic tolerance in neonatal rat brain. Ann Neurol 2000; 48(3):285–96.
39. Sheldon RA, Aminoff A, Lee CL, et al. Hypoxic preconditioning reverses protection after neonatal hypoxia-ischemia in glutathione peroxidase transgenic murine brain. Pediatr Res 2007;61(6):666–70.
40. Gidday JM, Fitzgibbons JC, Shah AR, et al. Neuroprotection from ischemic brain injury by hypoxic preconditioning in the neonatal rat. Neurosci Lett 1994; 168(1–2):221–4.
41. Vannucci RC, Towfighi J, Vannucci SJ, et al. Hypoxic preconditioning and hypoxic-ischemic brain damage in the immature rat: pathologic and metabolic correlates. J Neurochem 1998;71(3):1215–20.
42. Gustavsson M, Anderson MF, Mallard C, et al. Hypoxic preconditioning confers long-term reduction of brain injury and improvement of neurological ability in immature rats. Pediatr Res 2005;57(2):305–9.
43. Ran R, Xu H, Lu A, et al. Hypoxia preconditioning in the brain. Dev Neurosci 2005;27(2–4):87–92.
44. Villa P, Bigini P, Mennini T, et al. Erythropoietin selectively attenuates cytokine production and inflammation in cerebral ischemia by targeting neuronal apoptosis. J Exp Med 2003;198(6):971–5.
45. Wang L, Zhang Z, Wang Y, et al. Treatment of stroke with erythropoietin enhances neurogenesis and angiogenesis and improves neurological function in rats. Stroke 2004;35(7):1732–7.
46. Chong ZZ, Kang JQ, Maiese K, et al. Angiogenesis and plasticity: role of erythropoietin in vascular systems. J Hematother Stem Cell Res 2002;11(6): 863–71.
47. Juul SE, Yachnis AT, Rojiani AM, et al. Immunohistochemical localization of erythropoietin and its receptor in the developing human brain. Pediatr Dev Pathol 1999;2(2):148–58.

48. Shingo T, Sorokan ST, Shimazaki T, et al. Erythropoietin regulates the in vitro and in vivo production of neuronal progenitors by mammalian forebrain neural stem cells. J Neurosci 2001;21(24):9733–43.
49. Sola A, Wen TC, Hamrick SE, et al. Potential for protection and repair following injury to the developing brain: a role for erythropoietin? Pediatr Res 2005;57(5 Pt 2): 110R–7R.
50. Kumral A, Uysal N, Tugyan K, et al. Erythropoietin improves long-term spatial memory deficits and brain injury following neonatal hypoxia-ischemia in rats. Behav Brain Res 2004;153(1):77–86.
51. Sola A, Rogido M, Lee BH, et al. Erythropoietin after focal cerebral ischemia activates the Janus kinase-signal transducer and activator of transcription signaling pathway and improves brain injury in postnatal day 7 rats. Pediatr Res 2005; 57(4):481–7.
52. Chang YS, Mu D, Wendland M, et al. Erythropoietin improves functional and histological outcome in neonatal stroke. Pediatr Res 2005;58(1):106–11.
53. Gonzalez FF, Abel R, Almli CR, et al. Erythropoietin sustains cognitive function and brain volume after neonatal stroke. Dev Neurosci, in press.
54. Wen TC, Rogido M, Peng H, et al. Gender differences in long-term beneficial effects of erythropoietin given after neonatal stroke in postnatal day-7 rats. Neuroscience 2006;139(3):803–11.
55. Sun Y, Calvert JW, Zhang JH. Neonatal hypoxia/ischemia is associated with decreased inflammatory mediators after erythropoietin administration. Stroke 2005;36(8):1672–8.
56. Gonzalez FF, McQuillen P, Mu D, et al. Erythropoietin enhances long-term neuroprotection and neurogenesis in neonatal stroke. Dev Neurosci 2007;29(4–5): 321–30.
57. Plane JM, Liu R, Wang TW, et al. Neonatal hypoxic-ischemic injury increases forebrain subventricular zone neurogenesis in the mouse. Neurobiol Dis 2004; 16(3):585–95.
58. Lu D, Mahmood A, Qu C, et al. Erythropoietin enhances neurogenesis and restores spatial memory in rats after traumatic brain injury. J Neurotrauma 2005;22(9):1011–7.
59. Aher S, Ohlsson A. Late erythropoietin for preventing red blood cell transfusion in preterm and/or low birth weight infants. Cochrane Database Syst Rev 2006;(3): CD004868.
60. Demers EJ, McPherson RJ, Juul SE, et al. Erythropoietin protects dopaminergic neurons and improves neurobehavioral outcomes in juvenile rats after neonatal hypoxia-ischemia. Pediatr Res 2005;58(2):297–301.
61. McPherson RJ, Juul SE. High-dose erythropoietin inhibits apoptosis and stimulates proliferation in neonatal rat intestine. Growth Horm IGF Res 2007;17(5):424–30.
62. Juul SE, McPherson RJ, Bauer LA, et al. A phase I/II trial of high dose erythropoietin in extremely low birth weight infants: pharmacokinetics and safety. Pediatrics 2008;122(2):504–10.
63. Zachary I. Neuroprotective role of vascular endothelial growth factor: signalling mechanisms, biological function, and therapeutic potential. Neurosignals 2005; 14(5):207–21.
64. Palmer TD, Willhoite AR, Gage FH, et al. Vascular niche for adult hippocampal neurogenesis. J Comp Neurol 2000;425(4):479–94.
65. Krum JM, Rosenstein JM. VEGF mRNA and its receptor flt-1 are expressed in reactive astrocytes following neural grafting and tumor cell implantation in the adult CNS. Exp Neurol 1998;154(1):57–65.

66. Forstreuter F, Lucius R, Mentlein R, et al. Vascular endothelial growth factor induces chemotaxis and proliferation of microglial cells. J Neuroimmunol 2002;132(1–2):93–8.

67. Mu D, Jiang X, Sheldon RA, et al. Regulation of hypoxia-inducible factor 1alpha and induction of vascular endothelial growth factor in a rat neonatal stroke model. Neurobiol Dis 2003;14(3):524–34.

68. Jin K, Zhu Y, Sun Y, et al. Vascular endothelial growth factor (VEGF) stimulates neurogenesis in vitro and in vivo. Proc Natl Acad Sci U S A 2002;99(18):11946–50.

69. Yang X, Cepko CL. Flk-1, a receptor for vascular endothelial growth factor (VEGF), is expressed by retinal progenitor cells. J Neurosci 1996;16(19): 6089–99.

70. Maurer MH, Tripps WK, Feldmann RE Jr, et al. Expression of vascular endothelial growth factor and its receptors in rat neural stem cells. Neurosci Lett 2003; 344(3):165–8.

71. Bagnard D, Vaillant C, Khuth ST, et al. Semaphorin 3A-vascular endothelial growth factor-165 balance mediates migration and apoptosis of neural progenitor cells by the recruitment of shared receptor. J Neurosci 2001; 21(10):3332–41.

72. Raab S, Beck H, Gaumann A, et al. Impaired brain angiogenesis and neuronal apoptosis induced by conditional homozygous inactivation of vascular endothelial growth factor. Thromb Haemost 2004;91(3):595–605.

73. Zhang ZG, Zhang L, Jiang Q, et al. VEGF enhances angiogenesis and promotes blood-brain barrier leakage in the ischemic brain. J Clin Invest 2000;106(7): 829–38.

74. Hayashi T, Abe K, Itoyama Y, et al. Reduction of ischemic damage by application of vascular endothelial growth factor in rat brain after transient ischemia. J Cereb Blood Flow Metab 1998;18(8):887–95.

75. Harrigan MR, Ennis SR, Sullivan SE, et al. Effects of intraventricular infusion of vascular endothelial growth factor on cerebral blood flow, edema, and infarct volume. Acta Neurochir (Wien) 2003;145(1):49–53.

76. D'Ercole AJ, Ye P, Calikoglu AS, et al. The role of the insulin-like growth factors in the central nervous system. Mol Neurobiol 1996;13(3):227–55.

77. Johnston BM, Mallard EC, Williams CE, et al. Insulin-like growth factor-1 is a potent neuronal rescue agent after hypoxic-ischemic injury in fetal lambs. J Clin Invest 1996;97(2):300–8.

78. Pang Y, Zheng B, Fan LW, et al. IGF-1 protects oligodendrocyte progenitors against TNFalpha-induced damage by activation of PI3K/Akt and interruption of the mitochondrial apoptotic pathway. Glia 2007;55(11):1099–107.

79. Lin S, Fan LW, Rhodes PG, et al. Intranasal administration of IGF-1 attenuates hypoxic-ischemic brain injury in neonatal rats. Exp Neurol 2009; 217(2):361–70.

80. Cheng Y, Gidday JM, Yan Q, et al. Marked age-dependent neuroprotection by brain-derived neurotrophic factor against neonatal hypoxic-ischemic brain injury. Ann Neurol 1997;41(4):521–9.

81. Holtzman DM, Sheldon RA, Jaffe W, et al. Nerve growth factor protects the neonatal brain against hypoxic-ischemic injury. Ann Neurol 1996;39(1):114–22.

82. Husson I, Rangon CM, Lelievre V, et al. BDNF-induced white matter neuroprotection and stage-dependent neuronal survival following a neonatal excitotoxic challenge. Cereb Cortex 2005;15(3):250–61.

83. Cheng ET, Utley DS, Ho PR, et al. Functional recovery of transected nerves treated with systemic BDNF and CNTF. Microsurgery 1998;18(1):35–41.

84. Park KI, Teng YD, Snyder EY, et al. The injured brain interacts reciprocally with neural stem cells supported by scaffolds to reconstitute lost tissue. Nat Biotechnol 2002;20(11):1111–7.

85. Hoehn M, Kustermann E, Blunk J, et al. Monitoring of implanted stem cell migration in vivo: a highly resolved in vivo magnetic resonance imaging investigation of experimental stroke in rat. Proc Natl Acad Sci U S A 2002; 99(25):16267–72.

86. Park KI, Himes BT, Stieg PE, et al. Neural stem cells may be uniquely suited for combined gene therapy and cell replacement: evidence from engraftment of Neurotrophin-3-expressing stem cells in hypoxic-ischemic brain injury. Exp Neurol 2006;199(1):179–90.

87. Park KI, Hack MA, Ourednik J, et al. Acute injury directs the migration, proliferation, and differentiation of solid organ stem cells: evidence from the effect of hypoxia-ischemia in the CNS on clonal "reporter" neural stem cells. Exp Neurol 2006;199(1):156–78.

88. Capone C, Frigerio S, Fumagalli S, et al. Neurosphere-derived cells exert a neuroprotective action by changing the ischemic microenvironment. PLoS One 2007;2(4):e373.

89. Hicks AU, Hewlett K, Windle V, et al. Enriched environment enhances transplanted subventricular zone stem cell migration and functional recovery after stroke. Neuroscience 2007;146(1):31–40.

90. Imitola J, Raddassi K, Park KI, et al. Directed migration of neural stem cells to sites of CNS injury by the stromal cell-derived factor 1alpha/CXC chemokine receptor 4 pathway. Proc Natl Acad Sci U S A 2004;101(52):18117–22.

91. Mueller FJ, Serobyan N, Schraufstatter IU, et al. Adhesive interactions between human neural stem cells and inflamed human vascular endothelium are mediated by integrins. Stem Cells 2006;24(11):2367–72.

92. Modo M, Mellodew K, Cash D, et al. Mapping transplanted stem cell migration after a stroke: a serial, in vivo magnetic resonance imaging study. Neuroimage 2004;21(1):311–7.

93. Guzman R, Uchida N, Bliss TM, et al. Long-term monitoring of transplanted human neural stem cells in developmental and pathological contexts with MRI. Proc Natl Acad Sci U S A 2007;104(24):10211–6.

94. Rice HE, Hsu EW, Sheng H, et al. Superparamagnetic iron oxide labeling and transplantation of adipose-derived stem cells in middle cerebral artery occlusion-injured mice. AJR Am J Roentgenol 2007;188(4):1101–8.

95. Obenaus A, Robbins M, Blanco G, et al. Multi-modal magnetic resonance imaging alterations in two rat models of mild neurotrauma. J Neurotrauma 2007;24(7):1147–60.

96. Ferriero DM. Oxidant mechanisms in neonatal hypoxia-ischemia. Dev Neurosci 2001;23(3):198–202.

97. Fridovich I. Superoxide anion radical (O2-), superoxide dismutases, and related matters. J Biol Chem 1997;272(30):18515–7.

98. Halliwell B. Antioxidant defence mechanisms: from the beginning to the end (of the beginning). Free Radic Res 1999;31(4):261–72.

99. Taylor DL, Edwards AD, Mehmet H, et al. Oxidative metabolism, apoptosis and perinatal brain injury. Brain Pathol 1999;9(1):93–117.

100. Buonocore G, Perrone S, Bracci R, et al. Free radicals and brain damage in the newborn. Biol Neonate 2001;79(3–4):180–6.

101. Halliwell B. Oxidative stress and neurodegeneration: where are we now? J Neurochem 2006;97(6):1634–58.

102. Khan JY, Black SM. Developmental changes in murine brain antioxidant enzymes. Pediatr Res 2003;54(1):77–82.
103. Baud O, Li J, Zhang Y, et al. Nitric oxide-induced cell death in developing oligo-dendrocytes is associated with mitochondrial dysfunction and apoptosis-inducing factor translocation. Eur J Neurosci 2004;20(7):1713–26.
104. Volpe JJ. Brain injury in the premature infant. Neuropathology, clinical aspects, pathogenesis, and prevention. Clin Perinatol 1997;24(3):567–87.
105. Haynes RL, Baud O, Li J, et al. Oxidative and nitrative injury in periventricular leukomalacia: a review. Brain Pathol 2005;15(3):225–33.
106. Boucher JL, Moali C, Tenu JP. Nitric oxide biosynthesis, nitric oxide synthase inhibitors and arginase competition for L-arginine utilization. Cell Mol Life Sci 1999;55(8–9):1015–28.
107. Beckman JS, Koppenol WH. Nitric oxide, superoxide, and peroxynitrite: the good, the bad, and ugly. Am J Phys 1996;271(5 Pt 1):C1424–37.
108. Iadecola C, Zhang F, Casey R, et al. Delayed reduction of ischemic brain injury and neurological deficits in mice lacking the inducible nitric oxide synthase gene. J Neurosci 1997;17(23):9157–64.
109. Higuchi Y, Hattori H, Kume T, et al. Increase in nitric oxide in the hypoxic-ischemic neonatal rat brain and suppression by 7-nitroindazole and aminogua-nidine. Eur J Pharmacol 1998;342(1):47–9.
110. Ishida A, Trescher WH, Lange MS, et al. Prolonged suppression of brain nitric oxide synthase activity by 7-nitroindazole protects against cerebral hypoxic-ischemic injury in neonatal rat. Brain Dev 2001;23(5):349–54.
111. van den Tweel ER, van Bel F, Kavelaars A, et al. Long-term neuroprotection with 2-iminobiotin, an inhibitor of neuronal and inducible nitric oxide synthase, after cerebral hypoxia-ischemia in neonatal rats. J Cereb Blood Flow Metab 2005;25(1):67–74.
112. Black SM, Bedolli MA, Martinez S, et al. Expression of neuronal nitric oxide syn-thase corresponds to regions of selective vulnerability to hypoxia-ischaemia in the developing rat brain. Neurobiol Dis 1995;2(3):145–55.
113. Ferriero DM, Holtzman DM, Black SM, et al. Neonatal mice lacking neuronal ni-tric oxide synthase are less vulnerable to hypoxic-ischemic injury. Neurobiol Dis 1996;3(1):64–71.
114. Dawson VL, Dawson TM, Bartley DA, et al. Mechanisms of nitric oxide-mediated neurotoxicity in primary brain cultures. J Neurosci 1993;13(6):2651–61.
115. Ferriero DM, Sheldon RA, Black SM, et al. Selective destruction of nitric oxide synthase neurons with quisqualate reduces damage after hypoxia-ischemia in the neonatal rat. Pediatr Res 1995;38(6):912–8.
116. Marks KA, Mallard CE, Roberts I, et al. Nitric oxide synthase inhibition attenu-ates delayed vasodilation and increases injury after cerebral ischemia in fetal sheep. Pediatr Res 1996;40(2):185–91.
117. Ergenekon E, Gucuyener K, Erbas D, et al. Cerebrospinal fluid and serum nitric oxide levels in asphyxiated newborns. Biol Neonate 1999;76(4):200–6.
118. Groenendaal F, Vles J, Lammers H, et al. Nitrotyrosine in human neonatal spinal cord after perinatal asphyxia. Neonatology 2008;93(1):1–6.
119. Schreiber MD, Gin-Mestan K, Marks JD, et al. Inhaled nitric oxide in premature infants with the respiratory distress syndrome. N Engl J Med 2003;349(22):2099–107.
120. Ballard RA, Truog WE, Cnaan A, et al. Inhaled nitric oxide in preterm infants undergoing mechanical ventilation. N Engl J Med 2006;355(4):343–53.
121. Carloni S, Perrone S, Buonocore G, et al. Melatonin protects from the long-term consequences of a neonatal hypoxic-ischemic brain injury in rats. J Pineal Res 2008;44(2):157–64.

122. Koh PO. Melatonin attenuates the focal cerebral ischemic injury by inhibiting the dissociation of pBad from 14-3-3. J Pineal Res 2008;44(1):101–6.
123. Gitto E, Reiter RJ, Cordaro SP, et al. Oxidative and inflammatory parameters in respiratory distress syndrome of preterm newborns: beneficial effects of melatonin. Am J Perinatol 2004;21(4):209–16.
124. Gitto E, Reiter RJ, Sabatino G, et al. Correlation among cytokines, bronchopulmonary dysplasia and modality of ventilation in preterm newborns: improvement with melatonin treatment. J Pineal Res 2005;39(3):287–93.
125. Palmer C, Towfighi J, Roberts RL, et al. Allopurinol administered after inducing hypoxia-ischemia reduces brain injury in 7-day-old rats. Pediatr Res 1993;33 (4 Pt 1):405–11.
126. Clancy RR, McGaurn SA, Goin JE, et al. Allopurinol neurocardiac protection trial in infants undergoing heart surgery using deep hypothermic circulatory arrest. Pediatrics 2001;108(1):61–70.
127. Benders MJ, Bos AF, Rademaker CM, et al. Early postnatal allopurinol does not improve short term outcome after severe birth asphyxia. Arch Dis Child Fetal Neonatal Ed 2006;91(3):F163–5.
128. Mu D, Chang YS, Vexler ZS, et al. Hypoxia-inducible factor 1alpha and erythropoietin upregulation with deferoxamine salvage after neonatal stroke. Exp Neurol 2005;195(2):407–15.
129. Hamrick SE, McQuillen PS, Jiang X, et al. A role for hypoxia-inducible factor-1alpha in desferoxamine neuroprotection. Neurosci Lett 2005;379(2): 96–100.
130. Almli LM, Hamrick SE, Koshy AA, et al. Multiple pathways of neuroprotection against oxidative stress and excitotoxic injury in immature primary hippocampal neurons. Brain Res Dev Brain Res 2001;132(2):121–9.
131. Palmer C, Roberts RL, Bero C, et al. Deferoxamine posttreatment reduces ischemic brain injury in neonatal rats. Stroke 1994;25(5):1039–45.
132. Sarco DP, Becker J, Palmer C, et al. The neuroprotective effect of deferoxamine in the hypoxic-ischemic immature mouse brain. Neurosci Lett 2000;282(1–2): 113–6.
133. Aruoma OI, Halliwell B, Hoey BM, et al. The antioxidant action of N-acetylcysteine: its reaction with hydrogen peroxide, hydroxyl radical, superoxide, and hypochlorous acid. Free Radic Biol Med 1989;6(6):593–7.
134. Paintlia MK, Paintlia AS, Barbosa E, et al. N-acetylcysteine prevents endotoxin-induced degeneration of oligodendrocyte progenitors and hypomyelination in developing rat brain. J Neurosci Res 2004;78(3):347–61.
135. Brion LP, Bell EF, Raghuveer TS, et al. Vitamin E supplementation for prevention of morbidity and mortality in preterm infants. Cochrane Database Syst Rev 2003;(4):CD003665.
136. Olney JW. Excitotoxicity, apoptosis and neuropsychiatric disorders. Curr Opin Pharmacol 2003;3(1):101–9.
137. Gucuyener K, Atalay Y, Aral YZ, et al. Excitatory amino acids and taurine levels in cerebrospinal fluid of hypoxic ischemic encephalopathy in newborn. Clin Neurol Neurosurg 1999;101(3):171–4.
138. Kukley M, Capetillo-Zarate E, Dietrich D, et al. Vesicular glutamate release from axons in white matter. Nat Neurosci 2007;10(3):311–20.
139. Rossi DJ, Oshima T, Attwell D, et al. Glutamate release in severe brain ischaemia is mainly by reversed uptake. Nature 2000;403(6767):316–21.
140. Fern R, Moller T. Rapid ischemic cell death in immature oligodendrocytes: a fatal glutamate release feedback loop. J Neurosci 2000;20(1):34–42.

141. Cull-Candy S, Brickley S, Farrant M, et al. NMDA receptor subunits: diversity, development and disease. Curr Opin Neurobiol 2001;11(3):327–35.

142. Vannucci SJ, Hagberg H. Hypoxia-ischemia in the immature brain. J Exp Biol 2004;207(Pt 18):3149–54.

143. MacDonald JF, Jackson MF, Beazely MA, et al. Hippocampal long-term synaptic plasticity and signal amplification of NMDA receptors. Crit Rev Neurobiol 2006; 18(1–2):71–84.

144. Deng W, Wang H, Rosenberg PA, et al. Role of metabotropic glutamate receptors in oligodendrocyte excitotoxicity and oxidative stress. Proc Natl Acad Sci U S A 2004;101(20):7751–6.

145. Salter MG, Fern R. NMDA receptors are expressed in developing oligodendrocyte processes and mediate injury. Nature 2005;438(7071):1167–71.

146. Kinney HC, Back SA. Human oligodendroglial development: relationship to periventricular leukomalacia. Semin Pediatr Neurol 1998;5(3):180–9.

147. Karadottir R, Cavelier P, Bergersen LH, et al. NMDA receptors are expressed in oligodendrocytes and activated in ischaemia. Nature 2005;438(7071):1162–6.

148. Ikonomidou C, Turski L. Why did NMDA receptor antagonists fail clinical trials for stroke and traumatic brain injury? Lancet Neurol 2002;1(6):383–6.

149. Chen HS, Lipton SA. The chemical biology of clinically tolerated NMDA receptor antagonists. J Neurochem 2006;97(6):1611–26.

150. Chen HS, Wang YF, Rayudu PV, et al. Neuroprotective concentrations of the N-methyl-D-aspartate open-channel blocker memantine are effective without cytoplasmic vacuolation following post-ischemic administration and do not block maze learning or long-term potentiation. Neuroscience 1998;86(4):1121–32.

151. Manning S, Talos D, Zhou C, et al. NMDA receptor blockade with memantine attenuates white matter injury in a rat model of periventricular leukomalacia. J Neurosci 2008;28(26):6670–8.

152. Volbracht C, van Beek J, Zhu C, et al. Neuroprotective properties of memantine in different in vitro and in vivo models of excitotoxicity. Eur J Neurosci 2006; 23(10):2611–22.

153. Sfaello I, Baud O, Arzimanoglou A, et al. Topiramate prevents excitotoxic damage in the newborn rodent brain. Neurobiol Dis 2005;20(3):837–48.

154. Noh MR, Kim SK, Sun W, et al. Neuroprotective effect of topiramate on hypoxic ischemic brain injury in neonatal rats. Exp Neurol 2006;201(2):470–8.

155. Klein TW. Cannabinoid-based drugs as anti-inflammatory therapeutics. Nat Rev Immunol 2005;5(5):400–11.

156. Nagayama T, Sinor AD, Simon RP, et al. Cannabinoids and neuroprotection in global and focal cerebral ischemia and in neuronal cultures. J Neurosci 1999; 19(8):2987–95.

157. Panikashvili D, Shein NA, Mechoulam R, et al. The endocannabinoid 2-AG protects the blood-brain barrier after closed head injury and inhibits mRNA expression of pro-inflammatory cytokines. Neurobiol Dis 2006;22(2):257–64.

158. Benito C, Romero JP, Tolon RM, et al. Cannabinoid CB1 and CB2 receptors and fatty acid amide hydrolase are specific markers of plaque cell subtypes in human multiple sclerosis. J Neurosci 2007;27(9):2396–402.

159. Onaivi ES, Ishiguro H, Gong JP, et al. Brain neuronal CB2 cannabinoid receptors in drug abuse and depression: from mice to human subjects. PLoS One 2008; 3(2):e1640.

160. van der Stelt M, Veldhuis WB, van Haaften GW, et al. Exogenous anandamide protects rat brain against acute neuronal injury in vivo. J Neurosci 2001; 21(22):8765–71.

161. Fernandez-Lopez D, Pazos MR, Tolon RM, et al. The cannabinoid agonist WIN55212 reduces brain damage in an in vivo model of hypoxic-ischemic encephalopathy in newborn rats. Pediatr Res 2007;62(3):255–60.
162. Turkyilmaz C, Turkyilmaz Z, Atalay Y, et al. Magnesium pre-treatment reduces neuronal apoptosis in newborn rats in hypoxia-ischemia. Brain Res 2002; 955(1–2):133–7.
163. Marret S, Gressens P, Gadisseux JF, et al. Prevention by magnesium of excitotoxic neuronal death in the developing brain: an animal model for clinical intervention studies. Dev Med Child Neurol 1995;37(6):473–84.
164. Spandou E, Soubasi V, Papoutsopoulou S, et al. Neuroprotective effect of long-term MgSO4 administration after cerebral hypoxia-ischemia in newborn rats is related to the severity of brain damage. Reprod Sci 2007;14(7): 667–77.
165. Khashaba MT, Shouman BO, Shaltout AA, et al. Excitatory amino acids and magnesium sulfate in neonatal asphyxia. Brain Dev 2006;28(6):375–9.
166. Crowther CA, Hiller JE, Doyle LW, et al. Effect of magnesium sulfate given for neuroprotection before preterm birth: a randomized controlled trial. JAMA 2003;290(20):2669–76.
167. Groenendaal F, Rademaker CM, Toet MC, et al. Effects of magnesium sulphate on amplitude-integrated continuous EEG in asphyxiated term neonates. Acta Paediatr 2002;91(10):1073–7.
168. Levene M, Blennow M, Whitelaw A, et al. Acute effects of two different doses of magnesium sulphate in infants with birth asphyxia. Arch Dis Child Fetal Neonatal Ed 1995;73(3):F174–7.
169. Wu YW, Escobar GJ, Grether JK, et al. Chorioamnionitis and cerebral palsy in term and near-term infants. JAMA 2003;290(20):2677–84.
170. Wu YW, Colford JM Jr. Chorioamnionitis as a risk factor for cerebral palsy: a meta-analysis. JAMA 2000;284(11):1417–24.
171. Dammann O, Kuban KC, Leviton A, et al. Perinatal infection, fetal inflammatory response, white matter damage, and cognitive limitations in children born preterm. Ment Retard Dev Disabil Res Rev 2002;8(1):46–50.
172. Stirling DP, Koochesfahani KM, Steeves JD, et al. Minocycline as a neuroprotective agent. Neuroscientist 2005;11(4):308–22.
173. Dommergues MA, Patkai J, Renauld JC, et al. Pro-inflammatory cytokines and interleukin-9 exacerbate excitotoxic lesions of the newborn murine neopallium. Ann Neurol 2000;47(1):54–63.
174. Dommergues MA, Plaisant F, Verney C, et al. Early microglial activation following neonatal excitotoxic brain damage in mice: a potential target for neuroprotection. Neuroscience 2003;121(3):619–28.
175. Chen M, Ona VO, Li M, et al. Minocycline inhibits caspase-1 and caspase-3 expression and delays mortality in a transgenic mouse model of Huntington disease. Nat Med 2000;6(7):797–801.
176. Zhu S, Stavrovskaya IG, Drozda M, et al. Minocycline inhibits cytochrome c release and delays progression of amyotrophic lateral sclerosis in mice. Nature 2002;417(6884):74–8.
177. Pruzanski W, Greenwald RA, Street IP, et al. Inhibition of enzymatic activity of phospholipases A2 by minocycline and doxycycline. Biochem Pharmacol 1992;44(6):1165–70.
178. Machado LS, Kozak A, Ergul A, et al. Delayed minocycline inhibits ischemia-activated matrix metalloproteinases 2 and 9 after experimental stroke. BMC Neurosci 2006;7:56.

179. Wang J, Wei Q, Wang CY, et al. Minocycline up-regulates Bcl-2 and protects against cell death in mitochondria. J Biol Chem 2004;279(19):19948–54.
180. Scarabelli TM, Stephanou A, Pasini E, et al. Minocycline inhibits caspase activation and reactivation, increases the ratio of XIAP to smac/DIABLO, and reduces the mitochondrial leakage of cytochrome C and smac/DIABLO. J Am Coll Cardiol 2004;43(5):865–74.
181. Choi Y, Kim HS, Shin KY, et al. Minocycline attenuates neuronal cell death and improves cognitive impairment in Alzheimer's disease models. Neuropsychopharmacology 2007;32(11):2393–404.
182. Popovic N, Schubart A, Goetz BD, et al. Inhibition of autoimmune encephalomyelitis by a tetracycline. Ann Neurol 2002;51(2):215–23.
183. Du Y, Ma Z, Lin S, et al. Minocycline prevents nigrostriatal dopaminergic neurodegeneration in the MPTP model of Parkinson's disease. Proc Natl Acad Sci U S A 2001;98(25):14669–74.
184. Yrjanheikki J, Tikka T, Keinanen R, et al. A tetracycline derivative, minocycline, reduces inflammation and protects against focal cerebral ischemia with a wide therapeutic window. Proc Natl Acad Sci U S A 1999;96(23): 13496–500.
185. Wang CX, Yang T, Shuaib A, et al. Effects of minocycline alone and in combination with mild hypothermia in embolic stroke. Brain Res 2003;963(1–2): 327–9.
186. Arvin KL, Han BH, Du Y, et al. Minocycline markedly protects the neonatal brain against hypoxic-ischemic injury. Ann Neurol 2002;52(1):54–61.
187. Fox C, Dingman A, Derugin N, et al. Minocycline confers early but transient protection in the immature brain following focal cerebral ischemia-reperfusion. J Cereb Blood Flow Metab 2005;25(9):1138–49.
188. Cai Z, Lin S, Fan LW, et al. Minocycline alleviates hypoxic-ischemic injury to developing oligodendrocytes in the neonatal rat brain. Neuroscience 2006; 137(2):425–35.
189. Carty ML, Wixey JA, Colditz PB, et al. Post-insult minocycline treatment attenuates hypoxia-ischemia-induced neuroinflammation and white matter injury in the neonatal rat: a comparison of two different dose regimens. Int J Dev Neurosci 2008;26(5):477–85.
190. Wasserman JK, Zhu X, Schlichter LC, et al. Evolution of the inflammatory response in the brain following intracerebral hemorrhage and effects of delayed minocycline treatment. Brain Res 2007;1180:140–54.
191. Tsuji M, Wilson MA, Lange MS, et al. Minocycline worsens hypoxic-ischemic brain injury in a neonatal mouse model. Exp Neurol 2004;189(1):58–65.
192. Northington FJ, Ferriero DM, Graham EM, et al. Early neurodegeneration after hypoxia-ischemia in neonatal rat is necrosis while delayed neuronal death is apoptosis. Neurobiol Dis 2001;8(2):207–19.
193. Portera-Cailliau C, Price DL, Martin LJ, et al. Non-NMDA and NMDA receptor-mediated excitotoxic neuronal deaths in adult brain are morphologically distinct: further evidence for an apoptosis-necrosis continuum. J Comp Neurol 1997; 378(1):88–104.
194. Northington FJ, Graham EM, Martin LJ, et al. Apoptosis in perinatal hypoxic-ischemic brain injury: how important is it and should it be inhibited? Brain Res Brain Res Rev 2005;50(2):244–57.
195. Hu BR, Liu CL, Ouyang Y, et al. Involvement of caspase-3 in cell death after hypoxia-ischemia declines during brain maturation. J Cereb Blood Flow Metab 2000;20(9):1294–300.

196. Feng Y, Fratkin JD, LeBlanc MH, et al. Inhibiting caspase-8 after injury reduces hypoxic-ischemic brain injury in the newborn rat. Eur J Pharmacol 2003; 481(2–3):169–73.
197. Han BH, Xu D, Choi J, et al. Selective, reversible caspase-3 inhibitor is neuroprotective and reveals distinct pathways of cell death after neonatal hypoxicischemic brain injury. J Biol Chem 2002;277(33):30128–36.
198. Blomgren K, Zhu C, Wang X, et al. Synergistic activation of caspase-3 by m-calpain after neonatal hypoxia-ischemia: a mechanism of "pathological apoptosis"? J Biol Chem 2001;276(13):10191–8.
199. Ostwald K, Hagberg H, Andine P, et al. Upregulation of calpain activity in neonatal rat brain after hypoxic-ischemia. Brain Res 1993;630(1–2):289–94.
200. Kawamura M, Nakajima W, Ishida A, et al. Calpain inhibitor MDL 28170 protects hypoxic-ischemic brain injury in neonatal rats by inhibition of both apoptosis and necrosis. Brain Res 2005;1037(1–2):59–69.
201. Nunez J, Yang Z, Jiang Y, et al. 17beta-estradiol protects the neonatal brain from hypoxia-ischemia. Exp Neurol 2007;208(2):269–76.
202. Hagberg H, Wilson MA, Matsushita H, et al. PARP-1 gene disruption in mice preferentially protects males from perinatal brain injury. J Neurochem 2004; 90(5):1068–75.
203. Ducrocq S, Benjelloun N, Plotkine M, et al. Poly(ADP-ribose) synthase inhibition reduces ischemic injury and inflammation in neonatal rat brain. J Neurochem 2000;74(6):2504–11.
204. Dietrich WD, Busto R, Alonso O, et al. Intraischemic but not postischemic brain hypothermia protects chronically following global forebrain ischemia in rats. J Cereb Blood Flow Metab 1993;13(4):541–9.
205. Trescher WH, Ishiwa S, Johnston MV, et al. Brief post-hypoxic-ischemic hypothermia markedly delays neonatal brain injury. Brain Dev 1997;19(5): 326–38.
206. Ma J, Zhang GY. Lithium reduced N-methyl-D-aspartate receptor subunit 2A tyrosine phosphorylation and its interactions with Src and Fyn mediated by PSD-95 in rat hippocampus following cerebral ischemia. Neurosci Lett 2003; 348(3):185–9.
207. Dinse A, Fohr KJ, Georgieff M, et al. Xenon reduces glutamate-, AMPA-, and kainate-induced membrane currents in cortical neurones. Br J Anaesth 2005;94(4): 479–85.
208. Gruss M, Bushell TJ, Bright DP, et al. Two-pore-domain K^+ channels are a novel target for the anesthetic gases xenon, nitrous oxide, and cyclopropane. Mol Pharmacol 2004;65(2):443–52.
209. Ma D, Hossain M, Chow A, et al. Xenon and hypothermia combine to provide neuroprotection from neonatal asphyxia. Ann Neurol 2005;58(2):182–93.
210. Busto R, Globus MY, Dietrich WD, et al. Effect of mild hypothermia on ischemia-induced release of neurotransmitters and free fatty acids in rat brain. Stroke 1989;20(7):904–10.
211. Hobbs C, Thoresen M, Tucker A, et al. Xenon and hypothermia combine additively, offering long-term functional and histopathologic neuroprotection after neonatal hypoxia/ischemia. Stroke 2008;39(4):1307–13.
212. Khan M, Sekhon B, Jatana M, et al. Administration of N-acetylcysteine after focal cerebral ischemia protects brain and reduces inflammation in a rat model of experimental stroke. J Neurosci Res 2004;76(4):519–27.
213. Sekhon B, Sekhon C, Khan M, et al. N-Acetyl cysteine protects against injury in a rat model of focal cerebral ischemia. Brain Res 2003;971(1):1–8.

214. Jatana M, Singh I, Singh AK, et al. Combination of systemic hypothermia and N-acetylcysteine attenuates hypoxic-ischemic brain injury in neonatal rats. Pediatr Res 2006;59(5):684–9.
215. Alkan T, Kahveci N, Buyukuysal L, et al. Neuroprotective effects of MK 801 and hypothermia used alone and in combination in hypoxic-ischemic brain injury in neonatal rats. Arch Physiol Biochem 2001;109(2):135–44.
216. Liu Y, Barks JD, Xu G, et al. Topiramate extends the therapeutic window for hypothermia-mediated neuroprotection after stroke in neonatal rats. Stroke 2004;35(6):1460–5.

Neonatal Seizures: An Update on Mechanisms and Management

Frances E. Jensen, MD

KEYWORDS

- Epilepsy • Perinatal • Synapse • Neurotransmitter receptor
- Glutamate • γ-aminobutyric acid (GABA)

Neonatal seizures are an important example of an age-specific seizure syndrome. Compared with seizures at older ages, neonatal seizures differ in etiology, semiology, and electroencephalographic signature, and can be refractory to antiepileptic drugs (AEDs) that are effective in other age populations. Their unique pathophysiology has become the subject of many research studies from a basic and clinical perspective, and is leading the way to new therapies for this often refractory disorder.

EPIDEMIOLOGY AND ETIOLOGY

The risk of seizures is highest in the neonatal period (1.8–5/1000 live births in the United States). The relative incidence is higher in premature infants less than 30 weeks's gestation,[1] occurring in 3.9% of these neonates compared with 1.5% of older infants. In the neonate, a broad range of systemic and central nervous system (CNS) disorders can increase the risk of seizures (**Box 1**). Most neonatal seizures are symptomatic; they can be extremely difficult to control with currently available AEDs, and can lead to long-term neurologic sequelae. Benign forms include benign familial neonatal seizures and transient, treatable metabolic derangements; these forms are largely without significant long-term consequences.

The most common cause of symptomatic neonatal seizures is hypoxic/ischemic encephalopathy (HIE), which affects approximately 1 to 2 of 1000 live births.[2,3] About two-thirds of cases of neonatal seizures are caused by HIE.[4] These seizures can occur in the setting of birth asphyxia, respiratory distress, or as a complication of early-life extracorporeal membrane oxygenation (ECMO) or cardiopulmonary bypass for corrective cardiac surgery.[5] In the case of HIE, these seizures usually occur within the first 1 to 2 days of birth and often remit after a few days, but carry with them

The author acknowledges support from the National institutes of Health (grants RO1 NS31718 and DP1 OD003347, the Epilepsy Therapy Development Project, and a grant from Parents Against Childhood Epilepsy. Additional support was provided from the National institutes of Health Mental retardation and Developmental Disabilities Center (P30 HD18655).
Children's Hospital Boston, CLS 14073, 300 Longwood Avenue, Boston, MA 02115, USA
E-mail address: frances.jensen@childrens.harvard.edu

Clin Perinatol 36 (2009) 881–900
doi:10.1016/j.clp.2009.08.001
0095-5108/09/$ – see front matter © 2009 Elsevier Inc. All rights reserved.

Box 1
Diverse causes of neonatal seizures

Acute metabolic

Hypoglycemia

Hypocalcemia

Hypomagnesemia

Hypo- or hypernatremia

Withdrawal syndromes associated with maternal drug use

Iatrogenic associated with inadvertent fetal administration of local anesthetic

Rare inborn errors of metabolism (including pyridoxine responsive)

Cerebrovascular

Hypoxic/ischemic encephalopathy

Arterial and venous ischemic stroke

Intracerebral hemorrhage

Intraventricular hemorrhage

Subdural hemorrhage

Subarachnoid hemorrhage

CNS infection

Bacterial meningitis

Viral meningoencephalitis

Intrauterine ("TORCH") infections

Developmental

Multiple forms of cerebral dysgenesis

Other

Rare genetic syndromic disorders

Benign neonatal familial convulsions (sodium and potassium channel mutations identified)

Early myoclonic encephalopathy

---

a risk of long-term epilepsy and neurologic or cognitive deficits.[6,7] HIE is associated with a high incidence of seizures, reportedly in 40% to 60% of cases.[8,9] Other cerebrovascular disorders including arterial and venous stroke, intracerebral hemorrhage, and subarachnoid hemorrhage also frequently present clinically with seizures. Aside from HIE and cerebrovascular causes, the next most common causes of neonatal seizures are infections and malformations of cortical development. Common bacterial infectious causes include Group B streptococcus and *Escherichia coli*. Nonbacterial causes include intrauterine toxoplasmosis or cytomegalovirus infection, or neonatal encephalitis caused by toxoplasmosis, herpes simplex, coxsackie, or cytomegalovirus. Malformations of cortical development that frequently present with early-life seizures include lissencephaly, polymicrogyria, focal cortical dysplasia, and tuberous sclerosis. Metabolic disturbances responsible for neonatal seizures include hypoglycemia, hypocalcemia, hypomagnesemia, and abnormalities of other electrolytes and amino acids. Many metabolic causes are readily treatable (such as correction of glucose and electrolyte disturbances) and when such metabolic disturbances are the primary cause of neonatal seizures, they are rarely associated with significant long-term consequences. Pyridoxine-dependent seizures can present as unremitting and refractory seizures within the first days of life, but rapidly respond to intravenous pyridoxine. Inborn errors of amino or organic acid metabolism can also present with seizures in the first days of life, such as hyperglycinemia, type II glutaric aciduria, and urea cycle disorders.

Other less common causes of neonatal seizures include benign familial neonatal convulsions, an autosomal dominant disorder that presents within the first week of life and is associated with subsequent normal development. Genetic analysis has revealed these to be related to mutations in the neuronal potassium channels KCNQ2 or KCNQ3.[10–12] Another benign syndrome possibly associated with a mutation in KCNQ2 is that of "fifth day fits," which transiently occur for a day or so around the fifth or sixth postnatal day.[13]

Neonatal seizures can be refractory to AED therapy that is effective at later ages, especially when the seizures are symptomatic and a result of HIE. Conventional AEDs that are effective in older children and adults are largely inadequate, likely because seizures in the immature brain have unique mechanisms (see later discussion).

The outcome of prolonged neonatal seizures can include consequences in later life in more than 30% of survivors, with cognitive deficits ranging from learning disability (27%) to developmental delay and mental retardation (20%), and epilepsy later in life (27%).[6] The risk of mortality was reported previously as approximately 35%,[14] but recent studies of term infants with clinical seizures showed a lower neonatal mortality of less than 20% as a result of improvements in neonatal intensive care.[4,6] Despite improved survival, the long-term neurologic consequences remain high with studies reporting a range from 28%[4] to 46%.[6] Not all neonatal seizures portend the same risk, and it seems that worst prognosis is observed in those with symptomatic seizures caused by HIE or cerebral dysgenesis.[4] Better prognosis is also associated with milder electroencephalographic (EEG) abnormalities and no neuroimaging abnormalities.[15–17] As a result of advances in care, causes associated with more favorable outcome, such as hypocalcemic seizures, have decreased from accounting for approximately 30% of cases before the 1960s to less than 5% presently.[2] Currently, HIE predominates as the most common cause of refractory neonatal seizures.[4]

Although the term infant is at the highest risk for seizures, it is increasingly recognized that seizures can be a significant problem in preterm infants. According to a recent study, seizures can occur in 5.6% of very low birthweight infants; lower gestational age, male gender, and major systemic and neurologic injury, such as intraventricular hemorrhage or periventricular leukomalacia, are independent predictors of neonatal seizures.[18,19]

DIAGNOSIS

Neonatal seizures can be difficult to diagnose as there are often no clinical correlates of the electrographic seizures, a phenomenon called electroclinical dissociation. Regional interconnectivity, including interhemispheric and corticospinal, is not fully mature as a result of incomplete myelination of white matter tracts, leading to only modest behavioral manifestations of these seizures. Infants can show no signs or very subtle tonic or clonic movements, often limited to only 1 limb, making the diagnosis difficult to discern from myoclonus or other automatisms.[20] A recent study revealed that approximately 80% of EEG-documented seizures were not accompanied by observable clinical seizures.[21] Hence, EEG is essential for diagnosis and for assessing treatment efficacy in this group. Full 20-lead EEGs are most sensitive in detecting these often multifocal seizures (**Fig. 1**). As full-lead EEGs can be difficult to obtain on an emergent basis in many neonatal intensive care units, amplitude-integrated EEG (aEEG) devices are becoming increasingly used.[22] aEEG is usually obtained from a pair or limited number of leads, and is displayed as a fast Fourier spectral transform. With aEEG, seizures are detected by acute alterations in spectral width, and a raw EEG from the single channel can be accessed by the viewer for confirmation.[23] Several reports now indicate that aEEG has relatively high specificity but compromised sensitivity, detecting approximately 75% of that of conventional full-lead montage EEG.[22,24–28]

Once neonatal seizures are confirmed, treatable metabolic and symptomatic causes need to be identified. Serologic studies include blood and serologic studies of systemic infection, and metabolic derangements such as acidosis, hypocalcemia, hypomagnesemia, and hypoglycemia. The timing of the seizures can be a helpful indicator, such as in the case of "fifth day fits," caused by hypocalcemia. Pyridoxine-dependent seizures present as refractory early neonatal seizures that uniquely respond to parenteral pyridoxine administration.[29,30] Seizures that continue to be refractory in the setting of a history consistent with HIE manifest within the first 24 to 48 hours of life, persist for several days, then seem to gradually remit.

MR imaging provides an important assessment of risk in infants with neonatal seizures. Imaging can provide important information on cerebral dysgenesis and gross structural malformations, which can be associated with neonatal seizures such as tuberous sclerosis, hemimegalencephaly, or cortical dysplasia. For symptomatic seizures caused by HIE, abnormal T2, fluid attenuated inversion recovery, and diffusion signals can be used to pinpoint regional injury and severity.[31] Recent studies

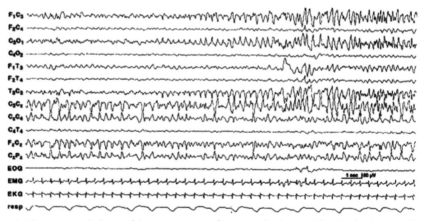

Fig. 1. Electroencephalographic appearance of neonatal seizures. Electrical seizure activity begins in the midline central region (CZ) and then shifts to the left central region (C3). Toward the end of the seizures, as the electrical activity persists in the left central region, the midline central region becomes uninvolved. This electrical seizure activity occurred in the absence of any clinical seizure activity in this 40-week gestational age female infant with hypoxic-ischemic encephalopathy. She was initially comatose and hypotonic and, at the time of EEG recording, had been treated with phenobarbital. (*Reprinted from* Mizrahi EM, Kellaway P. Characterization and classification of neonatal seizures. Neurology 1987;37(12):1837–44; with permission.)

show that magnetic resonance spectroscopy can be used to predict severity and outcome in patients. Miller and colleagues[17] reported that in HIE cases with seizures, an increased lactate to choline ratio, and reduced N-acetyl-aspartate levels, were more abnormal in patients with higher seizure burden. Another study of term infants with asphyxia and/or seizures by Glass and colleagues[16] showed that after adjusting for degree of MRI abnormality, seizure severity was associated with a higher risk of neuromotor abnormalities at 4 years of age than in those without seizures. These results suggest that neonatal seizures may independently worsen outcome even in the setting of documented MR lesions associated with HIE.

TREATMENT

Neonatal seizures can be extremely refractory to conventional AEDs, especially those associated with HIE. Early diagnosis should isolate metabolic or infectious causes and direct care to correcting the primary cause. However, the most refractory seizures are those caused by asphyxia and because of their short course (>72–96 hours) and poor prognosis, early treatment is essential and should be guided by EEG documentation of seizure activity. Current practices include early treatment with phenobarbital (doses ranging from 20–40 mg/kg),[32] with phenytoin (20 mg/kg), or fosphenytoin, and/or benzodiazepines such as lorazepam (0.05–0.1 mg/kg) as second-line adjuvant therapy for refractory seizures.[5] However, the consensus is that currently used AEDs are often ineffective for treatment of neonatal seizures.[33,34] Indeed, phenobarbital and phenytoin seem to be equally but incompletely effective, and either drug alone controls seizures in fewer than half of EEG-confirmed neonatal seizures.[35] As an alternative, second-line treatment with midazolam has variable efficacy, yet is less of a respiratory depressant than high dose barbiturates.[36,37] Lidocaine may be effective in refractory neonatal seizures, but its use may be limited by potential cardiac toxicity.[38] Newer AEDs such as topiramate and levetiracetam have been anecdotally reported to improve acute neonatal seizures.[39–41] It is also not known how long to continue treatment following the short course of neonatal seizures,[32] and how the length of treatment affects outcome.

In addition to pharmacologic therapy, neonates with HIE are also being increasingly treated with hypothermia. Recent clinical studies have led to a Cochrane review endorsement that early whole-body or limited cranial hypothermia improves neurologic outcome in treated neonates.[8,9,42,43] For whole-body hypothermia, current practice is to decrease core body temperature to 33.5°C for 72 hours.[8] Although aEEG is routinely employed to monitor brain activity during hypothermia, the effect of hypothermia on the incidence or severity of neonatal seizures is yet to be determined.[43]

PATHOPHYSIOLOGY

In response to the fact that neonatal seizures are refractory to conventional AEDs and can have severe consequences on long-term neurologic status, there is a growing body of active research directed at defining age-specific mechanisms of this disorder to identify new therapeutic targets and biomarkers. There have been substantial advances with regard to understanding pathophysiology, and, in particular, developmental stage-specific factors that influence mechanisms of seizure generation, responsiveness to anticonvulsants, and the impact on CNS development.[44] In addition, experimental data have raised concerns about the potential adverse effects of current treatments with barbiturates and benzodiazepines on brain development. Improved understanding of the unique age-specific mechanisms should yield new therapeutic targets with clinical potential. Indeed, to date, no novel compounds have been developed specifically or approved by the US Food and Drug Administration (FDA) for treatment of neonatal seizures.[33]

Developmental age-specific mechanisms influence the generation and phenotype of seizures, the impact of seizures on brain structure and function, and the efficacy of anticonvulsant therapy. Factors governing neuronal excitability conspire to create a relatively hyperexcitable state in the neonatal period, as shown by the extremely low threshold to seizures in general and by the fact that this is the period of highest incidence of seizures across the life span,[45,46] similarly, in the rodent, seizure susceptibility peaks in the second postnatal week in many models.[44,47,48] In addition, the incomplete development of neurotransmitter systems results in a lack of "target" receptors for conventional AEDs. The relatively minimal status of myelination in cortical and subcortical structures results in the multifocal nature or unusual behavioral correlates of seizures at this age.[49,50]

The neonatal period is a period of intense physiologic synaptic excitability, as synaptogenesis occurring at this time point is wholly dependent on activity.[44] In the human, synapse and dendritic spine density are both peaking around term gestation and into the first months of life.[51,52] In addition, the balance between excitatory versus inhibitory synapses is tipped in the favor of excitation to permit robust activity-dependent synaptic formation, plasticity, and remodeling.[44] Glutamate is the major excitatory neurotransmitter in the CNS, and γ-aminobutyric acid (GABA) is the major inhibitory neurotransmitter. There is considerable and growing evidence from animal models and human tissue studies that neurotransmitter receptors are highly developmentally regulated (**Fig. 2**).[44,47,53] Studies of cell morphology, myelination, metabolism, and more recently neurotransmitter receptor expression suggest that the first 1 to 2 weeks of life in the rodent is a roughly analogous stage to the human neonatal brain.

Enhanced Excitability of the Neonatal Brain

Glutamate receptors are critical for plasticity and are transiently overexpressed during development compared with adulthood in animal models and human tissue studies.[44] A relative overexpression of certain glutamate receptor subtypes in rodent and human developing cortex coincides with ages of increased seizure susceptibility (see **Fig. 2**).[47,54,55] Glutamate receptors include ligand-gated ion channels, permeable to sodium, potassium, and in some cases, calcium, and metabotropic subtypes.[56] They are localized to synapses and nonsynaptic sites on neurons, and are also expressed on glia. The ionotropic receptor subtypes are classified based on selective activation by specific ligands, N-methyl-D-aspartate (NMDA), α-amino-3-hydroxy-5-methyl-4-isoxazolepropionic acid (AMPA), and kainate.

NMDA receptors are heteromeric, including an obligate NR1 subunit, and their make-up is developmentally regulated. In the immature brain, the NR2 subunits are predominantly those of the NR2B subunit, with the functional correlate of longer current decay time compared with the NR2A subunit, which is the form expressed in later life on mature neurons.[57] Other developmentally regulated subunits with functional relevance include the NR2C, NR2D, and NR3A subunits. Rodent studies show that these are all increased in the first 2 postnatal weeks, that this period is associated with lower sensitivity to magnesium, the endogenous receptor channel blocker; these features in turn result in increased neuronal excitability (**Figs. 2 and 3**).[56,58] NMDA receptor antagonists administered to immature rat pups have been shown to be highly effective against various hypoxic/ischemic insults and seizures in the immature brain.[59-61] However, the clinical potential of NMDA antagonists may be limited because of their severe sedative effects and a potential propensity for inducing

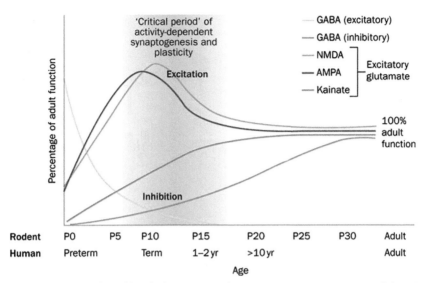

Fig. 2. Developmental profile of glutamate and GABA receptor expression and function. Equivalent developmental periods are displayed for rats and humans on the top and bottom x-axes, respectively. Activation of GABA receptors is depolarizing in rats early in the first postnatal week and in humans up to and including the neonatal period. Functional inhibition, however, is gradually reached over development in rats and humans. Before full maturation of GABA-mediated inhibition, the NMDA and AMPA subtypes of glutamate receptors peak between the first and second postnatal weeks in rats and in the neonatal period in humans. Kainate receptor binding is initially low and gradually rises to adult levels by the fourth postnatal week. Neonatal seizures emerge within the critical period of synaptogenesis and cerebral development. AMPA, α-amino-3-hydroxy-5-methyl-4-isoxazole propionate; GABA, γ-aminobutyric acid; NMDA, N-methyl-D-aspartate; P, postnatal day. (*Reprinted from* Rakhade SN, Jensen FE. Epileptogenesis in the immature brain: emerging mechanisms. Nat Rev Neurol 2009;5(7):380–91; with permission.)

apoptotic death in the immature brain.[62,63] Memantine, an agent currently in clinical use as a neuroprotectant in Alzheimer disease, may be an exception with fewer side effects, as a result of its use-dependent mechanism of action.[60,61,64]

Although the NMDA receptor has been reported to be selectively activated in processes related to plasticity and learning, the AMPA subtype of glutamate receptor is believed to subserve most fast excitatory synaptic transmission. In addition, unlike the NMDA receptor, most AMPA receptors (AMPAR) are not calcium permeable in the adult. AMPARs are heteromeric and made up of 4 subunits, including combinations of the GluR1, GluR2, GluR3, or GluR4 subunits.[56] However, in the immature rodent and human brain, AMPARs are calcium permeable because they lack the GluR2 subunit (see **Figs. 2** and **3**).[55,65] AMPAR subunits are developmentally regulated, with GluR2 expressed only at low levels until the third postnatal week in rodents and later in the first year of life in the human cortex.[54,66] Hence, AMPARs in the immature brain, because of their enhanced calcium permeability, may play an important role in contributing not only to excitability but also to activity-dependent signaling down stream of the receptor. NMDA and AMPARs are expressed at levels and with subunit composition that enhance excitability of neuronal networks around term in the human and in the first 2 postnatal weeks in the rodent (see **Fig. 2**).

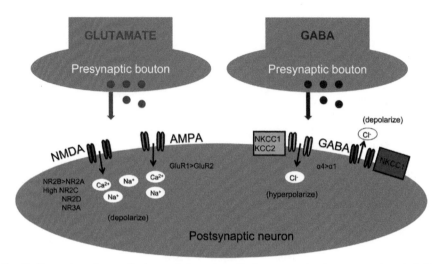

Fig. 3. Dynamics of synaptic transmission at cortical synapses in the neonatal period. Depicted are an excitatory glutamatergic synapse (*left panel*) and a GABAergic inhibitory synapse (*right panel*). Presynaptic release of glutamate results in depolarization (excitation) of the postsynaptic neuron (*left panel*) by activation of NMDA and AMPARs. In contrast, release of GABA (*right panel*) results in hyperpolarization (inhibition) when the postsynaptic neuron expresses sufficient quantities of the Cl⁻ transporter KCC2, but depolarization (excitation) when intracellular Cl⁻ accumulates as a result unopposed action of the Cl⁻ importer NKCC1. The immature glutamatergic receptors (*left panel*) are comprised of higher levels of NR2B, NR2C, NR2D, and NR3A subunits of the NMDA receptor, enhancing influx of Ca^{2+} and Na^{+} compared with mature synapses. In addition, AMPARs are relatively deficient in GluR2 subunits, resulting in increased Ca^{2+} permeability compared with mature synapses. Hence, specific NMDA receptor antagonists and AMPAR antagonists may prove to be age-specific therapeutic targets for treatment development. In addition, although $GABA_A$ receptor activation normally results in hyperpolarization and inhibition at mature synapses, because of the coexpression of NKCC1 and KCC2, the expression of KCC2 is low in the neonatal period compared with later in life and thus Cl⁻ levels accumulate intracellularly; opening of $GABA_A$ receptors allows the passive efflux of Cl⁻ out of the cell, resulting in paradoxic depolarization. $GABA_A$ receptor subunit expression in the immature brain is typified by higher levels of the α4 subunit, which is functionally associated with diminished benzodiazepine sensitivity. Both these attributes of the $GABA_A$ receptor make classic GABA agonists such as barbiturates and benzodiazepines less effective in the neonatal brain. The NKCC1 channel blocker bumetanide has anticonvulsant efficacy when administered with phenobarbital, suggesting a synergistic effect.

Rodent studies show that AMPAR antagonists seem to be potently effective against neonatal seizures, even superior to NMDA receptor antagonists or conventional AEDs and GABA agonists. Topiramate, which is approved by the FDA for seizure control in children and adults, has been shown to be an AMPAR antagonist, in addition to several other potential anticonvulsant mechanisms.[67] Topiramate has been shown to be effective in suppressing seizures and long-term neurobehavioral deficits in a rodent seizure model, even when administered following seizures.[68,69] In addition, topiramate in combination with hypothermia was found to be protective in a rodent neonatal stroke model.[70] The specific AMPAR antagonist, talampanel, currently in phase 2 trials for epilepsy and amyotrophic lateral sclerosis in children and adults, was recently shown to protect against neonatal seizures in a rodent model.[71]

Decreased Efficacy of Inhibitory Neurotransmission in the Immature Brain

Expression and function of the inhibitory GABA$_A$ receptors are also developmentally regulated. Rodent studies show that GABA receptor binding, synthetic enzymes, and overall receptor expression are lower in early life compared with later.[47,72] GABA receptor function is regulated by subunit composition, and the $\alpha 4$ and $\alpha 2$ subunits are relatively overexpressed in the immature brain compared with the $\alpha 1$ subunit (see **Fig. 3**).[73] When the $\alpha 4$ subunit is expressed the receptor is less sensitive to benzodiazepines compared with receptors containing $\alpha 1$,[74] and as is often the case clinically, seizures in the immature rat respond poorly to benzodiazepines.[75,76]

Receptor expression and subunit composition can partially explain the resistance of seizures in the immature brain to conventional AEDs that act as GABA agonists. However, in the mature brain, inhibition of neuronal excitability via GABA agonists relies on the ability of GABA$_A$ receptors to cause a net influx of chloride (Cl$^-$) from the neuron, resulting in hyperpolarization.[77] In the immature forebrain, GABA receptor activation can cause depolarization rather than hyperpolarization[78–80] because the Cl$^-$ gradient is reversed in the immature brain: intracellular Cl$^-$ levels are high in the immature brain because of a relative underexpression of the Cl$^-$ exporter KCC2 compared with mature brain (see **Figs. 2** and **3**).[81] Recent studies in human brain have shown that KCC2 is virtually absent in cortical neurons until late in the first year of life, and gradually increases thereafter, although the Cl$^-$ importer NKCC1 is overexpressed in the neonatal human brain and during early life in the rat when seizures are resistant to GABA agonists.[81] The NKCC1 inhibitor, bumetanide, shows efficacy against kainate-induced seizures in the immature brain[82]; this agent, already approved by the FDA as a diuretic, is currently under evaluation in a phase 1/2 trial as an add-on agent in the treatment of neonatal seizures (http://www.clinicaltrials.gov trial ID: NCT00830531).

Ion Channel Configuration Favors Depolarization in Early Life

Ion channels also regulate neuronal excitability and, like neurotransmitter receptors, are developmentally regulated. As stated earlier, mutations in the K$^+$ channels KCNQ2 and KCNQ3 are associated with benign familial neonatal convulsions.[83] These mutations interfere with the normal hyperpolarizing K$^+$ current that prevents repetitive action potential firing.[84] Hence, at the time when there is an overexpression of GluRs and incomplete network inhibition, a compensatory mechanism is not available in these mutations. Another K$^+$-channel superfamily member, the HCN (or h) channels, is also developmentally regulated. The h currents are important for maintenance of resting membrane potential and dendritic excitability,[85] and function is regulated by isoform expression. The immature brain has a relatively low expression of the HCN1 isoform, which serves to reduce dendritic excitability in the adult brain.[86] Hence, ion channel maturation can also contribute to the hyperexcitability of the immature brain, and can have a cumulative effect when occurring in combination with the aforementioned differences in ligand-gated channels. Recently, selective blockers of HCN channels have been shown to disrupt synchronous epileptiform activity in the neonatal rat hippocampus,[87] suggesting that these developmentally regulated channels may also represent a target for therapy in neonatal seizures. N- and P/Q-type voltage sensitive calcium channels regulate neurotransmitter release.[88] With maturation, this function is taken over exclusively by the P/Q-type channels, formed by Cav2.1 subunits, a member of the Ca^{2+} channel superfamily.[89] Mutations in Cav2.1 may be involved in absence epilepsy, suggesting a failure in the normal maturational profile.[90]

A Role for Neuropeptides in the Hyperexcitability of the Immature Brain

Neuropeptide systems are also dynamically fluctuating in the perinatal period. An important example is corticotrophin-releasing hormone (CRH), which elicits potent neuronal excitation.[91,92] Compared with later life, in the perinatal period CRH and its receptors are expressed at higher levels, specifically in the first 2 postnatal weeks in the rat.[93] CRH levels increase during stress, and thus seizure activity in the immature brain may exacerbate subsequent seizure activity. Adrenocorticotropic hormone, which has shown efficacy in infantile spasms, is also known to down-regulate CRH gene expression.[94] Hence, neuropeptide modulation may be an area of future clinical importance in developing novel neonatal seizure treatments.

Enhanced Potential for Inflammatory Response to Seizures in the Immature Brain

Neonatal seizures can occur in the setting of inflammation either because of an inter-current infection or secondary to hypoxic/ischemic injury. Experimental and clinical evidence exists for early microglial activation and inflammatory cytokine production in the developing brain in hypoxia/ischemia[95,96] and inflammation.[97,98] Microglia have been shown to be highly expressed in immature white matter in rodents and humans during cortical development.[99] Antiinflammatory compounds or agents that inhibit microglial activation, such as minocycline, have been reported to attenuate neuronal injury in models of excitotoxicity and hypoxia/ischemia.[100] During the term period, microglia density in deep gray matter is higher than at later ages, likely because of a migration of the population of cells en route to more distal cortical locations. Experimental models show microglia activation, as seen by morphologic changes and rapid production of proinflammatory cytokines occurring after acute seizures in different epilepsy animal models.[101,102] During brain development, microglia show maximal density simultaneous with the period of peak synaptogenesis.[103] During normal development and in response to injury, microglia participate in "synaptic stripping" by detaching presynaptic terminals from neurons.[104,105] The microglial inactivators minocycline and doxycycline have been shown to be protective against seizure-induced neuronal death[106] and in neonatal stroke models.[107,108]

Selective Neuronal Injury in the Developing Brain

Although many studies suggest that seizures, or status epilepticus, induce less death in the immature brain than in the adult, there is evidence that some neuronal populations are vulnerable. Similar to the sensitivity of subplate neurons, hippocampal neurons in the perinatal rodent have been shown to undergo selective cell death and oxidative stress following chemoconvulsant-induced cell death.[109] Stroke studies in neonatal rodents also suggest that there can be selective vulnerability of specific cell populations in early development.[110] Subplate neurons are present in significant numbers in the deep cortical regions during the preterm and neonatal period.[111] These neurons are critical for the normal maturation of cortical networks.[112,113] In humans and rodents these cells possess high levels of AMPARs and NMDARs.[49,54] These cells may also lack oxidative stress defenses present in mature neurons. Animal models have revealed that these neurons are selectively vulnerable compared with overlying cortex following a hypoxic/ischemic insult.[114] Indeed chemoconvulsant-induced seizures in rats, provoked by the convulsant kainate in early postnatal life, have produced a similar loss of subplate neurons, with consequent abnormal development of inhibitory networks.[112]

Several studies have shown that the application of clinically available antioxidants, such as eythropoetin (Epo), is protective against neuronal injury in neonatal stroke.[115,116] Recently, Epo was shown to decrease later increases in seizure susceptibility of hippocampal neurons following hypoxia-induced neonatal seizures in rats.[117]

Seizure-induced Neuronal Network Dysfunction: Potential Interaction Between Epileptogenesis and Development of Neurocognitive Disability

Given that there is minimal neuronal death in most models of neonatal seizures, the long-term outcome of neonatal seizures is believed to be caused by seizure-induced alterations in surviving networks of neurons. Evidence for this theory comes from several studies that reveal disordered synaptic plasticity and impaired long-term potentiation and impaired learning later in life in rodents following brief neonatal seizures.[118,119] The neonatal period represents a stage of naturally enhanced synaptic plasticity when learning occurs at a rapid pace.[120,121] A major factor in this enhanced synaptic plasticity is the predominance of excitation over inhibition, which also increases susceptibility to seizures, as mentioned earlier. However, seizures that occur during this highly responsive developmental window seem to access signaling events that have been found to be central to normal synaptic plasticity. There are rapid increases in synaptic potency that seem to mimic long-term potentiation, and this pathologic activation may contribute to enhanced epileptogenesis.[122] In addition, GluR-mediated molecular cascades associated with physiologic synaptic plasticity may be overactivated by seizures, especially in the developing brain.[122,123] Rodent studies show a reduction in synaptic plasticity in neuronal networks such as hippocampus following early-life seizures, suggesting that the pathologic plasticity may have occluded normal plasticity, contributing to the impaired learning observed after early-life seizures.[122] Many models reveal that neonatal seizures alter synaptic plasticity,[124] and recent studies are delineating the molecular signaling cascades that are altered following early-life seizures.[125,126] In addition to glutamate receptors, inhibitory $GABA_A$ receptors can also be affected by seizures in early life, resulting in long-term impairments in function. Early and immediate functional decreases in inhibitory GABAergic synapses mediated by post-translational changes in $GABA_A$ subunits are seen following hypoxia-induced seizures in rat pups.[125] Flurothyl-induced seizures result in a selective impairment of GABAergic inhibition within a week.[127] There is evidence that some of these changes may be downstream of Ca^{2+} permeable glutamate receptors and Ca^{2+} signaling cascades, and that early postseizure treatment with GluR antagonists or phosphatase inhibitors may interrupt these pathologic changes that underlie the long-term disabilities and epilepsy.[122,125]

ANTICONVULSANTS AND THE DEVELOPING BRAIN

Emerging identification of age-specific mechanisms for neonatal seizures is pointing to the use of novel therapeutic targets. Caution must be exercised when devising new therapies, as the target may indeed be essential for normal brain development, albeit a contributor to neuronal hyperexcitability. More than 2 decades ago, experimental data emerged showing that phenobarbital exposure had adverse effects on survival and morphology of cultured neurons, derived from fetal mouse tissue, and these observations raised concerns about risks of this drug for treatment of neonatal seizures.[128,129] Subsequent studies in neonatal rats showed that daily treatment with phenobarbital or diazepam in the first postnatal month resulted in measurable changes in regional cerebral metabolism and behavior.[130,131]

More recently, evidence emerged that brief systemic treatment with conventional AEDs such as phenobarbital, diazepam, phenytoin, and valproate all increase apoptotic neuronal death in normal immature rodents.[132] Similarly, NMDAR antagonists also induce an increase in constitutive apoptosis in the developing rodent brain.[62] Yet, the AMPAR antagonists NBQX and topiramate do not cause such adverse effects,[62,133] although the mechanism for this relative safety over the other agents is not understood. The novel AED levetiracetam also has no effect on apoptosis in the developing brain.[134]

Despite these data on adverse effects or lack thereof in rodents, no evidence of similar phenomena exists for other species, and it remains unknown if these toxicity mechanisms are relevant for human neonates. Moreover, interpretation of AED toxicity studies must be tempered by the consideration that these experiments are typically performed in normal animals, and that the impact of AED administration may well differ in normal animals and in those with seizures.

Table 1
Candidate potential targets and therapies from emerging experimental and clinical literature

Temporal Profile	Mechanism Targeted	Potential Therapeutic Options
Acute changes	Immediate early genes	Chromatin acetylation modifiers/ histone deacetylation inhibitors (valproate)
	NMDA receptors	NMDA receptor inhibitors (memantine, felbamate) NR2B-specific inhibitors (Ifenprodil)
	AMPARs	AMPAR antagonists (topiramate, talampanel, GYKI compounds)
	NKCC1 chloride transporters	NKCC1 inhibitor (bumetanide in combination with GABA agonists phenobarbital, benzodiazepines)
	GABA receptors	GABA receptor agonists (phenobarbital, benzodiazepines)
	Phosphatases (eg, calcineurin)	Phosphatase inhibitors (FK-506)
	Kinases (activation of PKA, PKC, CaMKII, Src kinases, and so forth)	Kinase inhibitors (CaMKII inhibitor KN-62, PKA inhibitor KT5720, PKC inhibitor chelerythrine)
Subacute changes	Inflammation	Antiinflammatory compounds (ACTH), microglial inactivators (minocycline, doxycycline)
	Neuronal injury	Erythropoietin, antioxidants, NO inhibitors, NMDAR antagonists (memantine)
	HCN channels	I(h)-blocker ZD7288
	CB1 receptor	CB1 receptor antagonists (SR 14176A, rimonabant)
Chronic changes	Sprouting	Protein synthesis inhibitors (rapamycin, cycloheximide)
	Gliosis	Antiinflammatory agents,(Cox-2 inhibitors, minocycline, doxycycline)

Reprinted from Rakhade SN, Jensen FE. Epileptogenesis in the immature brain: emerging mechanisms. Nat Rev Neurol 2009;5(7):380–91; with permission.

FUTURE DIRECTIONS AND NEW THERAPEUTIC TARGETS

Refractory neonatal seizures remain a significant clinical problem, and no new treatments for this condition have been introduced for decades. Many new mechanisms and components of neonatal seizures have been uncovered. These present important new possibilities for novel therapeutic strategies in the population of neonates at risk for acute and long-term neurologic damage from neonatal seizures. Several major classes of agents with possible age-specific effects have emerged and are summarized in **Table 1**. These include modulators of neurotransmitter receptors and ion channels and transporters, antiinflammatory compounds, neuroprotectants, and antioxidants. Interdisciplinary collaboration between neonatologists and neonatal neurologists is essential for the success of such studies. As basic research reveals new age-specific therapeutic targets, these targets can be validated with analysis of cell-specific gene and protein expression in human autopsy samples. Experimental data regarding the potential efficacy of agents such as bumetanide, topiramate, and levetiracetam are encouraging, but the duration of use of these agents may be limited by safety concerns related to their effects on long-term brain development. Animal model trials and human studies must be aligned to understand how safety and efficacy data from rodent and nonhuman primates predict human responses. Several early-life seizure models exist in which there are indeed long-term effects on learning, and these could also be employed to address the effects of treatment on brain and cognitive development. Clinical therapeutic trials in neonates would be greatly improved if there were accurate biomarkers of acute and chronic therapeutic efficacy, yet none exist other than the EEG. Measures of brain metabolic integrity such as magnetic resonance spectroscopy or near infrared spectroscopy, when combined with EEG data, may provide surrogate measures of treatment efficacy. Incorporation of continuous EEG monitoring into clinical studies of neonatal seizure therapy will be essential. Seizure cessation is an important therapeutic goal, yet improved neurodevelopmental outcome is clearly of critical importance.

REFERENCES

1. Scher MS, Aso K, Beggarly ME, et al. Electrographic seizures in preterm and full-term neonates: clinical correlates, associated brain lesions, and risk for neurologic sequelae. Pediatrics 1993;91:128–34.
2. Ronen GM, Penney S, Andrews W. The epidemiology of clinical neonatal seizures in Newfoundland: a population-based study. J Pediatr 1999;134(1): 71–5.
3. Saliba RM, Annegers JF, Waller DK, et al. Incidence of neonatal seizures in Harris County, Texas, 1992–1994. Am J Epidemiol 1999;150(7):763–9.
4. Tekgul H, Gauvreau K, Soul J, et al. The current etiologic profile and neurodevelopmental outcome of seizures in term newborn infants. Pediatrics 2006;117: 1270–80.
5. Volpe JJ. Neurology of the newborn. 5th edition. Philadelphia: Saunders/Elsevier; 2008.
6. Ronen GM, Buckley D, Penney S, et al. Long-term prognosis in children with neonatal seizures: a population-based study. Neurology 2007;69(19):1816–22.
7. Bergamasco B, Penna P, Ferrero P, et al. Neonatal hypoxia and epileptic risk: a clinical prospective study. Epilepsia 1984;25:131–46.
8. Shankaran S, Laptook AR, Ehrenkranz RA, et al. Whole-body hypothermia for neonates with hypoxic-ischemic encephalopathy. N Engl J Med 2005;353(15): 1574–84.

9. Gluckman PD, Wyatt JS, Azzopardi D, et al. Selective head cooling with mild systemic hypothermia after neonatal encephalopathy: multicentre randomised trial. Lancet 2005;365(9460):663–70.

10. Coppola G, Castaldo P, Miraglia del Giudice E, et al. A novel KCNQ2 K$^+$ channel mutation in benign neonatal convulsions and centrotemporal spikes. Neurology 2003;61(1):131–4.

11. Singh NA, Westenskow P, Charlier C, et al. KCNQ2 and KCNQ3 potassium channel genes in benign familial neonatal convulsions: expansion of the functional and mutation spectrum. Brain 2003;126(Pt 12):2726–37.

12. Coppola G, Veggiotti P, Del Giudice EM, et al. Mutational scanning of potassium, sodium and chloride ion channels in malignant migrating partial seizures in infancy. Brain Dev 2006;28(2):76–9.

13. Claes LR, Ceulemans B, Audenaert D, et al. De novo KCNQ2 mutations in patients with benign neonatal seizures. Neurology 2004;63(11):2155–8.

14. Holden KR, Mellits ED, Freeman JM. Neonatal seizures. I. Correlation of prenatal and perinatal events with outcomes. Pediatrics 1982;70(2):165–76.

15. McBride MC, Laroia N, Guillet R. Electrographic seizures in neonates correlate with poor neurodevelopmental outcome. Neurology 2000;55(4):506–13.

16. Glass HC, Glidden D, Jeremy RJ, et al. Clinical neonatal seizures are independently associated with outcome in infants at risk for hypoxic-ischemic brain injury. J Pediatr 2009;155(3):318–23.

17. Miller SP, Ramaswamy V, Michelson D, et al. Patterns of brain injury in term neonatal encephalopathy. J Pediatr 2005;146(4):453–60.

18. Kohelet D, Shochat R, Lusky A, et al. Risk factors for neonatal seizures in very low birthweight infants: population-based survey. J Child Neurol 2004;19(2): 123–8.

19. Kohelet D, Shochat R, Lusky A, et al. Risk factors for seizures in very low birthweight infants with periventricular leukomalacia. J Child Neurol 2006;21(11): 965–70.

20. Mizrahi EM, Kellaway P. Diagnosis and management of neonatal seizures. Philadelphia: Lippincott-Raven; 1998.

21. Clancy RR. Prolonged electroencephalogram monitoring for seizures and their treatment. Clin Perinatol 2006;33(3):649–65, vi.

22. Shellhaas RA, Soaita AI, Clancy RR. Sensitivity of amplitude-integrated electroencephalography for neonatal seizure detection. Pediatrics 2007;120(4): 770–7.

23. Lawrence R, Mathur A, Nguyen The Tich S, et al. A pilot study of continuous limited-channel aEEG in term infants with encephalopathy. J Pediatr 2009; 154(6):835–41 e1.

24. Tekgul H, Bourgeois BF, Gauvreau K, et al. Electroencephalography in neonatal seizures: comparison of a reduced and a full 10/20 montage. Pediatr Neurol 2005;32(3):155–61.

25. Navakatikyan MA, Colditz PB, Burke CJ, et al. Seizure detection algorithm for neonates based on wave-sequence analysis. Clin Neurophysiol 2006;117(6): 1190–203.

26. Shellhaas RA, Clancy RR. Characterization of neonatal seizures by conventional EEG and single-channel EEG. Clin Neurophysiol 2007;118(10):2156–61.

27. Clancy RR. Summary proceedings from the neurology group on neonatal seizures. Pediatrics 2006;117(3 Pt 2):S23–7.

28. de Vries LS, Toet MC. Amplitude integrated electroencephalography in the full-term newborn. Clin Perinatol 2006;33(3):619–32, vi.

29. Grillo E, da Silva RJ, Barbato JH Jr. Pyridoxine-dependent seizures responding to extremely low-dose pyridoxine. Dev Med Child Neurol 2001;43(6):413–5.
30. Baxter P. Pyridoxine-dependent and pyridoxine-responsive seizures. Dev Med Child Neurol 2001;43(6):416–20.
31. Grant PE, Yu D. Acute injury to the immature brain with hypoxia with or without hypoperfusion. Radiol Clin North Am 2006;44(1):63–77, viii.
32. Bartha A, Shen J, Katz KH, et al. Neonatal seizures: multi-center variability in current treatment practices. Pediatr Neurol Res 2007;37(2):85–90.
33. Sankar R, Painter MJ. Neonatal seizures: after all these years we still love what doesn't work. Neurology 2005;64(5):776–7.
34. Booth D, Evans DJ. Anticonvulsants for neonates with seizures. Cochrane Database Syst Rev 2004;(4):CD004218.
35. Painter MJ, Scher MS, Stein AD, et al. Phenobarbital compared with phenytoin for the treatment of neonatal seizures. N Engl J Med 1999;341(7):485–9.
36. Boylan GB, Young K, Panerai RB, et al. Dynamic cerebral autoregulation in sick newborn infants. Pediatr Res 2000;48(1):12–7.
37. Carmo KB, Barr P. Drug treatment of neonatal seizures by neonatologists and paediatric neurologists. J Paediatr Child Health 2005;41(7):313–6.
38. Malingre MM, Van Rooij LG, Rademaker CM, et al. Development of an optimal lidocaine infusion strategy for neonatal seizures. Eur J Pediatr 2006;165(9):598–604.
39. Silverstein FS, Ferriero DM. Off-label use of antiepileptic drugs for the treatment of neonatal seizures. Pediatr Neurol 2008;39(2):77–9.
40. Pellock J. Antiepileptic drugs trials: neonates and infants. Epilepsy Res 2006;68(1):42–5.
41. Hmaimess G, Kadhim H, Nassogne MC, et al. Levetiracetam in a neonate with malignant migrating partial seizures. Pediatr Neurol 2006;34(1):55–9.
42. Jacobs S, Hunt R, Tarnow-Mordi W, et al. Cooling for newborns with hypoxic ischaemic encephalopathy. Cochrane Database Syst Rev 2007;(4):CD003311.
43. Azzopardi D, Brocklehurst P, Edwards D, et al. The TOBY Study. Whole body hypothermia for the treatment of perinatal asphyxial encephalopathy: a randomised controlled trial. BMC Pediatr 2008;8:17.
44. Rakhade SN, Jensen FE. Epileptogenesis in the immature brain: emerging mechanisms. Nat Rev Neurol 2009;5(7):380–91.
45. Hauser WA, Annegers JF, Kurland LT. Incidence of epilepsy and unprovoked seizures in Rochester, Minnesota: 1935–1984. Epilepsia 1993;34:453–68.
46. Aicardi J, Chevrie JJ. Convulsive status epilepticus in infants and children. A study of 239 cases. Epilepsia 1970;11(2):187–97.
47. Sanchez RM, Jensen FE. Maturational aspects of epilepsy mechanisms and consequences for the immature brain. Epilepsia 2001;42:577–85.
48. Sanchez RM, Jensen FE, Pitanken A, et al. Modeling hypoxia-induced seizures and hypoxic encephalopathy in the neonatal period. Models of seizures and epilepsy. San Diego (CA): Elsevier; 2005.
49. Talos DM, Follett PL, Folkerth RD, et al. Developmental regulation of alpha-amino-3-hydroxy-5-methyl-4-isoxazole-propionic acid receptor subunit expression in forebrain and relationship to regional susceptibility to hypoxic/ischemic injury. II. Human cerebral white matter and cortex. J Comp Neurol 2006;497(1):61–77.
50. Haynes RL, Borenstein NS, DeSilva TM, et al. Axonal development in the cerebral white matter of the human fetus and infant. J Comp Neurol 2005;484(2):156–67.

51. Takashima S, Chan F, Becker LE, et al. Morphology of the developing visual cortex of the human infant: a quantitative and qualitative Golgi study. J Neuropathol Exp Neurol 1980;39(4):487–501.

52. Huttenlocher PR, deCourten C, Garey LJ, et al. Synaptogenesis in human visual cortex – evidence for synapse elimination during normal development. Neurosci Lett 1982;33:247–52.

53. Johnston MV. Neurotransmitters and vulnerability of the developing brain. Brain Dev 1995;17(5):301–6.

54. Talos DM, Fishman RE, Park H, et al. Developmental regulation of alpha-amino-3-hydroxy-5-methyl-4-isoxazole-propionic acid receptor subunit expression in forebrain and relationship to regional susceptibility to hypoxic/ischemic injury. I. Rodent cerebral white matter and cortex. J Comp Neurol 2006;497(1):42–60.

55. Sanchez RM, Koh S, Rio C, et al. Decreased glutamate receptor 2 expression and enhanced epileptogenesis in immature rat hippocampus after perinatal hypoxia-induced seizures. J Neurosci 2001;21(20):8154–63.

56. Hollmann M, Heinemann S. Cloned glutamate receptors. Annu Rev Neurosci 1994;17:31–108.

57. Jiang Q, Wang J, Wu X, et al. Alterations of NR2B and PSD-95 expression after early-life epileptiform discharges in developing neurons. Int J Dev Neurosci 2007;25(3):165–70.

58. Wong HK, Liu XB, Matos MF, et al. Temporal and regional expression of NMDA receptor subunit NR3A in the mammalian brain. J Comp Neurol 2002;450(4):303–17.

59. Stafstrom CE, Tandon P, Hori A, et al. Acute effects of MK801 on kainic acid-induced seizures in neonatal rats. Epilepsy Res 1997;26(2):335–44.

60. Mares P, Mikulecka A. Different effects of two N-methyl-D-aspartate receptor antagonists on seizures, spontaneous behavior, and motor performance in immature rats. Epilepsy Behav 2009;14(1):32–9.

61. Chen HS, Wang YF, Rayudu PV, et al. Neuroprotective concentrations of the N-methyl-D-aspartate open-channel blocker memantine are effective without cytoplasmic vacuolation following post-ischemic administration and do not block maze learning or long-term potentiation. Neuroscience 1998;86(4):1121–32.

62. Ikonomidou C, Bosch F, Miksa M, et al. Blockade of NMDA receptors and apoptotic neurodegeneration in the developing brain. Science 1999;283:70–4.

63. Bittigau P, Sifringer M, Ikonomidou C. Antiepileptic drugs and apoptosis in the developing brain. Ann N Y Acad Sci 2003;993:103–14 [discussion: 123–4].

64. Manning SM, Talos DM, Zhou C, et al. NMDA receptor blockade with memantine attenuates white matter injury in a rat model of periventricular leukomalacia. J Neurosci 2008;28(26):6670–8.

65. Kumar SS, Bacci A, Kharazia V, et al. A developmental switch of AMPA receptor subunits in neocortical pyramidal neurons. J Neurosci 2002;22(8):3005–15.

66. Talos DM, Follett PL, Folkerth RD, et al. Developmental regulation of alpha-amino-3-hydroxy-5-methyl-4-isoxazole-propionic acid receptor subunit expression in forebrain and relationship to regional susceptibility to hypoxic/ischemic injury. II. Human cerebral white matter and cortex. J Comp Neurol 2006;497(1):61–77.

67. Shank RP, Gardocki JF, Streeter AJ, et al. An overview of the preclinical aspects of topiramate: pharmacology, pharmacokinetics, and mechanism of action. Epilepsia 2000;41(Suppl 1):S3–9.

68. Koh S, Tibayan FD, Simpson J, et al. NBQX or topiramate treatment following perinatal hypoxia-induced seizures prevents later increases in seizure-induced neuronal injury. Epilepsia 2004;45(6):569–75.

69. Koh S, Jensen F. Topiramate blocks perinatal hypoxia- induced seizures in rat pups. Ann Neurol 2001;50(3):366–72.
70. Liu Y, Barks JD, Xu G, et al. Topiramate extends the therapeutic window for hypothermia-mediated neuroprotection after stroke in neonatal rats. Stroke 2004;35(6):1460–5.
71. Aujla PK, Fetell M, Jensen FE. Talampanel suppresses the acute and chronic effects of seizures in a rodent neonatal seizure model. Epilepsia 2009;50(4):694–701.
72. Swann JW, Brady RJ, Martin DL. Postnatal development of GABA-mediated synaptic inhibition in rat hippocampus. Neuroscience 1989;28(3):551–61.
73. Brooks-Kayal A, Jin H, Price M, et al. Developmental expression of GABA(A) receptor subunit mRNAs in individual hippocampal neurons in vitro and in vivo. J Neurochem 1998;70(3):1017–28.
74. Kapur J, Macdonald RL. Postnatal development of hippocampal dentate granule cell γ-aminobutyric acid A receptor pharmacological properties. Mol Pharmacol 1999;55:444–52.
75. Jensen FE, Alvarado S, Firkusny IR, et al. NBQX blocks the acute and late epileptogenic effects of perinatal hypoxia. Epilepsia 1995;36(10):966–72.
76. Swann J, Moshe SL, Engel J Jr, et al. Developmental issues in animal models epilepsy: a comprehensive textbook. Philadelphia: Lippincott-Raven Publishers; 1997. p. 467–80.
77. Dzhala VI, Staley KJ. Excitatory actions of endogenously released GABA contribute to initiation of ictal epileptiform activity in the developing hippocampus. J Neurosci 2003;23(5):1840–6.
78. Khazipov R, Khalilov I, Tyzio R, et al. Developmental changes in GABAergic actions and seizure susceptibility in the rat hippocampus. Eur J Neurosci 2004;19(3):590–600.
79. Loturco JJ, Owens DF, Heath MJ, et al. GABA and glutamate depolarize cortical progenitor cells and inhibit DNA synthesis. Neuron 1995;15(6):1287–98.
80. Owens DF, Boyce LH, Davis MB, et al. Excitatory GABA responses in embryonic and neonatal cortical slices demonstrated by gramicidin perforated-patch recordings and calcium imaging. J Neurosci 1996;16(20):6414–23.
81. Dzhala VI, Talos DM, Sdrulla DA, et al. NKCC1 transporter facilitates seizures in the developing brain. Nat Med 2005;11(11):1205–13.
82. Dzhala VI, Brumback AC, Staley KJ. Bumetanide enhances phenobarbital efficacy in a neonatal seizure model. Ann Neurol 2008;63(2):222–35.
83. Cooper EC, Jan LY. M-channels: neurological diseases, neuromodulation, and drug development. Arch Neurol 2003;60(4):496–500.
84. Yue C, Yaari Y. KCNQ/M channels control spike afterdepolarization and burst generation in hippocampal neurons. J Neurosci 2004;24(19):4614–24.
85. Pape HC. Queer current and pacemaker: the hyperpolarization-activated cation current in neurons. Annu Rev Physiol 1996;58:299–327.
86. Bender RA, Brewster A, Santoro B, et al. Differential and age-dependent expression of hyperpolarization-activated, cyclic nucleotide-gated cation channel isoforms 1–4 suggests evolving roles in the developing rat hippocampus. Neuroscience 2001;106(4):689–98.
87. Bender RA, Galindo R, Mameli M, et al. Synchronized network activity in developing rat hippocampus involves regional hyperpolarization-activated cyclic nucleotide-gated (HCN) channel function. Eur J Neurosci 2005;22(10):2669–74.
88. Iwasaki S, Momiyama A, Uchitel OD, et al. Developmental changes in calcium channel types mediating central synaptic transmission. J Neurosci 2000;20(1):59–65.

89. Noebels JL. The biology of epilepsy genes. Annu Rev Neurosci 2003;26: 599–625.

90. Chen Y, Lu J, Pan H, et al. Association between genetic variation of CACNA1H and childhood absence epilepsy. Ann Neurol 2003;54(2):239–43.

91. Baram TZ, Hatalski CG. Neuropeptide-mediated excitability: a key triggering mechanism for seizure generation in the developing brain. Trends Neurosci 1998;21(11):471–6.

92. Ju WK, Kim KY, Neufeld AH. Increased activity of cyclooxygenase-2 signals early neurodegenerative events in the rat retina following transient ischemia. Exp Eye Res 2003;77(2):137–45.

93. Brunson KL, Eghbal-Ahmadi M, Bender R, et al. Long-term, progressive hippo-campal cell loss and dysfunction induced by early-life administration of corticotropin-releasing hormone reproduce the effects of early-life stress. Proc Natl Acad Sci U S A 2001;98(15):8856–61.

94. Brunson KL, Khan N, Eghbal-Ahmadi M, et al. Corticotropin (ACTH) acts directly on amygdala neurons to down-regulate corticotropin-releasing hormone gene expression. Ann Neurol 2001;49(3):304–12.

95. Ivacko JA, Sun R, Silverstein FS. Hypoxic-ischemic brain injury induces an acute microglial reaction in perinatal rats. Pediatr Res 1996;39(1):39–47.

96. Dommergues MA, Plaisant F, Verney C, et al. Early microglial activation following neonatal excitotoxic brain damage in mice: a potential target for neuroprotection. Neuroscience 2003;121(3):619–28.

97. Debillon T, Gras-Leguen C, Leroy S, et al. Patterns of cerebral inflammatory response in a rabbit model of intrauterine infection-mediated brain lesion. Brain Res Dev Brain Res 2003;145(1):39–48.

98. Saliba E, Henrot A. Inflammatory mediators and neonatal brain damage. Biol Neonate 2001;79(3–4):224–7.

99. Billiards SS, Haynes RL, Folkerth RD, et al. Development of microglia in the cerebral white matter of the human fetus and infant. J Comp Neurol 2006; 497(2):199–208.

100. Tikka T, Fiebich BL, Goldsteins G, et al. Minocycline, a tetracycline derivative, is neuroprotective against excitotoxicity by inhibiting activation and proliferation of microglia. J Neurosci 2001;21(8):2580–8.

101. Shapiro LA, Wang L, Ribak CE. Rapid astrocyte and microglial activation following pilocarpine-induced seizures in rats. Epilepsia 2008;49(Suppl 2):33–41.

102. Vezzani A, Balosso S, Ravizza T. The role of cytokines in the pathophysiology of epilepsy. Brain Behav Immun 2008;22(6):797–803.

103. Dalmau I, Vela JM, Gonzalez B, et al. Dynamics of microglia in the developing rat brain. J Comp Neurol 2003;458(2):144–57.

104. Pfrieger FW, Barres BA. Synaptic efficacy enhanced by glial cells in vitro. Science 1997;277(5332):1684–7.

105. Stevens B, Allen NJ, Vazquez LE, et al. The classical complement cascade mediates CNS synapse elimination. Cell 2007;131(6):1164–78.

106. Heo K, Cho YJ, Cho KJ, et al. Minocycline inhibits caspase-dependent and -independent cell death pathways and is neuroprotective against hippo-campal damage after treatment with kainic acid in mice. Neurosci Lett 2006; 398(3):195–200.

107. Lechpammer M, Manning SM, Samonte F, et al. Minocycline treatment following hypoxic/ischaemic injury attenuates white matter injury in a rodent model of periventricular leucomalacia. Neuropathol Appl Neurobiol 2008;34(4): 379–93.

108. Jantzie LL, Cheung PY, Todd KG. Doxycycline reduces cleaved caspase-3 and microglial activation in an animal model of neonatal hypoxia-ischemia. J Cereb Blood Flow Metab 2005;25(3):314–24.
109. Wasterlain CG, Niquet J, Thompson KW, et al. Seizure-induced neuronal death in the immature brain. Prog Brain Res 2002;135:335–53.
110. Stone BS, Zhang J, Mack DW, et al. Delayed neural network degeneration after neonatal hypoxia-ischemia. Ann Neurol 2008;64(5):535–46.
111. Kinney HC, Haynes RL, Folkerth RD, et al. White matter lesions in the perinatal period. In: Golden JA, Harding B, editors. Pathology and genetics: acquired and inherited diseases of the developing nervous system. Basel (Switzerland): ISN Neuropathology Press; 2004.
112. Lein ES, Finney EM, McQuillen PS, et al. Subplate neuron ablation alters neurotrophin expression and ocular dominance column formation. Proc Natl Acad Sci U S A 1999;96(23):13491–5.
113. Kanold PO, Kara P, Reid RC, et al. Role of subplate neurons in functional maturation of visual cortical columns. Science 2003;301(5632):521–5.
114. McQuillen PS, Sheldon RA, Shatz CJ, et al. Selective vulnerability of subplate neurons after early neonatal hypoxia-ischemia. J Neurosci 2003;23(8):3308–15.
115. Chang YS, Mu D, Wendland M, et al. Erythropoietin improves functional and histological outcome in neonatal stroke. Pediatr Res 2005;58(1):106–11.
116. Gonzalez FF, McQuillen P, Mu D, et al. Erythropoietin enhances long-term neuroprotection and neurogenesis in neonatal stroke. Dev Neurosci 2007;29(4–5):321–30.
117. Mikati MA, El Hokayem JA, El Sabban ME. Effects of a single dose of erythropoietin on subsequent seizure susceptibility in rats exposed to acute hypoxia at P10. Epilepsia 2007;48(1):175–81.
118. Ben Ari Y, Holmes GL. Effects of seizures on developmental processes in the immature brain. Lancet Neurol 2006;5(12):1055–63.
119. Sayin U, Sutula TP, Stafstrom CE. Seizures in the developing brain cause adverse long-term effects on spatial learning and anxiety. Epilepsia 2004; 45(12):1539–48.
120. Silverstein FS, Jensen FE. Neonatal seizures. Ann Neurol 2007;62(2):112–20.
121. Maffei A, Turrigiano G. The age of plasticity: developmental regulation of synaptic plasticity in neocortical microcircuits. Prog Brain Res 2008;169:211–23.
122. Rakhade SN, Zhou C, Aujla PK, et al. Early alterations of AMPA receptors mediate synaptic potentiation induced by neonatal seizures. J Neurosci 2008; 28(32):7979–90.
123. Cornejo BJ, Mesches MH, Coultrap S, et al. A single episode of neonatal seizures permanently alters glutamatergic synapses. Ann Neurol 2007;61(5): 411–26.
124. Stafstrom CE, Moshe SL, Swann JW, et al. Models of pediatric epilepsies: strategies and opportunities. Epilepsia 2006;47(8):1407–14.
125. Sanchez RM, Dai W, Levada RE, et al. AMPA/kainate receptor-mediated downregulation of GABAergic synaptic transmission by calcineurin after seizures in the developing rat brain. J Neurosci 2005;25(13):3442–51.
126. Raol YH, Lund IV, Bandyopadhyay S, et al. Enhancing GABA(A) receptor alpha 1 subunit levels in hippocampal dentate gyrus inhibits epilepsy development in an animal model of temporal lobe epilepsy. J Neurosci 2006;26(44): 11342–6.
127. Isaeva E, Isaev D, Khazipov R, et al. Selective impairment of GABAergic synaptic transmission in the flurothyl model of neonatal seizures. Eur J Neurosci 2006;23(6):1559–66.

128. Bergey GK, Swaiman KF, Schrier BK, et al. Adverse effects of phenobarbital on morphological and biochemical development of fetal mouse spinal cord neurons in culture. Ann Neurol 1981;9(6):584–9.
129. Serrano EE, Kunis DM, Ransom BR. Effects of chronic phenobarbital exposure on cultured mouse spinal cord neurons. Ann Neurol 1988;24(3):429–38.
130. Pereira de Vasconcelos A, Colin C, Desor D, et al. Influence of early neonatal phenobarbital exposure on cerebral energy metabolism and behavior. Exp Neurol 1990;108(2):176–87.
131. Schroeder H, Humbert AC, Koziel V, et al. Behavioral and metabolic consequences of neonatal exposure to diazepam in rat pups. Exp Neurol 1995; 131(1):53–63.
132. Bittigau P, Sifringer M, Genz K, et al. Antiepileptic drugs and apoptotic neurodegeneration in the developing brain. Proc Natl Acad Sci U S A 2002;99(23): 15089–94.
133. Glier C, Dzietko M, Bittigau P, et al. Therapeutic doses of topiramate are not toxic to the developing rat brain. Exp Neurol 2004;187(2):403–9.
134. Manthey D, Asimiadou S, Stefovska V, et al. Sulthiame but not levetiracetam exerts neurotoxic effect in the developing rat brain. Exp Neurol 2005;193(2): 497–503.

The Long-Term Effects of Neonatal Seizures

Gregory L. Holmes, MD

KEYWORDS

- Epilepsy • Learning • Memory • Place cells
- EEG • Development

During the first months of life, children are at particularly high risk for seizures, with the largest number of new-onset seizure disorders occurring during this time.[1] Because of the birthing process, the infant is at risk for a number of insults that can result in seizures. These insults include birth trauma, hypoxic-ischemic insults, congenital and postnatally acquired infections, intracranial hemorrhages, and metabolic disturbances.

In addition to the immature brain's high risk for brain insults, there is considerable evidence that it is more susceptible to seizures than the mature brain. The propensity for seizures in the immature brain has been demonstrated in a number of experimental models, including kainic acid,[2,3] electrical stimulation,[4] hypoxia,[5] penicillin,[6] picrotoxin,[7] GABA(B) receptor antagonists,[8] and increased extracellular potassium.[9,10]

The underlying mechanisms responsible for this increased excitability have now been delineated. During the early postnatal period, at a time when the immature brain is highly susceptible to seizures,[10,11] γ-aminobutyric acid (GABA), which in the adult brain is the primary inhibitory neurotransmitter, exerts paradoxic excitatory action.[9,10] In the young brain, GABA is initially excitatory because of a larger intracellular concentration of chloride in immature neurons than mature ones (**Fig. 1**).[12–14] The shift from a depolarizing to a hyperpolarizing chloride current occurs in an extended period depending on the age and developmental stage of the structure. The shift is mediated by an active Na^+-K^+-$2Cl^-$ cotransporter (NKCC1) that facilitates the accumulation of chloride in neurons, and a delayed expression of a K^+-Cl^- cotransporter (KCC2) that extrudes chloride to establish adult concentrations of intracellular chloride.[15] The depolarization by GABA of immature neurons is sufficient to generate sodium action potentials and to remove the voltage-dependent Mg^{2+} blockade of N-methyl-D-aspartate (NMDA) channels and activate voltage-dependent calcium channels, leading to a large influx of calcium that in turn triggers long-term changes of synaptic efficacy. The synergistic action of GABA with NMDA and calcium channels is unique to

This article was supported by NIH grants (NINDS) NS0415951 and NS056170.
Department of Neurology, Dartmouth-Hitchcock Medical Center, Neuroscience Center at Dartmouth, Dartmouth Medical School, One Medical Center Drive, Lebanon, NH 03756, USA
E-mail address: gregory.l.holmes@dartmouth.edu

Clin Perinatol 36 (2009) 901–914
doi:10.1016/j.clp.2009.07.012
0095-5108/09/$ – see front matter © 2009 Elsevier Inc. All rights reserved.

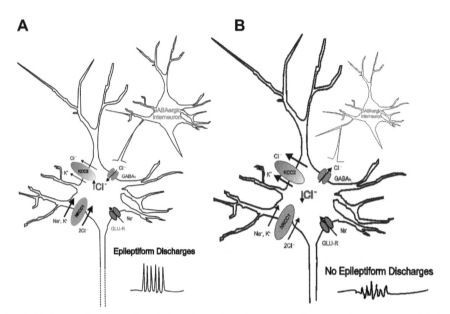

Fig. 1. Cartoons of an immature (*A*) and a mature (*B*) neuron. The immature neuron (*A*) is in a more excitable state than the mature neuron (*B*). Because NKCC1 is expressed and functions sooner than KCC2, there is an increase of chloride within immature neurons compared with mature neurons (*A*). The increase in intracellular chloride results in a depolarized chloride equilibrium potential. When the GABA channel is activated by GABA, there is a flow of chloride from inside the cell to outside the cell. Because chloride carries a negative charge, the exodus of chloride serves to depolarize the cell (excitation), making it more likely to discharge when sodium enters the cell. In the mature neuron (*B*), KCC2 is functional and balances the increase of chloride through NKCC1 with an outward flow of chloride. Because of lower intracellular chloride levels when the GABA receptor is activated, chloride enters the cell carrying a negative charge, thus resulting in hyperpolarization (inhibition).

the developing brain and has many consequences on the impact of GABAergic synapses on the network. In addition, agents that interfere with the transport of chloride exert an antiepileptogenic action.[15] With maturation, there is increasing function of KCC2 and decreasing function of NKCC1, a transporter that brings chloride into the cell that results in an inhibitory effect of GABA.

The lack of efficient time-locked inhibition, the delayed maturation of postsynaptic GABA(B)-mediated currents, and the high input resistance of immature neurons will facilitate the generation of action potentials and synchronized activities.[8,16] In addition, during the first few weeks of life there is enhanced excitation caused by an overabundance of NMDA and α-amino-3-hydroxyl-5-methyl-4-isoxazole-propionate receptors.[17,18] With maturation, axonal collaterals and attendant synapses regress.[19]

CLINICAL FEATURES OF NEONATAL SEIZURES

The clinical and electroencephalographic features of neonatal seizures differ considerably from these features in older children and adults. **Box 1** lists the clinical types of neonatal seizures. Some seizures can be quite subtle, making diagnosis difficult. Clonic seizures are usually easy to detect, and these seizures typically have a clear electroencephalogram (EEG) epileptiform discharge during the event. However,

Box 1
Behavioral features of neonatal seizures
Clonic
Focal
Lateralized
Multifocal
Tonic
Focal
Lateralized
Generalized
Myoclonic
Focal
Lateralized
Multifocal
Generalized
Discrete
Apnea
Automatisms (oral)
Autonomic phenomena
Ocular-nystagmus, eye deviation

some of the other behaviors listed in **Box 1** may not have clear EEG changes, raising the question of whether they are actual epileptic seizures. Perhaps more importantly, many neonates will have electroencephalographic seizures without any obvious clinical signs (**Fig. 2**).

Sometimes a disassociation between the EEG and behavioral features of the seizures occurs following administration of phenobarbital, wherein the EEG electrical seizures continue but the behavioral features of the seizures cease. As described earlier, during development activation of chloride-permeable GABA(A) receptors excites neurons as a result of elevated intracellular chloride levels. GABA becomes inhibitory as net outward neuronal transport of chloride develops in a caudal-rostral progression (i.e., GABA) becomes inhibitory in the brainstem before the cortex. Thus GABAergic drugs, such as phenobarbital, will inhibit brainstem activity, including the motor manifestations of seizures, while the cortex still generates electrical seizures.

Detecting electrographic seizures in the absence of behavior changes is imperative because data from animals suggest that even in the absence of behavioral changes, electroencephalographic seizures can result in brain damage.[20,21] Adolescent baboons who are paralyzed, artificially ventilated, and maintain normal blood pressure and glucose concentration develop brain damage when subjected to electroenceph-alographic seizures.[22] While extrapolating studies from animals to human infants is difficult, treating electrographic seizures as vigorously as behavioral seizures appears prudent.

		Rhythmic EEG Discharge	
		+	-
Clinical Signs	+	Electroclinical	Clinical
	-	Electrographic (occult, silent)	n/a

Fig. 2. Cartoon of relationship between EEG discharges and behavioral changes in neonates with suspected seizures. Electrical EEG changes may correspond with behavioral changes demonstrating the behavioral charges are epileptic seizures. Another scenario would be that there are behavioral events without EEG electrical changes. While it is possible that seizures involving a limited area of cortex are missed with surface EEG recordings, in most instances these events are not likely to be epileptic seizures. EEG ictal events without behavioral changes are typically seen in severely impaired infants, often suffering from hypoxic-ischemic encephalopathy, in infants pharmacologically paralyzed, or in infants given loading doses of barbiturates or benzodiazepines.

OUTCOME OF NEONATAL SEIZURES

Neonatal seizures are almost always symptomatic of an underlying neurologic condition. Consequently, the prognosis for the infants is usually poor. Death, postneonatal epilepsy, behavioral problems, and mental retardation are common outcomes.[23–27] However, outcome studies are somewhat difficult to interpret because of the uncertainty of diagnosis in some series. Some studies have used only behavioral seizures in making the diagnosis,[24] whereas other authors have required EEG confirmation of the seizures.[26,28–30] In the former case, some events are likely to be incorrectly classified as seizures, whereas in the later situation, reliance on recording ictal events on EEG may miss some infants with seizures.

To compare the outcome of neonates with seizures versus infants with similar neurologic conditions without seizures, McBride and colleagues[26] reviewed the EEG and outcome data from 68 infants who met at-risk criteria for neonatal seizures and underwent prolonged continuous EEG monitoring. Forty of the infants had electrical seizures on the EEG. The occurrence of electrical seizures was correlated with microcephaly, severe cerebral palsy, failure to thrive, and in the subgroup of infants with asphyxia, death. Those with the greatest number of electrical seizures were more likely to have these severe outcomes. In a similar study, Legido and colleagues[27] found that of 40 infants with neonatal seizures confirmed by EEG, there was a mortality rate of 33%, and 70% of the survivors had unfavorable outcome with high rates of postnatal epilepsy (56%), cerebral palsy (63%), and developmental delay (67%). Even in studies in which seizures are not confirmed by EEG, there is a high incidence of poor outcomes. Of 77 subjects who had observed behavioral neonatal seizures admitted to a tertiary care unit, 23 died (30%), 59% of the survivors had abnormal neurologic examinations, 40% were mentally retarded, 43% had cerebral palsy, and 21% had postnatal epilepsy.[24]

While it is widely recognized that the etiology of the seizures is the primary determinant of outcome, whether the occurrence of seizures themselves in the neonate contributes to the poor outcome is more controversial.[31,32] Separating the consequences of seizures from consequences of the underlying etiology is quite difficult. Miller and colleagues[33] used MRI and single-voxel (1)H-MRS to determine if neonatal seizures in children who had hypoxic-ischemic encephalopathy contributed to brain injury. The severity of the abnormality in the (1)H-MRS regions of interest was scored, and seizure severity was scored based on seizure frequency and duration, EEG findings, and antiepileptic drug administration. Multivariable linear regression tested the independent association of seizure severity with impaired cerebral metabolism, measured by the lactate/choline ratio, and compromised neuronal integrity, measured by N-acetylaspartate/choline. In 33 infants with neonatal seizures, the seizure severity was associated with an increased lactate/choline ratio in the intervascular boundary zone and the basal nuclei. Each increase in seizure score was independently associated with a 21% increase in lactate/choline in the intervascular boundary zone and a 15% increase in the basal nuclei. Seizure severity was independently associated with diminished N-acetylaspartate/choline in the intervascular boundary zone. The authors concluded that the severity of seizures in human newborns who have perinatal asphyxia is independently associated with brain injury and is not limited to structural damage detectable by MRI. While biochemical markers, such as lactate, may serve as a biomarker for cell injury, to date there are no long-term morbidity rates over the rate expected from the original brain insult.

Animal models have indicated that seizures can accelerate cell death in hypoxic-ischemic injuries. In a direct assessment of the effect of seizures on cell injury in the stressed brain, Dzhala and colleagues[34] used an intact hippocampus preparation from neonatal rats, which can be maintained *in vitro* for hours. The preparation allows pharmacologic and electrical studies in a hippocampus that maintains neuronal connections between cell layers.[35] In this preparation, prolonged episodes of anoxia/aglycemia induced rapid suppression of synaptic activity, followed sequentially by brief bursts of epileptiform activity and then by rapid anoxic depolarization. Anoxic depression is associated with irreversible neuronal damage manifested by irreversible loss of the membrane potential, synaptic responses, and neuronal degeneration. Aggravation of electrographic seizure activity during anoxic episodes accelerated anoxic depolarization and associated neuronal death by up to twofold, whereas blockade of seizure activity by the glutamate receptor antagonists or tetrodotoxin significantly delayed the onset of anoxic depolarization. This report provides direct evidence for the need to prevent seizures during neonatal brain hypoxia.

To definitively examine the effect of seizures on long-term neurocognitive development in neonates, a controlled trial would be needed in which neonates would be randomized to treatment versus no treatment and followed for several years. Because most clinicians consider it standard of care to treat children with antiepileptic drugs, designing such a study would be ethically challenging. Other obstacles to studying the role of seizures versus etiology in outcome in neonates is the lack of highly effective treatments in the neonatal period[26,36] and the possibly deleterious effects of antiepileptic drugs on brain development.[37,38]

Many of the inherent difficulties of separating the sequelae of seizures from the consequences of etiology and antiepileptic drugs can be overcome with animal studies. In the laboratory setting, many of the clinical variables, such as etiology, age of onset, drug therapy, and seizure frequency, duration, and intensity, can be controlled.

CONSEQUENCES OF RECURRENT SEIZURES IN IMMATURE ANIMALS

During development, the construction of cortical networks is associated with a sequential shift from an ensemble of immature cells with little or no organized communication devices to a highly active network composed of neurons endowed with thousands of active synapses. This shift is mediated by a series of sequences that includes intrinsic programs and extrinsic factors. The proposal made in several recent studies is that seizures, like other insults, will modify these sequences, leading to persistent deleterious sequels.

Our laboratory has extensively used the flurothyl model of recurrent seizures. In this model, the volatile agent flurothyl (bis-2, 2, 2-triflurothyl ether) is administered as an inhalant, and immature rats develop myoclonic, clonic, and tonic seizures within minutes of exposure. The seizures are easily elicited and are associated with a low mortality rate.[39] To mimic neonatal seizures, where infants have short but frequent seizures,[40] we subjected neonatal rats to multiple brief seizures daily during the first postnatal days.

In the adult animals, prolonged or frequent seizures cause neuronal loss in hippocampal fields CA1, CA3, and the dentate hilus.[41–44] Although the threshold for seizure generation is lower in immature brains than adult brains, developing neurons are less vulnerable in neuronal damage and cell loss than adult neurons to a wide variety of pathologic insults. For example, immature hippocampal neurons will continue responding to synaptic stimuli in a fully anoxic environment for longer durations than adult ones; likewise, longer anoxic episodes are required to irreversibly destroy the circuit in young animals.[45] Young animals are far less vulnerable to cell loss in the hippocampus following a prolonged seizure than are mature animals.[46–50] Likewise, recurrent seizures during the first 2 weeks of life result in no discernible cell loss.[51–53]

However, because neonatal seizures do not result in cell loss does not mean that seizures do not cause any morphologic damage. Recurrent seizures can result in spine loss in CA3 pyramidal cells[54] and synaptic reorganization of the axons and terminals of the mossy fibers of the dentate granule cells.[51,55–57] The mossy fiber sprouting differs significantly from the sprouting seen after status epilepticus in adult rats, occurring primarily in the CA3 pyramidal cell layer.[58]

Recurrent seizures in developing rats can adversely affect neurogenesis. McCabe and colleagues[59] studied the extent of neurogenesis in the granule cell layer of the dentate gyrus over multiple time points following a series of 25 flurothyl-induced seizures administered during the first 5 days of life. Rats with neonatal seizures had a significant reduction in the number of newly born neurons in the dentate gyrus and hilus compared with the control groups, with reductions in newly formed cells continuing for 6 days following the last seizure.

In addition to sprouting and impaired neurogenesis, recurrent early-life seizures have been shown to result in immunohistologic alterations of glutamate[57,60] and GABA subunit expression.[61] Neonatal seizures have been associated with a decrease in glutamate receptor 2 (GluR2) mRNA expression and protein levels,[62] and with selective reduction in the membrane pool of glutamate receptor 1 subunits and decreases in the total amount of NMDA receptor 2A.[63] In addition, the excitatory amino acid carrier 1 was reduced in rats with neonatal seizures compared with controls.[62] Animals with alterations in glutamate receptors have been shown to have deficits in a hippocampal-dependent radial arm water maze,[63] demonstrating the relationship between neonatal seizures and memory deficits with specific alterations in glutamatergic synaptic function.

Significant alterations in GABAergic function have also been reported following neonatal seizures. Rats subjected to lithium-pilocarpine-induced seizures at postnatal day 10 show long-term GABA(A) receptor changes, including a twofold increase in alpha1 subunit expression (compared with lithium-injected controls) and enhanced benzodiazepine augmentation, findings opposite to those seen after status epilepticus in adult rats.[64] Persistent decreases in GABA amplitude in the hippocampus in rats also occur following neonatal seizures.[65]

The alterations in the balance in excitation and inhibition following neonatal seizures also result in long-standing changes in seizure susceptibility when the animals are examined at an older age.[52,66]

Effects of Neonatal Seizures on Cognition

Using a variety of techniques to induce seizures, investigators have found that normal rats subjected to a series of recurrent seizures during the first weeks of life have considerable cognitive impairment when the animals are studied during adolescence or adulthood.[51,52,55–58,67,68]

A commonly used test to assess spatial memory is the Morris water maze, a test of hippocampal-dependent spatial memory. In this test, animals are placed in a 2-m diameter tank filled with water. Four points on the rim of the pool are designated north (N), south (S), east (E), and west (W), thus dividing the pool into four quadrants (NW, NE, SE, SW). An 8 × 8 cm plexiglass platform, onto which the rat can escape, is positioned in the center of one of the quadrants, 1 cm below the water's surface. Over multiple trials conducted over several days, the rat learns to find the submerged platform using cues around the tank that remain constant from trial to trial. After the end of the training the submerged platform is removed and the rat is placed in the swimming tank for 60 seconds. The time spent in the quadrant where the platform was previously located (called the target quadrant) is compared with time in the other quadrants. In this part of the task, called the probe test, normal rats spend most of their time swimming in the target quadrant. The probe test is a measure of the strength of spatial memory.

Following flurothyl-induced neonatal seizures, there is impairment of spatial memory in the water maze, with rats subjected to recurrent flurothyl seizures during

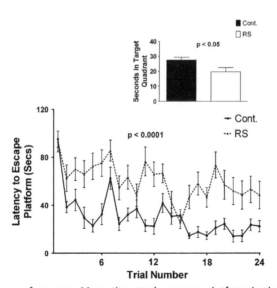

Fig. 3. Water maze performance. Mean time to the escape platform is plotted against trial number. Although both groups of rats reduced latencies to the escape platform across trials, rats with recurrent seizures (RS) during the first weeks of life were significantly slower in reaching the escape platform than the controls across all trials. The insert shows results from the probe test. Recurrent seizure rats spent significantly less time in the target quadrant than the controls. (*From* Karnam HB, Zhou JL, Huang LT, et al. Early life seizures cause long-standing impairment of the hippocampal map. Exp Neurol 2009;217:378–87; with permission.)

the neonatal period requiring longer times to find the platform than controls (**Fig. 3**).[51,52,55,69] This impairment occurs when the rats are tested either during adolescence or when fully mature. Likewise, recurrent pentylenetetrazol[56] and hyperthermic[67] seizures during early development result in subsequent impairment in visual-spatial memory. Animals subjected to recurrent flurothyl seizures between P15 to P20 also have impairment of auditory discrimination.[68]

To directly address the cellular concomitants of spatial memory impairment, we study firing patterns of single hippocampal neurons in freely moving rats. Certain cells are activated selectively when an animal moves through a particular location in space (the place field) (**Fig. 4**). Firing fields are stable over days to weeks as long as the

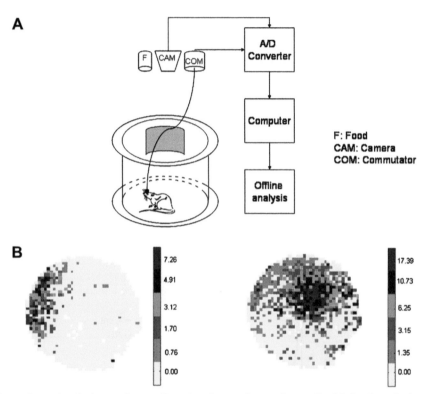

Fig. 4. Example of place cell recording chamber and two place cells. (*A*) Rat has diode on head which allows tracking of position. An orienting card is on the wall of the cylinder. The intracranial electrodes are attached to a cable with preamplifier in place. A food pellet dispenser is attached on the ceiling along with the camera and commutator. The recording system amplifies and digitizes the analog signal and allows the recording of single-cell action potentials while also recording position. Food pellets are dispensed randomly about the cylinder which causes the rat to visit all locations in the cylinder. (*B*) Color-coded firing rate maps were used to visualize firing distributions. Pixel rates were coded in the sequence: yellow, orange, red, green, blue, and purple. The firing rate was exactly zero for yellow pixels. Unvisited pixels in the cylinder and pixels outside the cylinder were coded white. In the left-hand figure, a place cell at approximately 11:00 is shown. In the right-hand figure, a place cell in the middle of the field was seen. (*From* Zhou JL, Shatskikh TN, Liu X, et al. Impaired single cell firing and long-term potentiation parallels memory impairment following recurrent seizures. Eur J Neurosci 2007;25:3667–77; with permission.)[83]

environment remains constant, suggesting that place cells retain information about location rather than creating it de novo each time the rat enters the environment.[70–72] Based on the finding that a considerable fraction (25%–50%) of the cell population of the hippocampus are place cells,[73,74] the hippocampus is proposed to function as a spatial map.[75] Hippocampal place cells have also been shown to code nonspatial information,[76–79] suggesting that the hippocampal map stores experiences associated with certain locations in the environment.[80] As shown by studies showing the association between place cell firing patterns and spatial performance,[81–84] place cell function appears to be a robust surrogate biologic marker for spatial memory.

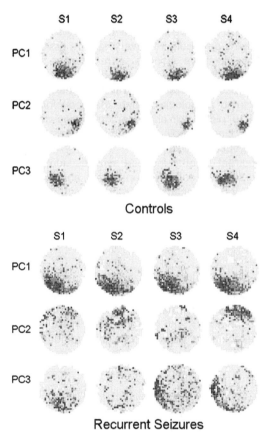

Fig. 5. Examples of place cells from controls and neonatal recurrent seizure rats. Color-coded firing rate maps were used to visualize firing distributions. Each row represents a single cell recorded during four sessions. The place cell firing fields were smoother and more precise in the controls than in the recurrent seizure rats. Cells from the recurrent seizure groups were noisier, with greater out-of-field firing than the controls. The firing fields were more stable across different testing sessions (S1, S2, S3, S4) in the controls than the recurrent seizure group. In the controls, none of the cells (PC1, PC2, PC3) changed position across sessions, whereas in the recurrent seizure group, the first cell (PC1) was stable but PC2 and PC3 were not stable. These findings suggest that place cells have a better memory for position in the controls than in the recurrent seizure group. (*From* Karnam HB, Zhou JL, Huang LT, et al. Early life seizures cause long-standing impairment of the hippocampal map. Exp Neurol 2007:217:378–87; with permission.)[69]

We recorded the activity of place cells from hippocampal subfield CA1 in freely moving rats subjected to 100 brief flurothyl-induced seizures during the first weeks of life, and then tested them in the Morris water maze followed by place cell testing. Compared with controls, rats with recurrent seizures had marked impairment in the Morris water maze. In parallel, there were substantial deficits in action potential firing characteristics of place cells, with two major defects: (1) the coherence, which provides a measure of the precision of the firing field, firing rate, and field size, was reduced compared with control cells; and (2) the fields were less stable than those in control place cells (**Fig. 5**). These results show that recurrent seizures during early development are associated with significant impairment in spatial learning, and that these deficits are paralleled by deficits in the hippocampal map.

This study thus provides a cellular explanation for how recurrent seizures during early development lead to cognitive impairment, and adds to the increasing evidence that seizures during early development have long-term adverse effects on cognitive function and that these cognitive changes are reflected at the single cell level. This study, and others,[81–83,85,86] confirms that abnormalities in place cell firing patterns can be associated with adverse cognitive consequences. The challenge is to determine which of the myriad of pathologic changes that occur following neonatal seizures mechanistically lead to place cell changes with associated spatial learning and memory disturbances. Understanding these mechanisms will be a critical step in designing novel therapeutic interventions.

In conclusion, recurrent flurothyl-induced seizures during early development in rodents result in long-standing cognitive impairment, aberrant, mossy fiber sprouting in the CA3 region of the hippocampus, reduced neurogenesis, alterations in the expression and distribution of glutamate and GABA receptors, and physiologic evidence for enhanced excitability.

SUMMARY

The outcome of neonatal seizures is most influenced by etiology of the seizures. While it is recognized that there are no definitive clinical studies indicating that seizures contribute to brain damage in the neonate, the evidence that seizures alter the brain in young animals is unequivocal. The challenge for clinicians and scientists is to find safe and effective therapies that prevent these seizure-induced brain alterations.

REFERENCES

1. Hauser WA. Epidemiology of epilepsy in children. Neurosurg Clin N Am 1995;6: 419–29.
2. Tremblay E, Nitecka L, Berger ML, et al. Maturation of kainic acid seizure-brain damage syndrome in the rat. I. Clinical, electrographic and metabolic observations. Neuroscience 1984;13(4):1051–72.
3. Khalilov I, Holmes GL, Ben-Ari Y. In vitro formation of a secondary epileptogenic mirror focus by interhippocampal propagation of seizures. Nat Neurosci 2003;6: 1079–85.
4. Moshe SL. The effects of age on the kindling phenomenon. Dev Psychobiol 1981; 14:75–81.
5. Jensen FE, Applegate CD, Holtzman D, et al. Epileptogenic effect of hypoxia in the immature rodent brain. Ann Neurol 1991;29:629–37.
6. Swann JW, Brady RJ. Penicillin-induced epileptogenesis in immature rats CA_3 hippocampal pyramidal cells. Brain Res 1984;12:243–54.

7. Gomez-Di Cesare CM, Smith KL, Rice FL, et al. Axonal remodeling during post-natal maturation of CA3 hippocampal pyramidal neurons. J Comp Neurol 1997; 384:165–80.
8. McLean HA, Caillard O, Khazipov R, et al. Spontaneous release of GABA activates GABAB receptors and controls network activity in the neonatal rat hippocampus. J Neurophysiol 1996;76:1036–46.
9. Dzhala VI, Staley KJ. Transition from interictal to ictal activity in limbic networks in vitro. J Neurosci 2003;23:7873–80.
10. Khazipov R, Khalilov I, Tyzio R, et al. Developmental changes in GABAergic actions and seizure susceptibility in the rat hippocampus. Eur J Neurosci 2004; 19:590–600.
11. Jensen FE, Baram TZ. Developmental seizures induced by common early-life insults: short- and long-term effects on seizure susceptibility. Ment Retard Dev Disabil Res Rev 2000;6:253–7.
12. Ben-Ari Y, Cherubini E, Corradetti R, et al. Giant synaptic potentials in immature rat CA3 hippocampal neurons. J Physiol 1989;416:303–25.
13. Ben-Ari Y. Excitatory actions of GABA during development: the nature of the nurture. Nat Rev Neurosci 2002;3:728–39.
14. Ben-Ari Y, Holmes GL. The multiple facets of gamma-aminobutyric acid dysfunction in epilepsy. Curr Opin Neurol 2005;18:141–5.
15. Dzhala VI, Talos DM, Sdrulla DA, et al. NKCC1 transporter facilitates seizures in the developing brain. Nat Med 2005;11:1205–13.
16. Gaiarsa JL, Tseeb V, Ben-Ari Y. Postnatal development of pre- and postsynaptic GABAB-mediated inhibitions in the CA3 hippocampal region of the rat. J Neurophysiol 1995;73:246–55.
17. Miller LP, Johnson AE, Gelhard RE, et al. The ontogeny of excitatory amino acid receptors in the rat forebrain - II. Kainic acid receptors. Neuroscience 1990;35: 45–51.
18. McDonald JW, Johnston MV, Young AB. Differential ontogenic development of three receptors comprising the NMDA receptor/channel complex in the rat hippocampus. Exp Neurol 1990;110:237–47.
19. Swann JW, Smith KL, Brady RJ. Age-dependent alterations in the operations of hippocampal neural networks. Ann N Y Acad Sci 1991;627:264–76.
20. Blennow G, Brierley JB, Meldrum BS, et al. Epileptic brain damage. The role of systemic factors that modify cerebral energy metabolism. Brain 1978;101: 687–700.
21. Ben-Ari Y, Tremblay E, Ottersen OP, et al. Evidence suggesting secondary epileptogenic lesions after kainic acid: pre-treatment with diazepam reduces distant but not local brain damage. Brain Res 1979;165:362–5.
22. Meldrum BS, Vigouroux RA, Brierley JB. Systemic factors and epileptic brain damage. Prolonged seizures in paralyzed artificially ventilated baboons. Arch Neurol 1973;29:82–7.
23. Scher MS, Aso K, Beggarly ME, et al. Electrographic seizures in preterm and full-term neonates: clinical correlates, associated brain lesions, and risk for neurologic sequelae. Pediatrics 1993;91:128–34.
24. Brunquell PJ, Glennon CM, DiMario FJ Jr, et al. Prediction of outcome based on clinical seizure type in newborn infants. J Pediatr 2002;140:707–12.
25. Scher MS, Painter MJ, Bergman I, et al. EEG diagnoses of neonatal seizures: clinical correlations and outcome. Pediatr Neurol 1989;5:17–24.
26. McBride MC, Laroia N, Guillet R. Electrographic seizures in neonates correlate with poor neurodevelopmental outcome. Neurology 2000;55:506–13.

27. Legido A, Clancy RR, Berman PH. Neurologic outcome after electroencephalographic proven neonatal seizures. Pediatrics 1991;88:583–96.
28. Rowe JC, Holmes GL, Hafford J, et al. Prognostic value of the electroencephalogram in term and preterm infants following neonatal seizures. Electroencephalogr Clin Neurophysiol 1985;60:183–96.
29. Rose AL, Lombroso CT. Neonatal seizure states. A study of clinical, pathological, and electroencephalographic features in 137 full-term babies with a long-term follow-up. Pediatrics 1970;45:404–25.
30. Clancy RR, Legido A. Postnatal epilepsy after EEG-confirmed neonatal seizures. Epilepsia 1991;32:69–76.
31. Mizrahi EM, Clancy RR. Neonatal seizures: early-onset seizure syndromes and their consequences for development. Ment Retard Dev Disabil Res Rev 2000;6:229–41.
32. Holmes GL, Ben-Ari Y. Seizures in the developing brain: perhaps not so benign after all. Neuron 1998;21:1231–4.
33. Miller SP, Weiss J, Barnwell A, et al. Seizure-associated brain injury in term newborns with perinatal asphyxia. Neurology 2002;58:542–8.
34. Dzhala V, Ben Ari Y, Khazipov R. Seizures accelerate anoxia-induced neuronal death in the neonatal rat hippocampus. Ann Neurol 2000;48:632–40.
35. Khalilov I, Esclapez M, Medina I, et al. A novel in vitro preparation: the intact hippocampal formation. Neuron 1997;19:743–9.
36. Painter MJ, Scher MS, Stein AD, et al. Phenobarbital compared with phenytoin for the treatment of neonatal seizures. N Engl J Med 1999;341:485–9.
37. Bittigau P, Sifringer M, Genz K, et al. Antiepileptic drugs and apoptotic neurodegeneration in the developing brain. Proc Natl Acad Sci U S A 2002;99:15089–94.
38. Mikati MA, Holmes GL, Chronopoulos A, et al. Phenobarbital modifies seizure-related brain injury in the developing brain. Ann Neurol 1994;36:425–33.
39. Zhao Q, Holmes GL. Repetitive seizures in the immature brain. In: Pitkänen A, Schwartzkroin PA, Moshé S, editors. Models of seizures and epilepsy. Elsevier Academic Press, Burlington, MA; 2006. p. 341–50.
40. Clancy RR, Legido A. The exact ictal and interictal duration of electroencephalographic neonatal seizures. Epilepsia 1987;28:537–41.
41. Nadler JV. Kainic acid as a tool for the study of temporal lobe epilepsy. Life Sci 1981;29:2031–42.
42. Ben-Ari Y. Cell death and synaptic reorganizations produced by seizures. Epilepsia 2001;42(Suppl 3):5–7.
43. Cavazos JE, Sutula TP. Progressive neuronal loss induced by kindling: a possible mechanism for mossy fiber synaptic reorganization and hippocampal sclerosis. Brain Res 1990;527:1–6.
44. Cavazos JE, Golarai G, Sutula TP. Mossy fiber synaptic reorganization induced by kindling: time course of development, progression, and permanence. J Neurosci 1991;11:2795–803.
45. Cherubini E, Ben-Ari Y, Krnjevic K. Anoxia produces smaller changes in synaptic transmission, membrane potential and input resistance in immature rat hippocampus. J Neurophysiol 1989;62:882–95.
46. Albala BJ, Moshé SL, Okada R. Kainic-acid-induced seizures: a developmental study. Brain Res 1984;13:139–48.
47. Holmes GL, Thompson JL. Effects of kainic acid on seizure susceptibility in the developing brain. Brain Res 1988;467:51–9.
48. Berger ML, Tremblay E, Nitecka L, et al. Maturation of kainic acid seizure-brain damage syndrome in the rat. III. Postnatal development of kainic acid binding sites in the limbic system. Neuroscience 1984;13:1095–104.

49. Sankar R, Shin DH, Liu H, et al. Patterns of status epilepticus-induced neuronal injury during development and long-term consequences. J Neurosci 1998;18: 8382–93.
50. Sankar R, Shin D, Mazarati AM, et al. Epileptogenesis after status epilepticus reflects age- and model-dependent plasticity. Ann Neurol 2000;48:580–9.
51. Holmes GL, Gairsa JL, Chevassus-Au-Louis N, et al. Consequences of neonatal seizures in the rat: morphological and behavioral effects. Ann Neurol 1998;44: 845–57.
52. Liu Z, Yang Y, Silveira DC, et al. Consequences of recurrent seizures during early brain development. Neuroscience 1999;92:1443–54.
53. Riviello P, de Rogalski Landrot I, Holmes GL. Lack of cell loss following recurrent neonatal seizures. Brain Res Dev Brain Res 2002;135:101–4.
54. Jiang M, Lee CL, Smith KL, et al. Spine loss and other persistent alterations of hippocampal pyramidal cell dendrites in a model of early-onset epilepsy. J Neurosci 1998;18:8356–68.
55. Huang L, Cilio MR, Silveira DC, et al. Long-term effects of neonatal seizures: a behavioral, electrophysiological, and histological study. Brain Res Dev Brain Res 1999;118:99–107.
56. Huang LT, Yang SN, Liou CW, et al. Pentylenetetrazol-induced recurrent seizures in rat pups: time course on spatial learning and long-term effects. Epilepsia 2002; 43:567–73.
57. Sogawa Y, Monokoshi M, Silveira DC, et al. Timing of cognitive deficits following neonatal seizures: relationship to histological changes in the hippocampus. Brain Res Dev Brain Res 2001;131:73–83.
58. de Rogalski Landrot I, Minokoshi M, Silveira DC, et al. Recurrent neonatal seizures: relationship of pathology to the electroencephalogram and cognition. Brain Res Dev Brain Res 2001;129:27–38.
59. McCabe BK, Silveira DC, Cilio MR, et al. Reduced neurogenesis after neonatal seizures. J Neurosci 2001;21:2094–103.
60. Bo T, Jiang Y, Cao H, et al. Long-term effects of seizures in neonatal rats on spatial learning ability and N-methyl-d-aspartate receptor expression in the brain. Brain Res Dev Brain Res 2004;152:137–42.
61. Ni H, Jiang YW, Bo T, et al. Long-term effects of neonatal seizures on subsequent N-methyl-d-aspartate receptor-1 and gamma-aminobutyric acid receptor A-alpha1 receptor expression in hippocampus of the Wistar rat. Neurosci Lett 2004;368:254–7.
62. Zhang G, Raol YS, Hsu FC, et al. Long-term alterations in glutamate receptor and transporter expression following early-life seizures are associated with increased seizure susceptibility. J Neurochem 2004;88:91–101.
63. Cornejo BJ, Mesches MH, Coultrap S, et al. A single episode of neonatal seizures permanently alters glutamatergic synapses. Ann Neurol 2007;61:411–26.
64. Zhang G, Raol YH, Hsu FC, et al. Effects of status epilepticus on hippocampal GABAA receptors are age-dependent. Neuroscience 2004;125:299–303.
65. Isaeva E, Isaev D, Khazipov R, et al. Selective impairment of GABAergic synaptic transmission in the flurothyl model of neonatal seizures. Eur J Neurosci 2006;23: 1559–66.
66. Villeneuve N, Ben-Ari Y, Holmes GL, et al. Neonatal seizures induced persistent changes in intrinsic properties of CA1 rat hippocampal cells. Ann Neurol 2000; 47:729–38.
67. Chang YC, Huang AM, Kuo YM, et al. Febrile seizures impair memory and cAMP response-element binding protein activation. Ann Neurol 2003;54:701–5.

68. Neill J, Liu Z, Sarkisian M, et al. Recurrent seizures in immature rats: effect on auditory and visual discrimination. Brain Res Dev Brain Res 1996;95:283–92.
69. Karnam HB, Zhou JL, Huang LT, et al. Early life seizures cause long-standing impairment of the hippocampal map. Exp Neurol 2009;217:378–87.
70. Muller RU, Kubie JL. The effects of changes in the environment on the spatial firing patterns of hippocampal complex-spike cells. J Neurosci 1987;7:1951–68.
71. Thompson LT, Best PJ. Place cells and silent cells in the hippocampus of freely-behaving rats. J Neurosci 1989;9:2382–90.
72. Thompson LT, Best PJ. Long-term stability of the place-field activity of single units recorded from the dorsal hippocampus of freely behaving rats. Brain Res 1990; 509:299–308.
73. Vazdarjanova A, McNaughton BL, Barnes CA, et al. Experience-dependent coincident expression of the effector immediate-early genes arc and Homer 1a in hippocampal and neocortical neuronal networks. J Neurosci 2002;22:10067–71.
74. Muller R. A quarter of a century of place cells. Neuron 1996;17:813–22.
75. O'Keefe J, Nadel L. The hippocampus as a cognitive map. Oxford(UK): Clarendon; 1978.
76. Ranck JB Jr. Studies on single neurons in dorsal hippocampal formation and septum in unrestrained rats. I. Behavioral correlates and firing repertoires. Exp Neurol 1973;41:461–531.
77. Young BJ, Fox GD, Eichenbaum H. Correlates of hippocampal complex-spike cell activity in rats performing a nonspatial radial maze task. J Neurosci 1994; 14:6553–63.
78. Hampson RE, Heyser CJ, Deadwyler SA. Hippocampal cell firing correlates of delayed-match-to-sample performance in the rat. Behav Neurosci 1993;107: 715–39.
79. Wood ER, Dudchenko PA, Eichenbaum H. The global record of memory in hippocampal neuronal activity. Nature 1999;397:613–6.
80. Colgin LL, Moser EI, Moser MB. Understanding memory through hippocampal remapping. Trends Neurosci 2008;31:469–77.
81. Lenck-Santini PP, Holmes GL. Altered phase precession and compression of temporal sequences by place cells in epileptic rats. J Neurosci 2008;28:5053–62.
82. Liu X, Muller RU, Huang LT, et al. Seizure-induced changes in place cell physiology: relationship to spatial memory. J Neurosci 2003;23:11505–15.
83. Zhou JL, Shatskikh TN, Liu X, et al. Impaired single cell firing and long-term potentiation parallels memory impairment following recurrent seizures. Eur J Neurosci 2007;25:3667–77.
84. Dube CM, Zhou JL, Hamamura M, et al. Cognitive dysfunction after experimental febrile seizures. Exp Neurol 2008;215:167–77.
85. Rotenberg A, Abel T, Hawkins RD, et al. Parallel instabilities of long-term potentiation, place cells, and learning caused by decreased protein kinase A activity. J Neurosci 2000;20:8096–102.
86. Rotenberg A, Mayford M, Hawkins RD, et al. Mice expressing activated lack low frequency LTP and do not form stable place cells in the CA1 region of the hippocampus. Cell 1996;87:1351–61.

Index

Note: Page numbers of article titles are in **bold face** type.

A

N-Acetylcysteine
   for hypoxic-ischemic encephalopathy, 844–845
   for neuroprotection, 865, 868
Activin A, in intraventricular hemorrhage, 742
Adolescence, preterm neurodevelopmental status at, 776
Adrenomedullin, in intraventricular hemorrhage, 742
Allopurinol, for neuroprotection, 863, 865
3-Aminobenzamide, for neuroprotection, 867
α-Amino-3-hydroxy-5-methylisoazole-4-propionic acid (AMPA) receptors
   in hypoxic-ischemic encephalopathy, 840–843
   in seizures, 886–888
Angiogenic agents, in intraventricular hemorrhage, 742–743
Anticoagulants, for intraventricular hemorrhage prevention, 752
Anti-inflammatory agents, for neuroprotection, 866–867
Antioxidants, for neuroprotection, 864–865
Apoptosis
   in hypoxic-ischemic encephalopathy, 836–839, 845–847
   inhibitors of, for neuroprotection, 867
Artifacts, in near-infrared spectroscopy, 825
Asphyxia, neuroprotection for. *See* Neuroprotection.
Auditory stimulation, for near-infrared spectroscopy, 824
Autism spectrum disorders, **791–805**
   definition of, 792
   earliest signs of, 792
   etiology of, 792–793
   prematurity and
      cerebellum role in, 797–800
      evidence for, 793–797
      neuroanatomic substrates for, 797–800
      risk factors for, 793
   societal impact of, 792
Autoregulation, cerebral
   in transitional period, 729–730
   near-infrared spectroscopy for, 808–817

B

Bcl-2 protein, in hypoxic-ischemic encephalopathy, 845
Benzodiazepines, for seizures, 885
Beta carotene, for neuroprotection, 864–865
Blood flow, cerebral. *See* Cerebral blood flow.
Blood volume, cerebral, near-infrared spectroscopy for, 808–817

Clin Perinatol 36 (2009) 915–922
doi:10.1016/S0095-5108(09)00102-X
0095-5108/09/$ – see front matter © 2009 Elsevier Inc. All rights reserved.
perinatology.theclinics.com

United States Postal Service

Statement of Ownership, Management, and Circulation
(All Periodicals Publications Except Requestor Publications)

1. Publication Title	2. Publication Number	3. Filing Date
Clinics in Perinatology	0 0 1 - 7 4 4	9/15/09

4. Issue Frequency	5. Number of Issues Published Annually	6. Annual Subscription Price
Mar, Jun, Sep, Dec	4	$217.00

7. Complete Mailing Address of Known Office of Publication (Not printer) (Street, city, county, state, and ZIP+4®)

Elsevier Inc.
360 Park Avenue South
New York, NY 10010-1710

Contact Person: Stephen Bushing
Telephone (Include area code): 215-239-3688

8. Complete Mailing Address of Headquarters or General Business Office of Publisher (Not printer)

Elsevier Inc., 360 Park Avenue South, New York, NY 10010-1710

9. Full Names and Complete Mailing Addresses of Publisher, Editor, and Managing Editor (Do not leave blank)

Publisher (Name and complete mailing address)

John Schreiber, Elsevier, Inc., 1600 John F. Kennedy Blvd. Suite 1800, Philadelphia, PA 19103-2899

Editor (Name and complete mailing address)

Carla Holloway, Elsevier, Inc., 1600 John F. Kennedy Blvd. Suite 1800, Philadelphia, PA 19103-2899

Managing Editor (Name and complete mailing address)

Catherine Bewick, Elsevier, Inc., 1600 John F. Kennedy Blvd. Suite 1800, Philadelphia, PA 19103-2899

10. Owner (Do not leave blank. If the publication is owned by a corporation, give the name and address of the corporation immediately followed by the names and addresses of all stockholders owning or holding 1 percent or more of the total amount of stock. If not owned by a corporation, give the names and addresses of the individual owners. If owned by a partnership or other unincorporated firm, give its name and address as well as those of each individual owner. If the publication is published by a nonprofit organization, give its name and address.)

Full Name	Complete Mailing Address
Wholly owned subsidiary of	4520 East-West Highway
Reed/Elsevier, US holdings	Bethesda, MD 20814

11. Known Bondholders, Mortgagees, and Other Security Holders Owning or Holding 1 Percent or More of Total Amount of Bonds, Mortgages, or Other Securities. If none, check box. ☐ None

Full Name	Complete Mailing Address
N/A	

12. Tax Status (For completion by nonprofit organizations authorized to mail at nonprofit rates) (Check one)
The purpose, function, and nonprofit status of this organization and the exempt status for federal income tax purposes:
☐ Has Not Changed During Preceding 12 Months
☐ Has Changed During Preceding 12 Months (Publisher must submit explanation of change with this statement)

PS Form 3526, September 2007 (Page 1 of 3 (Instructions Page 3)) PSN 7530-01-000-9931 PRIVACY NOTICE: See our Privacy policy in www.usps.com

---

13. Publication Title	14. Issue Date for Circulation Data Below
Clinics in Perinatology	June 2009

15. Extent and Nature of Circulation			Average No. Copies Each Issue During Preceding 12 Months	No. Copies of Single Issue Published Nearest to Filing Date
a. Total Number of Copies (Net press run)			3650	3400
b. Paid Circulation (By Mail and Outside the Mail)	(1)	Mailed Outside-County Paid Subscriptions Stated on PS Form 3541. (Include paid distribution above nominal rate, advertiser's proof copies, and exchange copies)	1955	1870
	(2)	Mailed In-County Paid Subscriptions Stated on PS Form 3541 (Include paid distribution above nominal rate, advertiser's proof copies, and exchange copies)		
	(3)	Paid Distribution Outside the Mails Including Sales Through Dealers and Carriers, Street Vendors, Counter Sales, and Other Paid Distribution Outside USPS®	801	719
	(4)	Paid Distribution by Other Classes Mailed Through the USPS (e.g. First-Class Mail®)		
c. Total Paid Distribution (Sum of 15b (1), (2), (3), and (4))		▶	2756	2589
d. Free or Nominal Rate Distribution (By Mail and Outside the Mail)	(1)	Free or Nominal Rate Outside-County Copies Included on PS Form 3541	99	76
	(2)	Free or Nominal Rate In-County Copies Included on PS Form 3541		
	(3)	Free or Nominal Rate Copies Mailed at Other Classes Through the USPS (e.g. First-Class Mail)		
	(4)	Free or Nominal Rate Distribution Outside the Mail (Carriers or other means)		
e. Total Free or Nominal Rate Distribution (Sum of 15d (1), (2), (3) and (4))		▶	99	76
f. Total Distribution (Sum of 15c and 15e)		▶	2855	2665
g. Copies not Distributed (See Instructions to publishers #4 (page #3))		▶	795	735
h. Total (Sum of 15f and g)		▶	3650	3400
i. Percent Paid (15c divided by 15f times 100)			96.53%	97.15%

16. Publication of Statement of Ownership

☐ If the publication is a general publication, publication of this statement is required. Will be printed in the December 2009 issue of this publication. ☐ Publication not required.

17. Signature and Title of Editor, Publisher, Business Manager, or Owner

[signature] Stephen R. Bushing – Subscription Services Coordinator

Date: September 15, 2009

I certify that all information furnished on this form is true and complete. I understand that anyone who furnishes false or misleading information on this form or who omits material or information requested on the form may be subject to criminal sanctions (including fines and imprisonment) and/or civil sanctions (including civil penalties).

PS Form 3526, September 2007 (Page 2 of 3)